Current Therapy for Acute Coronary Ischemia

edited by
Harold L. Lazar, MD
Associate Professor of Cardiothoracic Surgery
Boston University School of Medicine;
Attending Surgeon
Department of Cardiothoracic Surgery
The University Hospital;
Assistant Director of Thoracic Surgical Services
Boston City Hospital
Boston, Massachusetts;
Visiting Cardiothoracic Surgeon
Boston Veterans Administration Medical Center
Jamaica Plain, Massachusetts

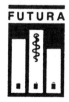

FUTURA

Futura Publishing Co., Inc.
Mount Kisco, NY

Library of Congress Cataloging-in-Publication Data

Current therapy for acute coronary ischemia / edited by Harold L.
   Lazar.
    p.   cm.
   Includes bibliographical references and index.
   ISBN 0-87993-555-3 (alk. paper)
   1. Coronary heart disease—Treatment. I. Lazar, Harold L.
   [DNLM: 1. Myocardial Ischemia—physiopathology. 2. Myocar-
dial Ischemia—drug therapy. 3. Myocardial Ischemia—surgery.
4. Thrombolytic Therapy. WG 300 C9767 1993]
RC685.C6C87 1993
616.1′2306—dc20
DNLM/DLC   93-14925
for Library of Congress   CIP

Copyright 1993
Futura Publishing Company, Inc.

Published by
Futura Publishing Company, Inc.
2 Bedford Ridge Road
Mount Kisco, New York 10549

LC #: 93-14925
ISBN #: 0-87993-555-3

Every effort has been made to ensure that the information in this
book is as up to date and as accurate as possible at the time of
publication. However, due to the constant developments in medicine, neither the author, nor the editor, nor the publisher can accept
any legal or any other responsibility for any errors or omissions that
may occur.

Printed in the United States of America.

This book is printed on acid-free paper.

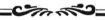

To my wife, Carol
     for her wisdom
     and understanding

And to Elizabeth, Michael, and Robert
     without whose support
     this book would not
     have been possible.

Contributors

Gabriel S. Aldea, MD
Assistant Professor, Cardiothoracic Surgery, Department of Cardiothoracic Surgery, Boston University Medical Center, Boston, Massachusetts

Jeffrey N. Berman, MD
Instructor in Medicine and Staff Cardiologist, Section of Cardiology, Department of Medicine, Boston University Medical Center, University Hospital, Boston, Massachusetts

Friedhelm Beyersdorf, MD
Associate Professor of Surgery, Department of Thoracic and Cardiovascular Surgery, Johann Wolfgang Goethe University, Frankfurt, Germany

Gerald D. Buckberg, MD
Professor of Surgery, Department of Cardiothoracic Surgery, UCLA School of Medicine, Los Angeles, California

Anthony J. Cannistra, MD, MSc
Fellow in Cardiology, The University Hospital, Boston University Medical Center, Boston, Massachusetts

Lawrence H. Cohn, MD
Professor of Surgery, Harvard Medical School, Chief of Cardiac Surgery, Brigham and Women's Hospital, Boston, Massachusetts

Matthew M. Cooper, MD
Instructor in Surgery, Columbia-Presbyterian Medical Center, Columbia University College of Physicians and Surgeons, New York, New York

David P. Faxon, MD
Professor of Medicine and Director of Interventional Cardiology, Section of Cardiology, Department of Medicine, Boston University Medical Center, University Hospital, Boston, Massachusetts

Alice K. Jacobs, MD
Associate Professor of Medicine, Boston University School of Medicine, and Director, Cardiac Catheterization Lab, The University Hospital, Boston, Massachusetts

Robert A. Kloner, MD, PhD
Director of Research, The Heart Institute, Hospital of the Good Samaritan, and Professor of Medicine, Division of Cardiology, University of Southern California, Los Angeles, California

Harold L. Lazar, MD
Associate Professor of Cardiothoracic Surgery, Boston University School of Medicine; Attending Surgeon, Department of Cardiothoracic Surgery, The University Hospital, Boston; Assistant Director of Thoracic Surgical Services, Boston City Hospital, Boston; Visiting Cardiothoracic Surgeon, Boston Veterans Administration Medical Center, Jamaica Plain, Massachusetts

Keith S. Naunheim, MD
Associate Professor of Surgery, Department of Surgery, St. Louis University Medical Center, St. Louis, Missouri

Michel Ovize, MD
Research Associate, The Heart Institute, Hospital of the Good Samaritan, and Research Fellow, Division of Cardiology, University of Southern California, Los Angeles, California

D. Glenn Pennington, MD
Professor of Surgery, Department of Surgery, St. Louis University Medical Center, St. Louis, Missouri

Karin Przyklenk, PhD
Assistant Director of Research and Director of Cardiac Function, The Heart Institute, Hospital of the Good Samaritan, and

Assistant Professor of Research Medicine, University of Southern California, Los Angeles, California

Eric A. Rose, MD
Associate Professor of Surgery, Department of Surgery, and Chief, Division of Cardiothoracic Surgery, Columbia University College of Physicians and Surgeons, New York, New York

Robert J. Rizzo, MD
Assistant Professor of Surgery, Harvard Medical School, and Attending Cardiac Surgeon, Brigham and Women's Hospital, Boston, Massachusetts

Nicholas A. Ruocco, Jr., MD
Assistant Professor of Medicine, Boston University School of Medicine; Associate Director, Cardiovascular Animal Research Laboratory, Boston University School of Medicine, Boston; Director, Cardiac Catheterization Laboratory, Norwood Hospital, Norwood, Massachusetts

Richard J. Shemin, MD
Professor and Chairman, Department of Cardiothoracic Surgery, Boston University Medical Center, Boston, Massachusetts

Marc T. Swartz, BA
Director of Circulatory Support, St. Louis University Medical Center, St. Louis, Missouri

Foreword

The understanding and management of myocardial ischemia has undergone a remarkable evolution over the past 20 years. It has been fascinating to watch the conceptual shift from the notion of pharmacological minimization of ischemic injury toward a strategy based on reperfusion supplemented with hemodynamic and pharmacological interventions. This strategic change was not a consequence of sudden insight or new pathophysiological discovery. It was, rather, the consequence of technology with thrombolytic therapy, angioplasty, and safer surgery constituting the three arms of a therapeutic triangle. Each of these points on the triangle has led to expanded knowledge and therapeutic ventures that have greatly altered the boundaries of the triangle.

Thrombolysis has stimulated study of the critical role of residual stenosis, residual ejection fraction, and elements fostering thrombosis in coronary arteries as critical determinants of long-term outcome from coronary artery disease. The potential for utilizing angioplasty in the acute treatment of myocardial infarction has allowed development of new catheters and arthrectomy devices, and has focused on the pharmacological and molecular basis for restenosis. The close relationship between the biology of restenosis and the more protracted process of atherosclerosis probably has mechanisms in common. Finally, at a time when options for interventions for acute ischemia were limited with the exception of direct operative revascularization, cardiac surgery played a critical role in the recognition and development of the notion of reperfusion injury. Even before the Gissi study demonstrating the efficacy of thrombolysis in acute myocardial infarction, the benefit of emergency operation in minimizing mortality from acute myocardial infarction and unstable angina had been demonstrated. Success of cardiac operations employed in these acutely ill patients mandated the development of pharmacological and mechanical modification of reperfusion conditions. Yet the long-term success of bypass surgery has been limited by progression of native coronary disease, graft atherosclerosis, and intimal hypertrophy. These latter processes are not dissimilar in their origin from events associated with fundamental genesis of atheroma and restenosis following angioplasty. The boundaries of the triangle are expanding rapidly. Perpendiculars to each of the sides of the triangle meet at areas of similar interest and discovery of solutions to common biological problems result in enhanced efficacy and safety of therapeutic interventions for acute myocardial ischemia.

Successful intervention in acute ischemic syndromes is of critical importance. Of those patients who survive an acute ischemic event, there is a long-term effect on both these individuals and society. Downstream problems of recurrent disease, congestive heart failure, disability, recurrent hospitalizations, and health care costs are all intertwined. As the mortality from acute myocardial infarction diminishes, the pool of patients in the population at risk for subsequent acute ischemic events increases exponentially. The efficacy of the original intervention in the acute ischemic state is of paramount importance. In this text, Dr. Lazar has drawn together a highly qualified and skilled multidisciplinary group to contribute to this highly focused problem.

Under one cover, the practicing physician may find the philosophy and strategy for each of the most currently applied approaches to acute myocardial ischemia. It is interesting that these approaches are applied without bias, but rather with the implication that thrombolysis, angioplasty, operation, ventricular support, and transplantation all have something to contribute to individualized patient care. Occasionally, it is by examination of that which is missing that one is able to direct future efforts. Clearly, in the field of management of acute myocardial ischemia, what is lacking is a uniform algorithm for patient management upon which there is universal agreement. This will be the task for the future and the challenge will be to do it at a time when individual management strategies are, themselves, moving targets. Constraints will be introduced by pathophysiology, cost, regionalization of care, rural versus urban settings in which myocardial ischemia occurs, and the evolution of technologies that are currently unpredictable. A management strategy that works well in the core of an urban environment with highly sophisticated and abundant tertiary care facilities may be highly impractical for the care of patients in rural areas serviced by few tertiary care facilities. Some tradeoff in most effective versus most economic care is an unfortunate but realistic part of future health care delivery systems. Future diagnostic modalities may allow enhanced specificity of care to be offered to patients with acute ischemic syndromes that may allow management 10 years from today to look rather different than it is currently applied. Certainly, one of the strengths of this book is to offer physicians today the opportunity to understand what is currently available and to provide the nidus for further reading that will allow intelligent and informed development of appropriate treatment strategies.

Andrew S. Wechsler, MD
Stuart McGuire Professor of Surgery
Professor of Physiology
Chairman, Department of Surgery
Chief, Division of Cardiothoracic Surgery
Medical College of Virginia/
Virginia Commonwealth University
Richmond, Virginia

Foreword

Perhaps nowhere else in clinical medicine is the role of the medical care specialist more intertwined with that of the surgical specialist than in the management of the patient with ischemic heart disease. It is, therefore, both timely and of considerable significance that Dr. Harold Lazar has assembled this compendium on *Current Therapy for Acute Coronary Ischemia* for the benefit of the internist, cardiologist, and the cardiac surgeon alike. There is also much in it for the cardiology fellow, thoracic surgical resident, anesthetist, and clinical nurse specialist as well.

For this clinician, the special merit of this monograph lies in the wealth of experimental data and basic investigation that has been succinctly summarized and neatly packaged within each chapter to provide the necessary pathophysiological background and scientific underpinnings that are so often difficult to find in the popular clinical literature. The opening chapter by Kloner and his colleagues clearly sets the stage for understanding reversible and irreversible myocardial injury and the importance as well as the limitations of quantifying the extent of myocardial damage. In a most readable fashion, these authors explain the meaning of myocardial stunning and introduce the reader to the important new concept of "preconditioning" of the myocardium through repetitive episodes of ischemia. With these concepts in place, the subsequent chapters devoted to reperfusion therapy, whether by fibrinolytic therapy or by direct angioplasty, are seen in perspective. An enormous clinical literature is nicely condensed in these latter two chapters, and they are clearly written by clinicians who have "labored in the trenches." Bracketing these two clinical chapters are two others written by accomplished investigators who have pioneered work in the area of coronary sinus interventions (Jacobs and Lazar) and performed the seminal work that established principles of myocardial protection during coronary bypass surgery (Buckberg and Beyersdorf).

It is also evident that the contributors to this book view angioplasty and bypass surgery as complementary techniques rather than competing strategies. Particularly germane to current-day practice is Lazar's personal assessment of the changing case mix in patients proposed for revascularization procedures and the impact this has on the outcome of backup surgery. The data are sobering and have clear implications for clinical decision making. It is equally clear that the role of the surgeon will continue to expand as greater success is achieved in the management of what not long ago were the incurable sequelae of acute myocardial infarction such as myocardial rupture and disruption of the mitral valve. The era of successful ventricular assist devices would appear to be "here and now" as described by Pennington and colleagues. Similarly, the every day success with cardiac transplantation holds new promise for those victims of acute ischemic syndromes who are left with terminally destroyed ventricles as outlined by Cooper and Rose.

This book successfully condenses an enormous volume of the scientific literature as it pertains to the invasive approach for the management of coronary ischemia. I believe it will move quickly to the high priority list of profitable reading for any clinician or cardiologist who is involved in the care of patients today.

Thomas J. Ryan, MD
Professor of Medicine
Chief of Cardiology
The University Hospital
Boston University Medical Center and
Boston University School of Medicine
Boston, Massachusetts

Preface

The Evolving Treatment of Acute Coronary Insufficiency: The Continued Efforts of Cardiologists and Cardiac Surgeons

Our understanding of ischemic coronary artery disease has evolved greatly during the past century. However, the past few decades have been distinguished by an explosion in the pathophysiological understanding of coronary artery disease. The creative development of medical technology has led to improved diagnosis and treatment. Currently we now have the most effective strategies to treat coronary insufficiency than have ever been possible. The close collaborative efforts between cardiologists and cardiac surgeons in the developing area of interventional cardiology has been essential and has contributed to the significant reduction in mortality from ischemic heart disease and myocardial infarction over the past few decades. However, in spite of these improvements, cardiovascular disease remains the primary cause of death in adults. Thus, much more needs to be done. This multiauthored text highlights the state of the art in the treatment of acute coronary insufficiency. It reviews what we know and how that knowledge has evolved. Finally, it attempts to forecast future directions of therapy and investigation.

The text begins with a thorough review of the pathophysiology of coronary ischemia and reperfusion. Our knowledge of the process of atherosclerosis and the complex interaction of blood elements with atherosclerotic plaque is critical to understanding unstable anginal syndromes and acute myocardial infarction. Furthermore, highly effective treatment strategies have developed from this information. The first two chapters of this text review this information in great detail.

Our understanding of the pathophysiology of reperfusion injury has led to creative techniques to modify the myocardium before reperfusion, thereby reducing myocardial injury. The coronary sinus has emerged as an alternative route for delivery of blood and medications to the ischemic myocardium. The role of coronary sinus interventions to treat acutely ischemic myocardium is thoroughly reviewed in the text.

The evolving role of percutaneous coronary angioplasty combined with thrombolytic therapy remains an area of active investigation. This topic is also well reviewed in the book. The surgical treatment of acute coronary artery insufficiency, myocardial infarction, surgery after a failed PTCA, and the principles of myocardial protection during myocardial ischemia and reperfusion is extensively covered in five chapters.

There are circumstances where massive myocardial injury results in end-stage ischemic congestive heart failure or cardiogenic shock and the only mode of therapy is mechanical circulatory support combined with conventional interventions such as PTCA, thrombolysis, or coronary bypass surgery. Often these treatments serve as a bridge to cardiac transplantation. The final two chapters of the text cover these heroic and increasingly successful therapeutic approaches.

The future advances in our technology appear to be unlimited. However, if our clinical approaches in the future are to equal the advances made in the past, the common denominator will require continued close collaboration among the surgeon, cardiologist, and basic scientist. These multidisciplinary efforts are the key to developing more effective therapies to treat the ischemic myocardium.

The time from coronary occlusion with initiation of infarction until irreversible necrosis is a very short window of opportunity for current therapy. Coordinated efforts in our clinical centers continue to challenge practitioners in this area. It is only through collaborative approaches that further breakthroughs will occur. It is essential that competition between various treatment strategies be thoroughly investigated to determine appropriate outcomes at a price our health care system can bear.

This book will be a valuable resource of our current knowledge from well-recognized experts in the fields of cardiology and cardiothoracic surgery for many years to come.

Richard J. Shemin, MD
Professor and Chairman
Department of Cardiothoracic Surgery
Boston University Medical Center
Boston, Massachusetts

Introduction

Despite significant reductions in the incidence of atherosclerotic heart disease due to better control and identification of risk factors, there has been a steady rise in the incidence of patients presenting with acute coronary insufficiency syndromes. Acute coronary ischemia and its sequelae remains the leading cause of death in the United States today. The past 10 years have seen the revolutionary development of interventional strategies aimed at decreasing the morbidity and mortality due to acute coronary insufficiency. These include thrombolytic therapy, percutaneous transluminal coronary artery angioplasty, retrograde coronary sinus perfusion, advances in techniques for coronary artery revascularization and myocardial preservation, and the introduction of ventricular assist devices and cardiac transplantation. This monograph was undertaken to provide the clinician with a comprehensive review and understanding of the latest treatment strategies for acute coronary insufficiency syndromes and how they can be applied most effectively in clinical practice. Since the treatment of acute coronary insufficiency requires the teamwork and cooperation of internists, invasive and diagnostic cardiologists, and cardiac surgeons, the book contains chapters written by both cardiologists and cardiac surgeons. Hence, this publication is unique in that it provides a reference for clinical practice for both medical and surgical practitioners.

The book covers all the significant aspects of the therapeutic management of acute coronary insufficiency syndromes. Five specific topics are addressed. These include: (1) the pathophysiology of acute coronary ischemia and reperfusion, (2) thrombolytic therapy, (3) the role of interventional cardiology, (4) surgical revascularization, and (5) ventricular assist devices and cardiac transplantation. The authors, each of whom is a recognized authority in his or her field, have emphasized that the treatment of acute coronary insufficiency is not merely to increase blood flow but to decrease infarct size and preserve ventricular function, thereby not only decreasing morbidity and mortality but also increasing the quality of life. In Chapter 1, Drs. Ovize, Przyklenk, and Kloner discuss the pathophysiology of acute coronary ischemia and reperfusion. In addition to characterizing the consequences of reversible and irreversible injuries, they describe the latest methods to quantify and determine infarct size. Reperfusion and myocardial stunning are reviewed and the role of "preconditioning" myocardium by repetitive episodes of ischemia is addressed. Drs. Cannistra and Ruocco review the role of thrombolytic therapy for acute coronary ischemia in Chapter 2. They discuss the indications, complications, and clinical results of thrombolytic therapy. In addition, the role of surgical intervention following thrombolytic therapy is detailed along with future trends and further pharmacological agents that may be used in clinical practice. Chapters 3 and 4 deal with the role of interventional cardiology in acute coronary ischemia. The role of coronary sinus interventions to reduce myocardial damage after acute coronary ischemia is reviewed by Drs. Jacobs and Lazar. They discuss the mechanisms and clinical applications of synchronized retroperfusion and pressure-controlled intermittent coronary sinus occlusion. Drs. Berman and Faxon discuss the current role of PTCA for acute coronary ischemic syndromes. They review the results of PTCA in patients with unstable angina, acute myocardial infarctions, cardiogenic shock, and after thrombolysis. Chapters 5 through 9 discuss the surgical therapy for acute coronary ischemia. In their chapter on principles of myocardial protection during acute coronary ischemia and reperfusion, Drs. Beyersdorf and Buckberg review their experimental and clinical experience with acute coronary revascularization. They discuss the importance of myocardial protection techniques including blood cardioplegia, substrate enhancement, warm induction, and controlled regional reperfusion in salvaging potentially irreversibly injured myocardium. In the chapters on emergency coronary artery bypass graft surgery after failed percutaneous transluminal coronary angioplasty and methods of reducing myocardial necrosis after failed PTCA in patients undergoing emergent CABG surgery, Dr. Lazar brings into focus the management of those patients who must undergo emergent CABG following a failed PTCA. This special type of acute coronary insufficiency has been a challenge for both the interventional cardiologist as well as for the cardiac surgeon. Dr. Lazar reviews the Boston University experience with this problem and discusses methods of reducing myocardial necrosis while these patients are being prepared for revascularization en route from the catheterization laboratory to the operating room. In their chapter on surgical revascularization for refractory unstable angina, Drs. Aldea and Shemin review the current surgical results of coronary bypass for unstable angina. These results are compared to standard medical therapy and PTCA. In addition to managing patients with unstable angina, today's practice of adult cardiac surgery requires that the surgeon be familiar with surgical techniques for patients with acute myocardial necrosis. In their chapter on the surgeon's role in the management of acute myocardial infarction, Drs. Rizzo and Cohn describe the role of surgical intervention for ventricular septal defects, mitral regurgitation, free wall ventricular ruptures, ventricular aneurysms, and coronary revascularization for patients with cardiogenic shock. Although the surgical morbidity and mortality is high in this group of patients, they are the group that stands the most to benefit from surgical intervention. Chapters 10 and 11 review the role of ventricular assist devices and cardiac transplantation during acute coronary ischemia. In their chapter on advanced mechanical circulatory support after acute coronary ischemia and infarction, Drs. Pennington, Swartz, and Naunheim review the current available devices and clinical indications for ventricular assist following acute myocardial infarctions. The results of VAD insertion for postcardiotomy support and as a bridge to transplantation is described. The role and results of cardiac transplantation for acute coronary ischemia are reviewed by Drs. Cooper and Rose. They discuss patient selection and clinical outcomes and attempt to predict the future directions of cardiac transplantation in this difficult group of patients.

I am grateful to the many outstanding authors for their hard work and enthusiasm in contributing to the preparation of this book. Each has described his or her area of expertise by presenting both the experimental and clinical data by which their interventions have been developed. It is hoped that the internists, cardiologists, and surgeons who read these chapters will use this knowledge to base their clinical decision making in what has become one of the most challenging and exciting areas of medicine today.

Harold L. Lazar, MD
Department of Cardiothoracic Surgery
Boston University Medical Center
Boston Massachusetts

Contents

Contributors: v

Foreword: *Andrew S. Wechsler* ix

Foreword: *Thomas J. Ryan* xiii

Preface: *Richard J. Shemin* xv

Introduction: *Harold L. Lazar* xvii

1 • Pathophysiology of Acute Coronary Ischemia
and Reperfusion
*Michel Ovize, Karin Przyklenk,
and Robert A. Kloner* 1

2 • The Role of Thrombolytic Therapy for Acute Coronary
Ischemia
Anthony J. Cannistra and Nicholas A. Ruocco, Jr 33

3 • The Role of Coronary Sinus Interventions to Reduce
Myocardial Damage After Acute Coronary Ischemia
Alice K. Jacobs and Harold L. Lazar 63

4 • The Current Role of Percutaneous Transluminal Coronary
Angioplasty for Acute Coronary Ischemic Syndromes
Jeffrey N. Berman and David P. Faxon 85

5 • Principles of Myocardial Protection During Acute
Coronary Ischemia and Reperfusion
Friedhelm Beyersdorf and Gerald D. Buckberg 111

6 • Emergency Coronary Artery Bypass Graft Surgery After
Failed Percutaneous Transluminal Coronary Angioplasty
Harold L. Lazar 149

7 • Methods of Reducing Myocardial Necrosis After Failed
Percutaneous Transluminal Coronary Angioplasty in
Patients Undergoing Emergent Coronary Artery Bypass
Surgery
Harold L. Lazar 167

8 • Surgical Revascularization for Refractory Unstable
Angina
Gabriel S. Aldea and Richard J. Shemin 187

9 • The Surgeon's Role in the Management of Acute
Myocardial Infarction
Robert J. Rizzo and Lawrence H. Cohn 205

10 • Advanced Mechanical Circulatory Support After Acute
Coronary Ischemia and Infarction
*D. Glenn Pennington, Marc T. Swartz,
and Keith S. Naunheim* 229

11 • Cardiac Transplantation and Mechanical Bridge
to Transplantation for Acute Coronary Ischemia
Matthew M. Cooper and Eric A. Rose 257

• Index 285

Chapter 1

Pathophysiology of Acute Coronary Ischemia and Reperfusion

Michel Ovize, Karin Przyklenk,
and Robert A. Kloner

Introduction

Much of our understanding of the pathophysiology of myocardial ischemia relates to clinical and experimental acute myocardial infarction. During the past two decades, the development of cardiac bypass surgery, thrombolysis, and angioplasty also has led to further understanding of the pathophysiology of myocardial reperfusion. It is now accepted that reperfusion is the only consistently effective treatment of acute myocardial infarction.[1-4] However, there is also a large body of evidence that suggests that reperfusion may be associated with deleterious effects on cardiac rhythm, myocardial perfusion and metabolism, and ventricular function.[5,6]

This chapter reviews the consequences of myocardial ischemia and the beneficial effects of reperfusion, and then focuses on some of

Lazar HL (editor): *Current Therapy for Acute Coronary Ischemia,* © Futura Publishing Co., Inc., Mount Kisco, NY, 1993.

the detrimental aspects of reperfusion (i.e., "reperfusion injury"), including reperfusion arrhythmias, vascular damage, and myocardial stunning.

Myocardial Ischemic Injury

What Is Myocardial Ischemia?

Myocardial ischemia is simply defined as a lack of blood perfusion, sufficient to result in a conversion from aerobic to anaerobic metabolism. From a dynamic point of view, it represents an imbalance between myocardial oxygen supply and demand. Although reduction of oxygen supply, caused by obstructive (atheroma) and/or dynamic (spasm) coronary artery flow reduction is its common cause, myocardial ischemia can also be caused by an increase in oxygen demand (as occurs during left ventricular hypertrophy, tachycardia, or exercise).

In the clinical setting, myocardial ischemia may involve either a limited region of the heart (acute myocardial infarction) or the whole cardiac muscle (cardiac surgery, hypotensive shock). Although global and regional ischemia undoubtedly are different, many aspects of the ischemic process are similar and therefore will be discussed together.

Consequences of Myocardial Ischemia

Ischemic injury is a *dynamic* phenomenon dependent on both the duration and severity of ischemia.

Reversible Ischemic Injury

Within seconds after the onset of ischemia, a dramatic reduction of contractile activity occurs: active shortening/thickening is replaced by passive bulging/thinning. Anaerobic conditions develop within the ischemic myocyte due to the reduction or cessation of adenosine triphosphate (ATP) production from oxidative phosphorylation in the mitchondria. Although greatly accelerated at the onset of ischemia, anaerobic glycolysis is a far less efficient provider of ATP than aerobic respiration.[7,8] As a result of this deficit in energy production, a loss of control of transmembrane ionic gradients occurs and osmotic changes lead to cellular water accumulation and cell swelling that may contribute to further cell membrane damage.[9,10] Ultrastructural changes that characterize reversibly injured tissue include a loss of glycogen granules, development of intracellular edema, and nuclear clumping and margination (Fig. 1).

For several minutes, the ischemic damage is fully reversible: if coronary blood flow is restored, there will be no ischemia-induced myocyte necrosis. In the canine model, when reperfusion occurs within 15 minutes after coronary artery occlusion, no necrosis develops; rather, the previously ischemic cells recover fully in terms of contractile function and metabolism in the hours to days following reflow.

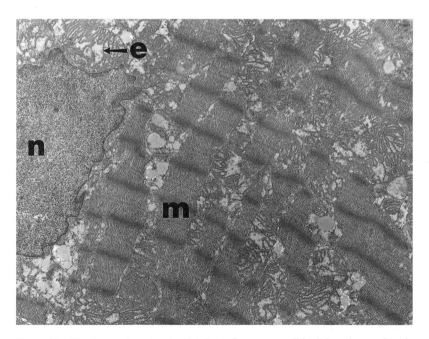

Figure 1: Electron micrograph obtained from reversibly injured, previously ischemic subepicardium of an anesthetized dog. Note intramitochondrial edema (e); myofilaments (m) and nucleus (n) appear intact.

Irreversible Ischemic Injury

If ischemia is more prolonged (i.e., more than 20 min in the canine model), reversibly injured myocytes become irreversibly injured or necrotic. Because the subendocardium has a higher sensitivity to ischemia and receives less collateral blood flow from the adjacent normally perfused myocardium, subendocardial myocytes become necrotic first. After 40 to 60 minutes of coronary artery occlusion, the inner third of the ischemic myocardium becomes necrotic. When the duration of coronary artery occlusion is extended to 3 hours and is followed by reperfusion, necrosis develops into the midmyocardium and the inner part of the subepicardium. In the canine model, reperfusion instituted between 3 and 6 hours after coronary artery occlusion provides very little salvage of myocardial tissue. Thus, as the duration of ischemia is increased, the necrosis

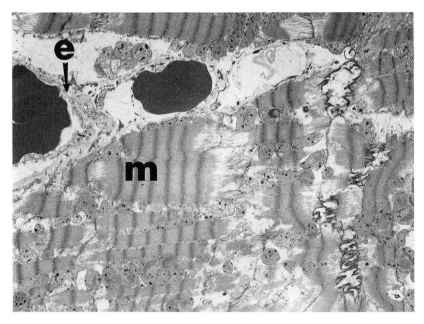

Figure 2A: Electron micrograph obtained from the previously ischemic endocardium of an anesthetized dog that underwent 2 hr of left anterior descending coronary artery occlusion followed by 4 hr of reperfusion. Both the myocytes (m) and the vascular endothelial cells (e) are severely damaged (approximate magnification, × 5100).

progressively extends toward the subepicardium: this has been termed the "wavefront phenomenon" by Reimer and Jennings.[11]

Morphological hallmarks of irreversible injury include the presence of mitochondrial dense bodies, membrane rupture (i.e., sarcolemmal blebs and gaps), and, in the worst instances, total architectural disruption (Fig. 2). Obviously, this tissue will never show functional or metabolic recovery.

Determinants of Infarct Size

At any time during the necrotic process, the size of the infarct depends on the following determinants: the size of the risk region (i.e., the ischemic area), the amount of collateral blood flow (i.e.,

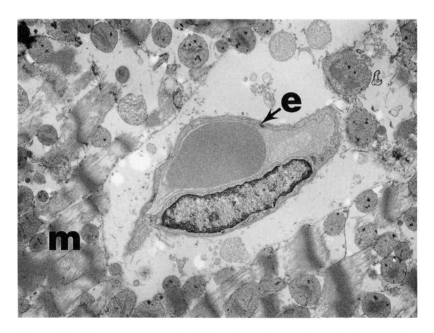

Figure 2B: Electron micrograph obtained from the previously ischemic endocardium of a dog that received SOD + catalase, a potent scavenger of oxygen-derived free radicals, at the time of reperfusion. The myocytes (m) are irreversibly injured, but the vascular endothelium (e) has been preserved (approximate magnification, ×3100). Reprinted with permission of the American Heart Association.[46]

blood flow persisting in the ischemic area after the coronary artery has been occluded), and the metabolic demand of the ischemic heart. Thus, to compare accurately the efficiency of therapies aimed at reducing infarct size, these determinants must be measured.

The Risk Region

Not surprisingly, the larger the occluded bed, the larger the infarct[12] (Fig. 3). Risk region is easily measured in experimental preparations by in vivo or ex vivo injection of dye into the coronary circulation. Quantitation of the area at risk by these methods involves postmortem examination of the heart. Obviously, this is not applicable to clinical situations and the evaluation of the risk region

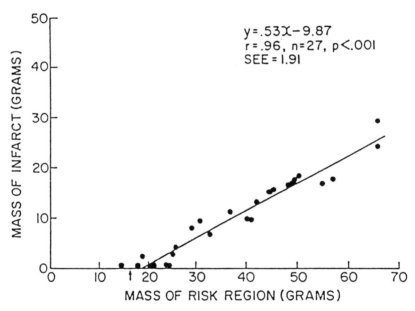

Figure 3: Area at risk as a determinant of infarct size. Infarct size (expressed as a percentage of the left ventricular weight) is plotted as a function of area at risk (expressed as a percentage of the left ventricular weight). Risk region was determined from radiograms of barium gel–injected dogs hearts. It is apparent that infarct size decreases with decreasing size of the area at risk, and that for a small area at risk (less than approximately 20 g in this model), the amount of necrosis is very small or nonexistent. Reprinted with permission of the American Heart Association.[12]

in humans remains difficult. Identification of an area of contractile dysfunction (i.e., by echocardiography or ventriculography) lacks accuracy because of the difficulty in delineating the boundaries between dysfunctional and normally contracting tissue. A promising technique is single photon emission computerized tomography (SPECT) imaging, using isotopes such as Tc-sestamibi, that have proven in experimental preparations to be good perfusion markers.[13–16] The major advantage of this isotope as compared to thallium is the absence of myocardial redistribution once injected. It can, for example, be administered at the time of hospital admission, without delaying thrombolytic therapy and nevertheless allowing delayed imaging.[17] Experimental evidence indicates that the accuracy of the measurement of risk region by this technique is good.[18,19] Moreover, when injected after reperfusion, Tc-sestamibi behaves as a marker of viability.[18,20,21] In fact, it has been shown to delineate accurately the area of necrosis in experimental models.[22]

Collateral Blood Flow

It is well established that infarct size is inversely related to the amount of collateral blood flow during coronary artery occlusion[12,23] (Fig. 4). The large variability in collateral development in some animal species such as dogs (or humans) makes it mandatory to measure this parameter if one wants to assess accurately the effects of therapies aimed at reducing infarct size.

Measurement of collateral flow in human heart remains a major problem. The radioactive microsphere technique, which is a very accurate method to quantitate myocardial blood flow in animals, unfortunately has no equivalent in humans. Angiography is not accurate enough, and is not consistently performed during the course of acute myocardial infarction. Positron emission tomography (PET) could be a useful tool in the measurement of blood flow, but because of its costs, is not widely available.

Myocardial Metabolic Demand

Although less important than risk region or collateral blood flow as a determinant of infarct size, metabolic demand plays some role in myocardial ischemic injury. Higher myocardial oxygen demand during ischemia results in a larger infarct. Oxygen demand

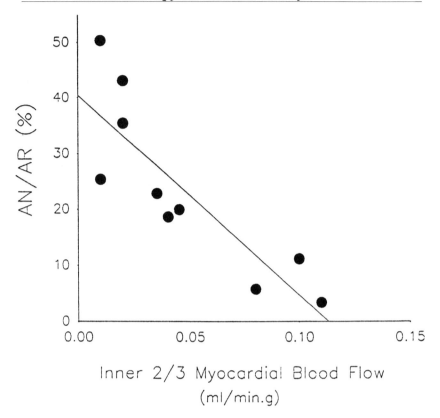

Figure 4: Collateral flow as a determinant of infarct size. Infarct size (expressed as a percentage of the area at risk) is plotted as a function of myocardial blood flow in the inner two-thirds of the left ventricular wall during a 60-min coronary artery occlusion. Infarct size is inversely related to collateral flow during ischemia. Adapted with permission of the American Heart Association.[97]

usually is estimated by the rate-pressure product (RPP = systolic blood pressure × heart rate), a gross index that can be used in all species (including man). Another index of metabolic demand in the canine model is myocardial blood flow (as measured by the radioactive microsphere technique) perfusing the nonischemic zone during ischemia in a remote territory.

Thus, although our clinical approach in assessing infarct size and its determinants has clearly improved, it remains imprecise. As a consequence, interpretation of trials using therapies aimed at reducing infarct size must be done cautiously unless very large numbers of patients are included to override the large variability in the major determinants of infarct size.

Quantitation of Infarct Size

The quantitation of infarct size has been the subject of numerous experimental and clinical investigations in the past years. Its measurement in in situ experimental preparations is now determined typically by either incubation of heart slices in triphenyl-tetrazolium chloride solution or by histologic determination.[24]

Although enzymatic determination (measurement of creatine kinase isoforms in the blood) is still used widely in clinical settings, its lack of accuracy is a concern. In addition, interpretation of creatine kinase curves in the setting of reperfusion is complicated by the fact that reperfusion causes a rapid washout of this enzyme from the necrotic tissue. There has been a constant quest for more precise methods of infarct size determination in the past years. Aside from SPECT imaging previously cited, magnetic resonance imaging (MRI) also appears promising.[25–28] The recent use of paramagnetic and superparamagnetic contrast agents permits a more accurate quantitation of infarct size and still is completely noninvasive.[29–32] Furthermore, recent advances allow left ventricular regional wall motion analysis by cine-MRI. However, further investigations are warranted to ascertain the usefulness of these techniques in daily clinical practice.

Reperfusion of the Ischemic Myocardium

Reperfusion-Induced Myocardial Salvage

Coronary reperfusion has proven to be the *only* reliable method to reduce infarct size consistently in the experimental as well as in the clinical setting. With the advent of thrombolysis, angioplasty, and bypass surgery, early reperfusion has become clinically feasible. In fact, reperfusion is the treatment of choice for acute myocardial infarction.

Due to the progressive nature of necrosis, the time frame for tissue salvage is critical. Although it is not defined accurately in man, most clinical studies suggest that myocardial salvage may occur when thrombolysis is started within 4 to 6 hours after the onset of chest pain.

Reperfusion Injury: Does It Exist?

There is no doubt that early reperfusion is the only way to salvage ischemic myocardium. However, there is ongoing debate whether reflow per se after an ischemic insult may inflict myocyte injury, which differs from that due to ischemia. That is, despite its benefits, reperfusion may be a "double-edged sword."[5]

This concept first arose from investigations by Jennings et al., who reported using the canine model that reperfusion was accompanied by an apparent acceleration of the necrotic process.[33] Hearse further demonstrated, using the isolated rat heart model, that reoxygenation resulted in massive release of enzymes and morphological damages ("oxygen paradox") that were much more significant than if hypoxia were maintained.[34]

There is considerable confusion as to the definition of "reperfusion injury." In fact, the existence of "reperfusion injury" is largely a matter of how this phenomenon is defined. In our opinion, "reperfusion injury" should refer to an event associated with reperfusion that either is entirely new, or an event that can be attenuated or prevented by an intervention given only at the time of reperfusion. Accordingly, four possible forms of reperfusion injury may be distinguished and will be reviewed here: reperfusion arrhythmias, vascular damage and no-reflow, reperfusion necrosis, and myocardial stunning.

Reperfusion Arrhythmias

Reperfusion arrhythmias are considered to be a form of reperfusion injury because they are induced rapidly by reperfusion. They have been observed in all species and include single ventricular extrasystoles, accelerated idioventricular rhythm, ventricular tachycardia, and ventricular fibrillation. Although there is no question of their existence, their clinical relevance is debatable. This is mainly due to a lower incidence of ventricular fibrillation after reperfusion by thrombolysis in humans than after reperfusion of acute coronary artery occlusion in experimental preparations.[35] This discrepancy is likely the consequence of a different speed of reflow: sudden reperfusion used in most experimental studies results in a greater incidence of ventricular fibrillation than the gradual reperfusion that typically occurs with thrombolysis. The timing of reperfusion also may play a role, as the incidence of ventricular fibrillation in the canine model is higher when reflow occurs after 15 minutes of ischemia than when it occurs after 90 minutes of ischemia. Although the mechanism for reperfusion arrhythmias remains unresolved, both excess intracellular Ca^{2+} oscillations and membrane damage induced by oxygen-derived free radicals are thought to play a role.[36,37]

Vascular Damage and No-Reflow

The no-reflow phenomenon is defined as the inability to reperfuse regions of previously ischemic myocardium after removal of a coronary occlusion.[38] In an early study, anesthetized open-chest dogs underwent 90 minutes of ischemia followed by reperfusion.[38] Thioflavin S (a fluorescent dye staining endothelial cells) was injected intravenously at the onset of reperfusion. Subendocardial areas were not penetrated by the dye, indicating that they had not been reperfused (Fig. 5). This was confirmed indirectly by a marked reduction in myocardial blood flow (measured by radioactive microspheres) in the unstained tissue. Ambrosio et al. later suggested that no-reflow in this canine model may worsen as reperfusion evolves, since the area of no-reflow markedly increased between 2 minutes and 3.5 hours after reperfusion.[39]

Several morphological abnormalities can be observed in areas of no-reflow: decreased endothelial pinocytotic vesicles, endothelial gaps, endothelial blebs, fibrin tactoids, rouleaux formation, and on occasion, microthrombi[40] (Fig. 2A). Hemorrhage, indicating endothelial damage, is confined always within the necrotic area. Swollen myocytes actually compressing capillaries, sometimes believed to be responsible for no-reflow, actually are sparse. Moreover, obstruction of microvessels by fibrin tactoids do not seem crucial since neither streptokinase nor tissue plasminogen activator prevented no-reflow.[40,41] It has also been proposed that polymorphonuclear neutrophil plugging in capillaries may contribute to no-reflow.[42] However, neutrophils are not present in the subendocardium during

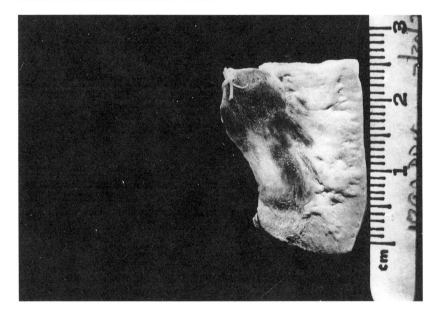

Figure 5: Posterior papillary muscle subjected to 90 min of ischemia (circumflex coronary occlusion) followed by 5 min of coronary reperfusion. Thioflavin S, a fluorescent dye, was injected during reperfusion. Regions of the subendocardium are nonfluorescent, representing areas of no-reflow. Reprinted with permission of the American Society for Clinical Investigation.[38]

the first minutes after reperfusion, whereas no-reflow already exists.[43] Furthermore, no-reflow occurs in isolated perfused hearts that are devoid of neutrophils.[44,45]

Przyklenk and Kloner recently demonstrated that superoxide dismutase (SOD) and catalase, potent free radical scavengers, significantly attenuated no-reflow and preserved the integrity of the vascular endothelium in dogs subjected to 2 hours of coronary artery occlusion[46] (Fig. 2B). This suggests that no-reflow may be a consequence of free radicals, generated at the time of reflow, by neutrophils or other pathways.

Whether no-reflow can contribute to myocardial injury is doubtful. Histologic examination reveals that areas of no-reflow are always smaller than, and included well within, areas of necrosis.[41] Nevertheless, lack of perfusion of infarcted tissue may be detrimental. Late coronary reperfusion may favor the healing process and limit infarct expansion. In this regard, although no-reflow appears to be a secondary phenomenon, therapeutic agents aimed at reducing its extent might have long-term beneficial effects.

"Low-reflow" is an extension of the concept of no-reflow. It describes a mild reduction in myocardial perfusion that occurs in previously ischemic but *still* viable tissue (as opposed to no-reflow that occurs in necrotic tissue). Its pathophysiology remains unclear.

Another feature of reperfusion-induced vascular injury is a deterioration in coronary vasodilator reserve. Several studies have demonstrated that coronary flow reserve is decreased transiently in viable reperfused tissue.[47–52] Specifically, reactivity to endothelium-dependent vasodilators (such as acetylcholine, bradykinin, adenosine diphosphate [ADP]) is decreased, whereas reactivity to endothelium-independent vasodilators (such as nitroprusside, nitroglycerin) may be decreased or remain unchanged.[47,49,50] This phenomenon may be due to endothelial injury mediated by oxygen radicals generated upon reperfusion, since it can be attenuated by scavengers of these reactive oxygen species.[51,52]

Reperfusion Necrosis

The concept of "reperfusion necrosis" remains highly controversial. In our opinion, "reperfusion necrosis" represents the reperfusion-induced death of myocytes that otherwise (i.e., if ischemia had persisted) would have survived. Importantly, this rigorous definition of reperfusion necrosis differs from the concept, introduced by Jennings, that reperfusion may hasten death of myocytes already destined to die by severe ischemia.

One way to prove reperfusion-induced necrosis is to reduce infarct size with an intervention given at the time of reperfusion. To address this issue, many investigators have administered free radical scavengers at the onset of reperfusion in various experimental models of myocardial infarction. The results are controversial: some studies have reported a significant reduction in infarct size, whereas others did not. For example, Ambrosio et al. found that recombinant human SOD given at the time of reflow in the canine model significantly reduced infarct size produced by 90 minutes of ischemia and 48 hours of reperfusion.[53] In contrast, Przyklenk and Kloner found that SOD + catalase administered 1 minute before reperfusion in the anesthetized dogs did not reduce infarct size caused by 2 hours of coronary occlusion followed by 4 hours of reflow.[46] So far, there is no consensus for a consistently positive effect on infarct size of oxygen-derived free radical scavengers, or any other treatment, given after reperfusion. Consequently, definitive evidence for the existence of "reperfusion necrosis" awaits further careful investigation.

Myocardial Stunning

Stunned myocardium initially was described and defined as reperfused myocardium that exhibits prolonged postischemic dysfunction despite the absence of irreversible damage.[54] The important aspect of this definition is that this contractile dysfunction applies to viable tissue, and the functional abnormality is fully reversible. Stunned myocardium is clearly a consequence of the preceding ischemic insult but, as it can be modified by agents given only at the time of reflow, it is considered as a manifestation of "reperfusion injury." This profound but transient postischemic dysfunction—both systolic and diastolic—has been documented extensively in ischemic canine myocardium reperfused after a 5- to 15-minute coronary artery occlusion.[55,56]

Although initially described in the canine model of brief ischemia, postischemic contractile dysfunction has also been demonstrated in experimental and clinical instances of viable, peri-infarct tissue.[56] Its specific evolution or response to therapy, however, is more difficult to assess in these models of prolonged occlusion, as the contractile performance of the salvaged myocardium is influenced by factors such as tethering to underlying dead tissue or healing of the necrotic myocardium, infarct expansion, or ventricular myocyte hypertrophy. Other clinical evidence of stunning includes left ventricular dysfunction after angioplasty, cardiopulmonary bypass, or episodes of angina.[57]

Time Course

Several studies have assessed the time course of recovery of contractile function after a reversible ischemic insult.[55,58] Results depend on the model (conscious or anesthetized animals), the severity and duration of the ischemic insult, and the layer of myocardium being studied. In the canine model, regional wall motion abnormalities usually persist for hours to days after reperfusion following 5 to 15 minutes of coronary artery occlusion (Fig. 6). If

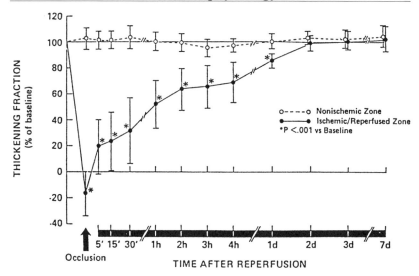

Figure 6: Time course of postischemic dysfunction after a reversible ischemic insult in conscious dogs. Changes in systolic wall thickening during a 15-min left anterior descending coronary artery occlusion and at selected times after reperfusion in the nonischemic and ischemic/reperfused canine myocardium. Thickening fraction is expressed as percentage of baseline values. Data are means ± SD (n = 21). Function in reperfused myocardium recovered slowly: on average, wall thickening still was significantly depressed at 1 day after reflow, but returned to baseline at 2 days after reperfusion. Reprinted with permission of the American Physiological Society.[58]

the duration of ischemia is extended and subendocardial necrosis occurs, then recovery of function is slower.[59] Although difficult to assess, the time course of stunning is likely comparable in humans since, after thrombolytic therapy, 10 to 16 days often elapse before improved wall motion can be detected by 2D echocardiography or angiography.

Severity of Myocardial Stunning

The severity of stunning depends mainly on two factors: the duration and severity of ischemia.

It is clear that at least 3 to 5 minutes of ischemia are necessary to induce stunning in the canine model[55,60,61]: one episode of 2 minutes of coronary artery occlusion is insufficient to create postischemic systolic dysfunction.[60] In the conscious dog, the degree of myocardial dysfunction after reperfusion is correlated in an exponential manner with the magnitude of blood flow reduction during the preceding ischemic insult[56] (Fig. 7). This relationship, however, is weaker in the anesthetized open-chest model. We found that severe ischemia is required to create stunning in the anesthetized dog. In this model, the degree of stunning is a function of the degree of dyskinesis during the preceding ischemic episode.[62] Thus, the severity of stunning appears to be determined by the severity of the initial ischemic insult. In this regard, although stunning is likely to

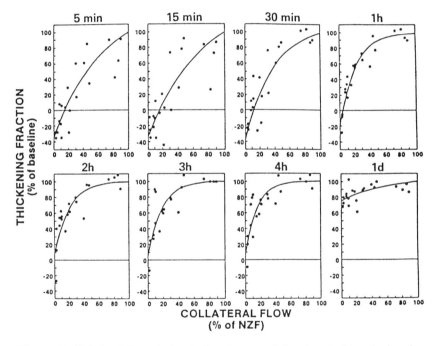

Figure 7: Collateral flow during ischemia as a determinant of postischemic recovery of contractile function in the conscious dog. Relationship between mean transmural collateral flow to the ischemic region during a 15-min coronary occlusion and systolic wall thickening at various intervals after reperfusion (n = 21). Collateral flow is expressed as a percentage of simultaneous nonischemic zone flow (NZF); thickening fraction is expressed as percentage of baseline values. Thickening fraction is related in an exponential manner to collateral flow. Note that small differences in collateral flow may result in large differences in recovery of function after reperfusion. Reprinted with permission of the American Physiological Society.[58]

be a form of reperfusion injury, any therapeutic improvement of the antecedent ischemic injury is likely to reduce the postischemic dysfunction.

Mechanism of Myocardial Stunning

Several hypotheses have been proposed to explain myocardial stunning including: depletion of myocardial ATP content, altered intracellular Ca^{2+} metabolism, generation of oxygen-derived free radicals, and damage to the collagen matrix.

Myocardial ATP Depletion: A similar time course of recovery of ATP stores and contractile function first suggested a cause and effect relationship between these two parameters.[63-65] Striking observations to the contrary, however, have eliminated this theory. First, inotropic stimulation markedly improved stunning without affecting ATP content.[66] Similarly, Przyklenk and Kloner observed that whereas SOD + catalase, potent scavengers of oxygen-derived free radicals, improved contractile function, they did not restore myocardial ATP levels.[46] Finally, increasing ATP stores by metabolic precursors failed to alter mechanical activity,[66] whereas decreasing ATP/adenine nucleotide pool—to values lower than those observed in the stunned myocardium—does not necessarily result in contractile dysfunction.[67-69] Thus, reduced energy production is not the cause of myocardial stunning.

Altered Intracellular Ca^{2+} Metabolism: Several studies have suggested a role of altered Ca^{2+} homeostasis in myocardial stunning.

In vitro investigations suggest that *subtle* alterations in intracellular Ca^{2+} homeostasis at reperfusion (as opposed to massive Ca^{2+} overload associated with the reperfusion of necrotic tissue) play a role in the pathogenesis of the stunned myocardium. Using the isolated globally ischemic ferret heart model, Kusuoka et al. have demonstrated that reperfusion with solutions containing low Ca^{2+} concentrations results in significantly improved recovery of function.[70] They also suggest that postischemic contractile dysfunction is related to both a decreased maximal force of contraction and a reduced Ca^{2+} sensitivity of the myofilaments. Also, exposure of nonischemic isolated hearts to Ca^{2+} overload induces contractile abnormalities similar to stunning.[6]

However, the role of Ca^{2+} overload in in vivo models of myocardial stunning is unclear. In the canine model, Krause et al.

observed that sarcoplasmic reticulum of myocardium stunned by repeated 5-minute coronary artery occlusions exhibited a decreased activity of the Ca^{2+}-Mg^{2+}-ATPase and decreased ability to take up Ca^{2+}.[71] This could further lead to reduced release of Ca^{2+} into the cytosol and limited availability of Ca^{2+} for contractile proteins. However, this is not in agreement with in vitro studies showing no alteration of intracellular Ca^{2+} transients in stunning. Another option is that the responsiveness of contractile proteins may be altered during reperfusion so that more free Ca^{2+} becomes necessary to achieve a given force of contraction.[72] Further investigations are required to determine if this applies to the in vivo model of myocardial stunning.

Oxygen-Derived Free Radicals: Oxygen-derived free radicals likely play an important role in the pathogenesis of myocardial stunning.

Studies using electron paramagnetic resonance spectroscopy have demonstrated that these oxygen species are produced mainly during the first seconds after a brief reversible ischemic insult.[73,74] Moreover, Bolli et al. showed that N-(2-mercaptopropionyl)-glycine, administered 1 minute before reperfusion, prevented the production of oxygen-derived free radicals at the onset of reperfusion and consequently attenuated stunning.[75] In contrast, when this oxygen scavenger was administered 1 minute after reperfusion, the burst of oxygen-derived free radicals was blunted only slightly and stunning persisted.

Numerous investigations have demonstrated that various oxygen scavengers or antioxidants administered before or during a reversible ischemic insult protect postischemic contractile function.[46,74,76] In addition, Przyklenk et al. recently reported that infusion of xanthine oxidase + purine + iron-loaded transferrin (a combination of solutions that generate oxygen-derived free radicals) into a coronary vein in dogs resulted in systolic contractile dysfunction mimicking stunning.[77] Thus, there is a large body of evidence suggesting that oxygen-derived free radicals are, at least in part, responsible for myocardial stunning.

The precise mechanisms whereby these toxic species may induce stunning remain unclear. One attractive possibility suggests that alterations of Ca^{2+} homeostasis and production of oxygen-derived free radicals are interrelated. The latter can cause lipid peroxidation of myocyte membranes (mainly sarcolemma and sarcoplasmic reticulum), resulting in altered delivery of Ca^{2+} to contractile proteins. Confirmation of this hypothesis awaits further investigation.

Damage to Collagen Matrix: It has been hypothesized that stunning may be partly due to alteration of the collagen matrix. In fact, repeated brief coronary artery occlusions are associated with rupture of the collagen fibers.[78] However, Whittaker et al. recently demonstrated that, although multiple episodes of ischemia damage the collagen framework, one single 15-minute ischemic insult results in stunning but does not alter collagen structure.[79] This strongly suggests that collagen damage may be a consequence, but not a cause, of stunning. Furthermore, the usual recovery of function seen within hours or days after a 5- to 15-minute ischemic insult, and recovery of function with inotropic stimulation, seems incompatible with repair of such structural damage. However, damage to the collagen matrix may be a very important long-term consequence in case of recurrent ischemia (as occurs in patients with unstable angina).

In summary, the pathophysiology of myocardial stunning remains unclear, although production of oxygen-derived free radicals and alteration of Ca^{2+} homeostasis are likely to play an important role in this phenomenon.

"Therapies" for Stunned Myocardium

In the canine model, myocardial stunning after a single 15-minute coronary artery occlusion is amenable to pharmacological interventions.

However, one must distinguish agents that limit myocardial injury during ischemia (i.e., administered before or during coronary artery occlusion) from those affecting postischemic contractile dysfunction per se. For example, beta blockers attenuate stunning by reducing energy demand during ischemia.[80] However, they do not improve stunning when given after reperfusion.[81]

Inotropic agents (dopamine, dobutamine, and isoproterenol) administered after reperfusion dramatically improve postischemic contractile function, thereby confirming that contractile reserve of stunned myocardium is intact.[82,83] Different types of Ca^{2+} antagonists, even when given at or after reperfusion, restore systolic function independently of an effect on hemodynamics or coronary perfusion[84–86] (Fig. 8). Angiotensin-converting enzyme (ACE) inhibitors, administered either before coronary artery occlusion or

% SEGMENT SHORTENING
Ischemic LAD Bed

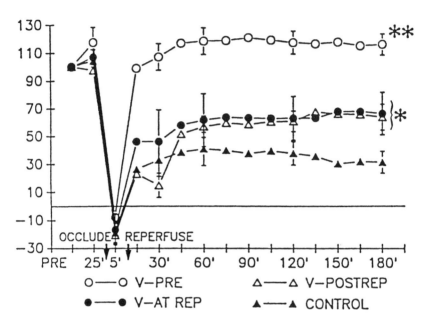

Figure 8: Effect of verapamil on postischemic contractile function after a 15-min myocardial ischemic insult in the anesthetized dog. Segment shortening (expressed as a percentage of baseline values) in the ischemic left anterior descending coronary artery bed is presented during coronary occlusion and at different time points after reperfusion. Verapamil given before coronary occlusion ablated myocardial stunning. When given at or after reperfusion, verapamil significantly attenuated postischemic contractile dysfunction. V-PRE = verapamil given before occlusion; V-AT REP = verapamil given at reperfusion; V-POST REP = verapamil given 30 min after reperfusion. $^*p<0.05$ vs. control, $^{**}p<0.01$ vs. control. Reprinted with permission of the American College of Cardiology.[84]

after reperfusion, have been reported to improve stunning (Fig. 9). Their mechanism of action is uncertain, although Przyklenk and Kloner recently suggested that some ACE inhibitors may act through enhanced prostanoid production.[87]

The fact that all these pharmacological agents can improve postischemic contractile function further confirm that stunning is a transient and fully reversible phenomenon.

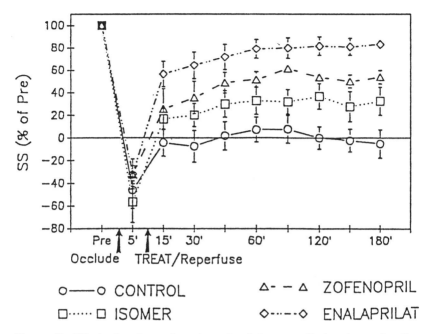

o——o CONTROL   Δ– – Δ ZOFENOPRIL

□······□ ISOMER   ◇·····◇ ENALAPRILAT

Figure 9: Effect of zofenopril and enalaprilat on postischemic contractile function after a 15-min ischemic insult in the anesthetized dog. Segment shortening (expressed as a percentage of baseline values) in the ischemic left anterior descending coronary artery bed is presented during coronary occlusion and at different time points after reperfusion. Zofenopril is a sulfhydryl-containing ACE inhibitor; enalaprilat is a nonsulfhydryl-containing ACE inhibitor; SQ 14,534 is a stereoisomer of captopril that contains the sulfhydryl group but has no ACE inhibitor properties. Both enalaprilat and zofenopril, given at the time of reperfusion, enhanced recovery of contractile function as a consequence of their property to inhibit angiotensin-converting enzyme. In contrast, the beneficial effect of SQ 14,534 on recovery of postischemic contractile function was likely due to antioxidant properties of this compound. Reprinted with permission of the American Heart Journal.[87]

Recurrent Episodes of Ischemia/Reperfusion: The "Preconditioning" Phenomenon

As patients with coronary artery disease often suffer recurrent episodes of angina and/or silent myocardial ischemia, the effects of these multiple ischemic insults on myocyte metabolism and function have been the subject of considerable investigation in the past decades.

Studies of repeated brief ischemia have revealed minimal myocardial damage or necrosis and little cumulative effect on tissue adenine nucleotide content. Also, postischemic contractile dysfunction was not exacerbated after repeated occlusions.[88] Thus, repeated episodes of brief ischemia did not appear to worsen myocardial injury and the resultant contractile dysfunction does not appear to be additive.

Recently, Murry et al. extended this concept by an intriguing observation.[89] They reported that one or several brief (i.e., reversible) ischemic episodes reduced infarct size produced by a subsequent sustained period (i.e., irreversible) of ischemia. They named this phenomenon "ischemic preconditioning." These data demonstrate that brief ischemia/reperfusion episodes are protective and render the myocardium more tolerant to subsequent ischemia. This observation has now been confirmed in all animal species in which it has been studied: dogs, rats, pigs, and rabbits.[90–92] However, its mechanism remains unknown, although recent evidence suggests that it may be mediated by adenosine.[93]

One major question is the clinical relevance of myocardial preconditioning. Extrapolation of the concept of preconditioning to the clinical setting of spontaneous occlusion/reperfusion is confounded by the fact that the progressive occlusion of a stenosed coronary artery by an active thrombus formed on damaged endothelium is quite different from the sudden mechanical occlusion followed by abrupt reperfusion commonly used in the experimental setting. Deutsch et al. (using anginal discomfort, ST segment modifications, and lactate production as criteria of ischemia) recently reported that, during angioplasty, ischemia was tolerated significantly better during the second balloon inflation than during the first one.[94] They attributed this to a preconditioning effect.

Using the canine model, we recently addressed the issue that unstable angina may precondition the heart.[95] We used the model described by Folts where repeated formation and dislodgment of a thrombus on a stenosed and endothelially injured coronary artery result in recurrent brief episodes of ischemia/reperfusion. Comparison of brief ischemia by thrombosis versus brief ischemia by mechanical coronary occlusion revealed no difference in terms of infarct size: repeated coronary thrombus formation preconditioned the heart as effectively as mechanical occlusion (Fig. 10). In other words, endothelial injury, severe coronary stenosis, and thrombus formation, all major components of the pathogenesis of unstable

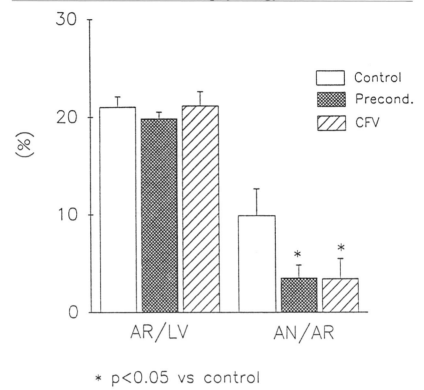

* p<0.05 vs control

Figure 10: Protective effect of coronary cyclic flow variations on infarct size after a subsequent 60-min ischemic insult. The area at risk (AR), expressed as a percentage of the left ventricular weight, was similar in all three groups. Area of necrosis (AN), expressed as a percentage of the area at risk, was significantly reduced in both CFV and mechanically preconditioned dogs ($p<0.05$ vs. control). Thus, repeated coronary thrombus formation "preconditions" the ischemic myocardium. Reprinted with permission of the American Heart Association.[95]

angina in humans, did not interfere with the mechanism of preconditioning. Although any extrapolation must be made with caution, this suggests that unstable angina may precondition the human myocardium undergoing myocardial infarction.

Preconditioning, although it dramatically reduced infarct size, neither improved contractile function during the sustained ischemia nor attenuated myocardial stunning during the first hours of reperfusion[95] (Fig. 11). Thus, preconditioning does not seem to protect myocardial function, at least during the early hours of

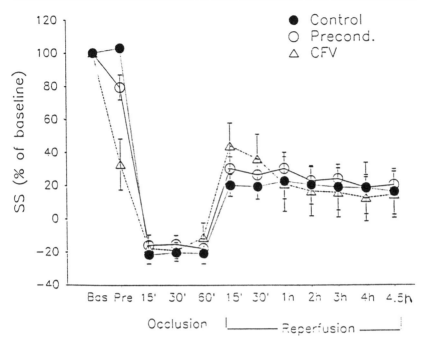

Figure 11: Effects of coronary cyclic flow variations on contractile function. Segment shortening (expressed as a percentage of baseline values) in ischemic left anterior descending coronary artery bed of dogs submitted to four episodes of brief coronary occlusion/reperfusion followed by 60 min of coronary occlusion and 4.5 hr of reperfusion. Data was obtained at baseline (Bas), at the end of the preconditioning period (Pre), and at multiple time points throughout sustained occlusion and after reperfusion. No statistical difference existed among groups during the sustained occlusion and after reperfusion, indicating that preconditioning neither preserved contractile function during ischemia nor attenuated stunning in the peri-infarct tissue during the first hours of reperfusion. Reprinted with permission of the American Heart Association.[95]

reperfusion, in the canine model. This observation confirms previous investigations indicating that the mechanisms of preconditioning and stunning likely are not related.[96] Preliminary data from our laboratory also suggest that preconditioning does not protect the vascular endothelium or protect against loss of vasodilator reserve after sustained ischemia/reperfusion.

Obviously, further investigations are needed to ascertain the existence of preconditioning in humans. If preconditioning does occur in humans, it could represent a useful form of preventive therapy to protect ischemic myocardium during angioplasty or cardiac surgery.

Summary

Clinical and experimental studies investigating myocardial ischemia and reperfusion have contributed to our understanding of a very complex set of phenomena. It is clear that coronary reperfusion, provided it is instituted relatively early after coronary occlusion, salvages ischemic myocardium. In fact, reperfusion by thrombolysis, angioplasty, or bypass surgery is the treatment of choice for acute myocardial infarction. However, the unquestionable benefit of reperfusion on tissue salvage is accompanied by some potentially deleterious effects within both the necrotic and viable tissue. The no-reflow phenomenon, confined to the irreversibly injured tissue, appears as a secondary event and should not act as a deterrent to treatment with reperfusion. Myocardial tissue that has been salvaged by reperfusion may exhibit reversible abnormalities in ultrastructure, biochemistry, and function. Full recovery may take days to weeks, but finally occurs. Interestingly, brief ischemia/reperfusion (which often occurs in patients suffering from angina pectoris) recently has been shown in experimental preparations to induce tolerance to further prolonged ischemia. Further investigations are needed to determine the clinical relevance of this phenomenon termed "preconditioning."

References

1. Ganz W, Buchbinder N, Marcus M, Mondkar H, Maddahi J, et al. Intracoronary thrombolysis in evolving myocardial infarction. Am Heart J 1981; 101:4–13.
2. Rentrop KP, Blanke H, Karsch KR. Effects of nonsurgical coronary reperfusion on the left ventricle in human subjects compared with conventional treatment: study of 18 patients with acute myocardial infarction treated with intracoronary infusion of streptokinase. Am J Cardiol 1983; 49:1–8.
3. Kennedy JW, Ritchie JL, Davis KB, Fritz JK. Western Washington randomized Trial of Intracoronary Streptokinase in Acute Myocardial Infarction. N Engl J Med 1983; 309:1977–1982.
4. Laffel GL, Braunwald E. Thrombolytic therapy. A new strategy for the treatment of acute myocardial infarction. N Engl J Med 1984; 311:710–717, 770–776.

5. Braunwald E, Kloner RA. Myocardial reperfusion: a double-edged sword? J Clin Invest 1985; 76:1713–1719.
6. Opie LH. Reperfusion injury and its pharmacological modification. Circulation 1989; 80:1049–1062.
7. Neely JR, Grotyohann LW. Role of glycolytic products in damage to ischemic myocardium. Dissociation of adenosine triphosphate levels and recovery of function of reperfused ischemic hearts. Circ Res 1984; 55:816–824.
8. Opie L. Myocardial ischemia: metabolic pathways and implications of increased glycolysis. Cardiovasc Drugs Ther 1990; 4:777–790.
9. Jennings RB, Reimer KA, Hill ML, Mayer SE. Total ischemia in dog hearts, in vitro: 1. Comparison of high energy phosphate production, utilization, and depletion, and of adenine nucleotide catabolism in total ischemia in vitro vs severe ischemia in vivo. Circ Res 1981; 49:892–900.
10. Jennings RB, Reimer KA, Hill ML. Total ischemia in dog hearts, in vitro: 2. High energy phosphate depletion and associated defects in energy metabolism, cell volume regulation, and sarcolemmal integrity. Circ Res 1981; 49:901–911.
11. Reimer KA, Jennings RB. The "wavefront phenomenon" of myocardial cell death. II. Transmural progression of necrosis within the framework of ischemic bed size (myocardium at risk) and collateral flow. Lab Invest 1979; 40:633–644.
12. Jugdutt BI, Hutchins GM, Bullkley BH, Becker LC. Myocardial infarction in the conscious dog: three-dimensional mapping of infarct, collateral flow and region at risk. Circulation 1979; 60:1141–1150.
13. Machac J. Technetium-99m Isonitrile: a perfusion or a viability agent? J Am Coll Cardiol 1989; 14:1685–1688.
14. Mousa SA, Cooney JM, Williams SJ. Relationship between regional myocardial blood flow and the distribution of 99mTc-sestamibi in the presence of total coronary occlusion. Am Heart J 1990; 119:842–847.
15. Marshall RC, Leidholdt EM, Zhang DY, Barnett CA. Technetium-99m hexakis 2-methoxy-2-isobutyl isonitrile and Thallium-201 extraction, washout, and retention at varying coronary flow rates in rabbit heart. Circulation 1990; 82:998–1007.
16. Beanlands RSB, Dawood F, Wen WH, Mclaughlin PR, Butany J, et al. Are the kinetics of Technetium-99m Methoxyisobutyl isonitrile affected by cell metabolism and viability? Circulation 1990; 82:1802–1814.
17. Gibbons RJ, Verani MS, Behrenbeck T, Pellikka PA, O'Connor MK, et al. Feasibility of tomographic 99m-Tc-Hexakis-2-Methoxy-2-Methylpropyl-isonitrile imaging for the assessment of myocardial area at risk and the effect of treatment in acute myocardial infarction. Circulation 1989; 80:1277–1286.
18. Sinusas AJ, Trautman KA, Bergin JD, Watson DD, Ruiz M, et al. Quantification of area at risk during coronary occlusion and degree of myocardial salvage after reperfusion with Technetium-99m Methoxyisobutyl isonitrile. Circulation 1990; 82:1424–1437.
19. De Coster PM, Winjs W, Cauwe F, Robert A, Beckers C, Melin JA. Area at risk determination by Technetium-99m Hexakis-2-Methoxyisobutyl

isonitril in experimental reperfused myocardial infarction. Circulation 1990; 82:2152–2162.

20. Rocco TP, Dilsizian V, Strauss W, Boucher CA. Technetium-99m Isonitrile myocardial uptake at rest. II. Relation to clinical markers of potential viability. J Am Coll Cardiol 1989; 14:1678–1684.
21. Christian TF, Gibbons RJ, Gersch BJ. Effect of infarct location on myocardial salvage assessed by Technetium-99m Isonitrile. J Am Coll Cardiol 1991; 17:1303–1308.
22. Verani MS, Jeroudi MO, Mahmarian JJ, Boyce TM, Borges-Neto S, et al. Quantification of myocardial infarction during coronary occlusion and myocardial salvage after reperfusion using cardiac imaging with Technetium-99m Hexakis-2-Methoxyisobutyl Isonitrile. J Am Coll Cardiol 1988; 12:1573–1581.
23. Bishop SP, White FC, Bloor CM. Regional myocardial blood flow during acute myocardial infarction in the conscious dog. Circ Res 1976; 38:429–438.
24. Bishop SP. How well can we measure coronary flow, risk zones, and infarct size? In: Hearse DJ, Yellon DM, eds. Therapeutic Approaches to Myocardial Infarct Size Limitation. New York: Raven Press. 1984; pp 139–162.
25. Goldman MR, Brady TJ, Pykett IL, Burt CT, Buonanno FS, et al. Quantification of experimental myocardial infarction using nuclear magnetic resonance imaging and paramagnetic ion contrast enhancement in excised canine hearts. Circulation 1982; 66:1012–1016.
26. Wesbey G, Higgins CB, Lanzer P, Botvinick E, Lipton MJ. Imaging and characterization of acute myocardial infarction in vivo by gated nuclear magnetic resonance. Circulation 1984; 69:125–130.
27. Pfugfelder PN, Wisenberg G, Prato FS, Caroll SE, Turner KL. Early detection of canine myocardial infarction by magnetic resonance imaging in vivo. Circulation 1985; 71:587–594.
28. Tscholakoff D, Higgins CB, McNamara MT, Derugin N. Early-phase myocardial infarction: evaluation by MR imaging. Radiology 1986; 159:667–672.
29. Schaefer S, Malloy CR, Katz J, Parkey RW, Buja LM, et al. Gadolinium-DTPA-enhanced nuclear magnetic resonance imaging of reperfused myocardium: identification of the myocardium bed at risk. J Am Coll Cardiol 1988; 12:1064–1072.
30. Schouman-claeys E, Frija G, Revel D, Doucet D, Donadieu AM. Canine acute myocardial infarction. In vivo detection by MRI with gradient echo technique and contribution of Gd DOTA. Invest Radiol 1988; 23:S254–S257.
31. Ovize M, Revel D, de Lorgeril M, Pichard JB, Dandis G, et al. Quantification of reperfused myocardial infarction by Gd-DOTA-enhanced magnetic resonance imaging. An experimental study. Invest Radiol 1991; 26:1065–1070.
32. Rozenman Y, Xueming Z, Kantor HL. Cardiovascular MR imaging with iron oxide particles: utility of superparamagnetic contrast agent and the role of diffusion in signal loss. Radiology 1990; 175:655–659.
33. Jennings RB, Sommers HM, Smyth GA, Flack HA, Linn H. Myocardial

necrosis induced by temporary occlusion of the coronary artery in dog. Arch Pathol 1960; 70:68–78.

34. Hearse DJ. Reperfusion of ischemic myocardium. J Mol Cell Cardiol 1977; 9:605–616.
35. Marras P, Della Grazia E, Klugmann S. Reperfusion ventricular arrhythmias during thrombolysis. Eur Heart J 1986; 7(Suppl A): 23–30.
36. Hearse DJ, Tosaki A. Free radicals and calcium: simultaneous interacting triggers as determinants of vulnerability to reperfusion-induced arrhythmias in the rat heart. J Mol Cell Cardiol 1988; 20:213–223.
37. Allen DG, Lee JA, Smith GL. The effect of simulated ischemia on intracellular calcium and tension in isolated ferret ventricular muscle. J Physiol (Lond) 1988; 401:81P.
38. Kloner RA, Ganote CE, Jennings RB. The "no-reflow" phenomenon following temporary coronary occlusion in the dog. J Clin Invest 1974; 54:1496–1508.
39. Ambrosio G, Weisman HF, Becker LC. The "no-reflow" phenomenon: a misnomer? Circulation 1986; 74(Suppl II):II–260.
40. Kloner RA, Alker KJ, Campbell C, Figures G, Eisenhauer A, Hale S. Does tissue-type plasminogen activator have direct beneficial effects on the myocardium independent of its ability to lyse intracoronary thrombi? Circulation 1989; 79:1125–1136.
41. Kloner RA, Alker KJ. The effect of streptokinase on intramyocardial hemorrhage, infarct size, and the no-reflow phenomenon during coronary reperfusion. Circulation 1984; 70:513–521.
42. Engler RL, Schmidt-schoenbein GW, Pavelec RS. Leukocyte capillary plugging in myocardial ischemia and reperfusion in the dog. Am J Pathol 1983; 111:98–111.
43. Go LO, Murry CE, Richard VJ, Weischedel GR, Jennings RB, Reimer RA. Myocardial neutrophil accumulation during reperfusion after reversible or irreversible ischemic injury. Am J Physiol 1988; 255:H1188–H1198.
44. Humphrey SM, Gavin JB, Herdson PB. The relationship of ischemic contracture to vascular reperfusion in the isolated rat heart. J Mol Cell Cardiol 1980; 12:1397–1406.
45. Watts JA, Whipple JP, Hatley AA. A low concentration of nisoldipine reduces ischemic heart injury: enhanced reflow and recovery of contractile function without energy preservation during ischemia. J Mol Cell Cardiol 1987; 19:809–817.
46. Przyklenk K, Kloner RA. "Reperfusion injury" by oxygen-derived free radicals? Effect of superoxide dismutase + catalase, given at the time of reperfusion, on myocardial infarct size, contractile function, coronary microvasculature and regional myocardial blood flow. Circ Res 1989; 64:86–96.
47. Vanhaecke J, Flameng W, Borgers M, Ik-Kyung J, Van de Werf F, De Geest H. Evidence for decreased coronary flow reserve in viable postischemic myocardium. Circ Res 1990; 67:1201–1210.
48. Headrick JP, Angello DA, Berne RM. Effects of brief coronary occlusion

and reperfusion on porcine coronary artery reactivity. Circulation 1990; 82:2163–2169.

49. Quillen JE, Sellke FW, Brooks LA, Harrison DG. Ischemia-reperfusion impairs endothelium-dependent relaxation of coronary microvessels but does not affect large arteries. Circulation 1990; 82:586–594.

50. Tsao PS, Aoki N, Lefer DJ, Johnson G III, Lefer AM. Time course of endothelial dysfunction and myocardial injury during myocardial ischemia and reperfusion in the cat. Circulation 1990; 82:1402–1412.

51. Dauber IM, Lefnesky EJ, Van Benthuysen KM, Weil JV, Horwitz LD. Reactive oxygen metabolite scavengers decrease functional coronary microvascular injury due to ischemia-reperfusion. Am J Physiol 1991; 260:H42–H49.

52. Mehta JL, Nichols WW, Donnelly WH, Lawson DL, Thompson L, et al. Protection by superoxide dismutase from myocardial dysfunction and attenuation of vasodilator reserve after coronary occlusion and reperfusion in dog. Circ Res 1989; 65:1283–1295.

53. Ambrosio G, Becker LC, Hutchins GM, Weisman HF, Weisfeld ML. Reduction in experimental infarct size by recombinant human superoxide dismutase: insights into the pathophysiology of reperfusion injury. Circulation 1986; 74:1424–1433.

54. Braunwald E, Kloner RA. The stunned myocardium: prolonged, postischemic ventricular dysfunction. Circulation 1982; 66:1146–1149.

55. Heyndrickx GR, Millard RW, McRitchie RJ, Maroko PR, Vatner SF. Regional myocardial functional and electrophysiological alterations after brief coronary artery occlusion in conscious dogs. J Clin Invest 1975; 56:978–985.

56. Bolli R. Mechanism of myocardial "stunning." Circulation 1990; 82:723–738.

57. Kloner RA, Przyklenk K, Patel B. Altered myocardial states. The stunned and hibernating myocardium. Am J Med 1989; 86(Suppl IA):14–19.

58. Bolli R, Zhu WX, Thornby JI, O'Neill PG, Roberts R. Time-course and determinants of recovery of function after reversible ischemia in conscious dogs. Am J Physiol 1988; 254:H102–H114.

59. Ellis SG, Henschke CI, Sandor T, Wynne J, Braunwald E, Kloner RA. Time course of functional and biochemical recovery of myocardium salvaged by reperfusion. J Am Coll Cardiol 1983; 1:1047–1055.

60. Warner KG, Khuri SF, Marston W, Sharma S, Butler MD, et al. Significance of the transmural diminution in regional hydrogen ion production after repeated coronary artery occlusions. Circ Res 1989; 64:616–628.

61. Kloner RA, Ellis SG, Lange R, Braunwald E. Studies of experimental coronary artery reperfusion: effects of infarct size, myocardial function, biochemistry, ultrastructure, and microvascular damage. Circulation 1983; 68(Suppl I):I8–I15.

62. Przyklenk K, Kloner RA. What factors predict recovery of contractile function in the canine model of the stunned myocardium? Am J Cardiol 1989; 64:18F–26F.

63. DeBoer FWV, Ingwall JS, Kloner RA, Braunwald E. Prolonged derangements of canine myocardial purine metabolism after a brief coronary artery occlusion not associated with anatomic evidence of necrosis. Proc Natl Acad Sci USA 1980; 77:5471–5475.

64. Reimer KA, Hill ML, Jennings RB. Prolonged depletion of ATP and of the adenine nucleotide pool due to delayed resynthesis of adenine nucleotides following reversible myocardial injury in dogs. J Mol Cell Cardiol 1981; 13:229–239.

65. Swain JL, Sabina RL, McHale PA, Greenfield JC Jr, Holmes EW. Prolonged myocardial nucleotide depletion after brief ischemia in the open-chest dog. Am J Physiol 1982; 242:H818–H826.

66. Arnold JMO, Braunwald E, Sandor T, Kloner RA. Inotropic stimulation of reperfused myocardium with dopamine: effects on infarct size and myocardial function. J Am Coll Cardiol 1985; 6:1026–1034.

67. Ambrosio G, Jacobus WE, Mitchell MC, Litt MR, Becker LC. Effects of ATP precursors on ATP and free ADP content and functional recovery of postischemic hearts. Am J Physiol 1989; 256:H560–H566.

68. Kupriyonov VV, Lakomkin VL, Kapelko VI, Steinschneider AY, Ruuge EK, Saks VA. Dissociation of adenosine triphosphate levels and contractile function in isovolumetric hearts perfused with 2-deoxyglucose. J Mol Cell Cardiol 1987; 19:729.

69. Zucchi R, Limbruno U, di Vincenzo A, Mariani M, Ronca G. Adenine nucleotide depletion and contractile dysfunction in the "stunned" myocardium. Cardiovasc Res 1990; 24:440.

70. Kusuoka H, Porterfield JK, Weisman HF. Pathophysiology and pathogenesis of stunned myocardium: depressed Ca^{2+}-activation of contraction as a consequence of reperfusion-induced cellular Ca^{2+} overload in ferrets hearts. J Clin Invest 1987; 79:950–961.

71. Krause SM, Jacobus WE, Becker LC. Alterations in cardiac sarcoplasmic reticulum calcium transport in the postischemic "stunned" myocardium. Circ Res 1989; 65:526–530.

72. Morgan JP. Abnormal intracellular modulation of calcium as a major cause of cardiac contractile dysfunction. N Engl J Med 1991; 325:625–632.

73. Zweier JL, Flaherty JT, Weisfeld ML. Direct measurement of free radical generation following reperfusion of ischemic myocardium. Proc Natl Acad Sci USA 1987; 84:1404–1407.

74. Bolli R, Patel BS, Jeroudi MO, Lai EK, McKay PB. Demonstration of free radical generation in "stunned" myocardium of intact dogs with the use of spin trap alpha-phenyl N-tertbutyl nitrone. J Clin Invest 1988; 82:476–485.

75. Bolli R, Jeroudi MO, Patel BS, Aruoma Oi, Halliwell B, et al. Marked reduction of free radical generation and contractile dysfunction by antioxidant therapy begun at the time of reperfusion. Evidence that myocardial stunning is a manifestation of reperfusion injury. Circ Res 1989; 65:607–622.

76. Bolli R. Oxygen-derived free radicals and postischemic dysfunction ("stunned" myocardium). J Am Coll Cardiol 1988; 12:239–249.

77. Przyklenk K, Whittaker P, Kloner RA. In vivo injection of oxygen free

radical substrate causes myocardial systolic, but not diastolic function. Am Heart J 1990; 119:807–815.

78. Zhao M, Zhang H, Robinson TF, Factor SM, Sonnenblick EH, Eng C. Profound structural alterations of the extracellular collagen matrix in postischemic ("stunned") but viable myocardium. J Am Coll Cardiol 1987; 10:1322–1334.

79. Whittaker P, Boughner DR, Kloner RA, Przyklenk K. Stunned myocardium and myocardial collagen damage: differential effects of single and repeated occlusions. Am Heart J 1991; 121:434–441.

80. Lange R, Kloner RA, Braunwald E. First ultra short-acting beta adrenergic blocking agent: its effect on size and segmental wall dynamics of reperfused myocardial infarcts in dogs. Am J Cardiol 1983; 51:1759–1767.

81. Przyklenk K, Kloner RA. Is "stunned myocardium" a protective mechanism? Effect of acute recruitment and acute beta-blockage on recovery of contractile function and high energy phosphate stores at 1 day post reperfusion. Am Heart J 1989; 118:480–489.

82. Arnold JMO, Braunwald E, Sandor T, Kloner RA. Inotropic stimulation of reperfused myocardium with dopamine: effects on infarct size and myocardial function. J Am Coll Cardiol 1985; 6:1026–1034.

83. Ellis SG, Wynne J, Braunwald E, Henschke CI, Sandor T, Kloner RA. Inotropic stimulation of reperfused myocardium with dopamine: effects on infarct size and myocardial function. J Am Coll Cardiol 1985; 6:1026–1034.

84. Przyklenk K, Kloner RA. Effect of verapamil on postischemic "stunned" myocardium: importance of the timing of treatment. J Am Coll Cardiol 1988; 11:614–623.

85. Przyklenk K, Ghafari GB, Eitzman DT, Kloner RA. Nifedipine administered after reperfusion ablates systolic contractile dysfunction of postischemic "stunned" myocardium. J Am Coll Cardiol 1989; 13:1176–1183.

86. Taylor AL, Golino P, Eckels R, Pastor P, Buja M, Willerson JT. Differential enhancement of postischemic segmental systolic thickening by diltiazem. J Am Coll Cardiol 1990; 15:737–747.

87. Przyklenk K, Kloner RA. Angiotensin converting enzyme inhibitors improve contractile function of stunned myocardium by different mechanisms of action. Am Heart J 1991; 121:1319–1330.

88. Lange R, Ware J, Kloner RA. Absence of cumulative deterioration of regional function during three repeated 5 or 15 minute coronary occlusions. Circulation 1984; 69:400–408.

89. Murry CE, Jennings RB, Reimer KA. Preconditioning with ischemia: a delay of lethal cell injury in ischemic myocardium. Circulation 1986; 5:1124–1136.

90. Schott RJ, Rohmanns S, Brau ER, Schaper W. Ischemic preconditioning reduces infarct size in swine myocardium. Circ Res 1990; 66:1133–1142.

91. Thornton J, Striplin S, Liu GS, Swafford A, Stanley AWH, et al. Inhibition of protein synthesis does not block myocardial protection afforded by preconditioning. Am J Physiol 1990; 259:H1822–H1825.

92. Shiki K, Hearse DJ. Preconditioning of ischemic myocardium: reperfusion-induced arrhythmias. Am J Physiol 1987; 253:H1470–H1476.
93. Liu GS, Thornton J, Van Winckle DM, Stanley AWH, Olsson RA, Downey JM. Protection against infarction afforded by preconditioning is mediated by A_1 adenosine receptors in rabbit heart. Circulation 1991; 84:350–356.
94. Deutsch E, Berger M, Kussmaul WG, Hirshfeld JW Jr, Herrmann HC, Laskey WK. Adaptation to ischemia during percutaneous transluminal coronary angioplasty. Clinical, hemodynamic, and metabolic features. Circulation 1990; 82:2044–2051.
95. Ovize M, Kloner RA, Hale SH, Przyklenk K. Coronary cyclic flow variations precondition ischemic myocardium. Circulation 1992; 85:779–789.
96. Murry CE, Richard VJ, Jennings RB, Reimer KA. Myocardial protection is lost before contractile function recovers from ischemic preconditioning. Am J Physiol 1991; 260:H796–H804.
97. Ovize M, Przyklenk K, Hale SL, Kloner RA. Preconditioning does not attenuate myocardial stunning. Circulation 1992; 85:2247–2254.

Chapter 2

The Role of Thrombolytic Therapy for Acute Coronary Ischemia

Anthony J. Cannistra and Nicholas A. Ruocco, Jr.

Introduction

Thrombolytic therapy has revolutionized the management of acute myocardial infarction (AMI). Over the last decade, several large trials have demonstrated that intravenous administration of thrombolytic agents early in the course of an AMI help to re-establish perfusion of acutely ischemic myocardium, limit infarct size, and minimize left ventricular dysfunction. Both early and late mortality rates for AMI have been reduced significantly.[1–8]

This chapter provides an overview of thrombosis and thrombolysis. The basic differences that exist between the three main thrombolytic agents that have been extensively studied is discussed, and data supporting the efficacy of thrombolytic therapy are presented. Indications, contraindications, and complications of lytic therapy, as

Lazar HL (editor): *Current Therapy for Acute Coronary Ischemia,* © Futura Publishing Co., Inc., Mount Kisco, NY, 1993.

well as controversial subgroups and difficult management decisions, are emphasized. Myocardial rupture also is reviewed. The potential role of percutaneous transluminal coronary angioplasty (PTCA) in combination with thrombolytic therapy for the management of AMI also is considered.

Coronary artery bypass surgery often is necessary when a patient has evidence of recurrent or persistent coronary ischemia despite aggressive medical management with thrombolytic agents. The incidence and indications for bypass are discussed. Finally, future trends in clinical thrombolytic research are reviewed.

Pathophysiology of Acute Coronary Syndromes

The treatment of acute coronary ischemia in general and myocardial infarction in particular has changed dramatically over the last 12 years. This evolution has occurred because of a better understanding of the pathophysiology of acute coronary ischemia and myocardial infarction. A review of the pathophysiology of acute coronary ischemia will provide insight into why thrombolytic therapy, which has revolutionized therapy for AMI, is a rational and effect treatment. In 1980, DeWood et al.,[9] utilizing coronary angiography, established that total coronary artery occlusion played a major role in the development and evolution of an acute, transmural myocardial infarction. In this study, patients with symptoms and signs of AMI were evaluated within 4 hours of symptom onset. Eighty-seven percent of patients were found to have complete absence of blood flow in the infarct-related vessel and angiographic evidence of coronary artery thrombosis. Of interest, 10% to 20% of patients evaluated were found to have spontaneously patent infarct-related vessels. These findings supported early theories by Herrick[10] and others[11,12] that coronary thrombosis at the sight of an atherosclerotic plaque is the inciting event leading to myocardial infarction.

The actual physiological or mechanical events that trigger the development of thrombus at the site of a previously stable atherosclerotic plaque are not well understood. Potential mechanisms leading to plaque rupture and thrombus formation include a) thinning of the fibrous cap overlying the lipid core, b) release of enzymes or oxygen free radicals that may destroy collagen and elastin leading to plaque rupture, c) rheologic factors secondary to shear stress, turbulence, and hemodynamic changes at the stenosis, and d) rupture of the vaso-vasorum, and hemorrhage within the plaque.[13,14] Although one can only hypothesize about the triggers initiating plaque rupture, the events that occur at the surface of the plaque after rupture have been studied in detail.

Folts et al. developed an animal model that simulates the pathophysiology of an unstable plaque.[15] The Folts' model involves placing an occluder on the left anterior descending artery of a dog creating a severe stenosis. The endothelium is then damaged with a balloon at the site of the stenosis. Once the endothelium is damaged thrombus begins to form. It is important to emphasize the role of the endothelium as a natural barrier to thrombus formation.[13,14] If the endothelium is left intact, even in the presence of a severe stenosis, thrombus formation does not occur. A healthy endothelium is capable of synthesizing a number of substances that prevent the development of thrombus. These include both potent antiplatelet substances such as prostacycline, endothelial relaxing factor, and adenosine and potent antithrombin substances such as heparin and tissue plasminogen activator (t-PA).[13,14] However, if the endothelium is damaged, a sequence of events occur that lead to the development of a stable occlusive thrombus.

The initial event in this sequence is platelet mediated. Utilizing membrane receptors IIb + IIIa as well as von Willebrand's factor, platelets adhere to subendothelial collagen. This is followed by platelet activation and the release of thromboxane and serotonin leading to further platelet activation and the formation of a platelet plug. The platelet plug or aggregate is unstable and often embolizes, resulting in fluctuations of coronary blood flow referred to as cyclic flow reductions.[15] Cyclic flow reductions can go on for hours before the platelet plug is stabilized. Stabilization of the platelet aggregate is secondary to the simultaneous activation of the coagulation system at the sight of plaque rupture and the conversion of prothrombin to thrombin. Thrombin, in turn, converts circulating soluble fibrinogen into insoluble fibrin, which stabilizes the platelet aggregate and results in the formation of an occlusive thrombus.[16,17] This complex pathophysiological process occurring at the level of the atherosclerotic plaque is associated clinically with the familiar syndromes of unstable angina and AMI.

A clear understanding of this pathophysiological process promotes prompt administration of appropriate medical therapy. Early administration of antiplatelet agents such as aspirin or antithrombin agents such as heparin to a patient presenting with acute coronary ischemia may prevent the formation of an occlusive thrombus and the development of a myocardial infarction. Clinical studies have documented the efficacy of herapin and aspirin therapy in the treatment of unstable angina patients.[18] The Folts' model has made major contributions to our understanding of how and why present therapy for unstable angina works. Heparin and aspirin have become the primary weapons in the battle to stabilize unstable angina patients. However, if therapy is not administered in time to prevent the formation of an occlusive thrombus, there are currently three methods available to restore blood flow and limit the extent of myocardial infarction. These options include thrombolytic therapy to lyse the occlusive thrombus, angioplasty to dilate the total occlusion, and emergency coronary bypass surgery to bypass the obstructed vessel.

Thrombolysis and Thrombolytic Agents

With an understanding of the pathophysiology of an acute myocardial infarction, the administration of thrombolytic therapy to lyse the thrombus and restore coronary blood flow appears to be a rational and potentially efficacious therapy. As outlined above, rupture of an atherosclerotic plaque is associated with a potent thrombotic stimulus in the coronary artery. Interestingly, an endogenous thrombolytic system also exists that is activated in response to thrombogenesis and can lead to spontaneous lysis of the occlusive thrombus.[19] Unfortunately, as documented by DeWood et al.,[9] spontaneous lysis with restoration of flow is time dependent and frequently occurs too late to salvage a significant amount of myocardium. Agents are now available to accelerate the endogenous thrombolytic system and restore flow in time to salvage myocardium and reduce mortality.

The factor central to the endogenous thrombolytic system is the proenzyme plasminogen. Plasminogen becomes bound to recently formed thrombus in addition to existing in an unbound circulating form. The endogenous plasminogen activator, t-PA, catalyzes the conversion of plasminogen to plasmin. The active enzyme plasmin causes the insoluble fibrin network to breakdown, which leads to the dissolution of the thrombus. Genetically engineered recombinant t-PA as well as other pharmacological plasminogen activators can now be administered to accelerate the conversion of plasminogen to plasmin, leading to rapid clot lysis, restoration of coronary blood flow, and myocardial salvage.

There are two broad categories of plasminogen activators or thrombolytic agents: fibrin selective and nonselective (Table 1). Nonselective agents activate plasminogen indiscriminately in the circulation and at the site of the thrombus, whereas selective agents require the presence of fibrin for maximal activity and therefore act primarily at the site of the thrombus. There are potential advantages and disadvantages of each category. The nonselective agents, because of their indiscriminate activation of plasminogen, produce what is referred to as a "systemically lytic" state.[20–22] Systemic activation of plasminogen leads to systemic fibrinolysis and fibrinogenolysis, which depletes circulating fibrinogen and produces high levels of fibrin degradation products. Fibrin degradation products have anticoagulant activity and fibrinogen depletion leads to prolongation of thrombin, prothrombin, and activated partial thromboplastin times, essentially knocking out the patient's coagulation system for approximately 24 to 48 hours.[23,24] The potential benefit of

Table 1

Pharmacological Characteristics

Characteristic	SK	APSAC	rt-PA
Plasminogen binding	Indirect	Indirect	Direct
Fibrin selectivity	No	No	Yes
Fibrinogen breakdown	Extensive	Extensive	Moderate
Time dependency (>3 hr)	Yes	Yes	No
Half-life (min)	18	95	4
Antigenicity	Yes	Yes	No
Hypotension	Yes	Yes	No
Dose/administration	1.5 mill. units >1 hr	30 units >5 min	100 mg*
Cost	$320	$1,650	$2,200

*Standard—3-hr IV infusion.
Accelerated—90-min IV infusion.
SK = streptokinase; APSAC = anisoylated plasminogen streptokinase activator; rt-PA = recombinant tissue plasminogen activator.

this systemic lytic state is a decreased risk of vessel reocclusion; data are available to support this hypothesis.[25] The potential risk involves an increased likelihood of significant bleeding.

Recombinant t-PA (rt-PA) is the only fibrin selective agent currently approved for use. It is a human serine protease produced by vascular endothelium that can be manufactured in large quantities through recombinant DNA technology. rt-PA has very little activity in the circulation; however, after binding to fibrin at the site of a thrombus its ability to activate plasmin increases 1000-fold.[26] Its activity is therefore concentrated at the site of the clot with limited systemic activation of plasmin and degradation of circulating fibrinogen. The potential benefits of fibrin selectivity include more rapid clot lysis since therapy is concentrated at the thrombus. Catheterization data support this hypothesis.[1,27,28] Also, it was felt initially that since production of a systemically lytic state was rare, that bleeding would be less with a fibrin selective agent compared to a nonselective agent. This has not turned out to be the case as large randomized trials have demonstrated similar bleeding complications for both categories.[3,5] The potential risk with a selective agent is an increased incidence of reocclusion due to an intact coagulation system once the enzymatic effects of rt-PA have dissipated. Indeed, data suggest that reocclusion occurs more frequently after rt-PA than after a nonselective agent. However, the administration of aspirin and systemic heparin appear to decrease this risk significantly.[29–31]

The major thrombolytic agents currently available are outlined in Table 1. All have been shown to be effective for the treatment of AMI.[5] As indicated above, each agent has particular strengths and weaknesses. rt-PA appears to open more vessels in a shorter amount of time but is expensive and is associated with an increased risk of reocclusion and perhaps more bleeding. Streptokinase (SK) is inexpensive and is associated with a lower incidence of reocclusion and perhaps less bleeding. However, SK also opens fewer vessels and takes longer to achieve patency. Anisoylated plasminogen streptokinase activator (APSAC) is a pharmacological modification of SK that gives it a long half-life and allows for the ease of bolus administration. It has some of the attributes and weaknesses of both rt-PA and SK.

Based on the available data from head to head comparisons of these agents in extremely large patient populations, there is no clear-cut superiority of one agent over another with regard to reduction of mortality.[5] The results are so comparable that the major distinguishing feature among the agents comes down to cost (Table 1). Based on the clear-cut cost advantages, SK is the current agent of choice in eligible patients. This is not to say that the issue has been settled. There are some design concerns regarding the large European trials that mainly revolve around the route of administration of heparin and its influence on the efficacy of rt-PA. This has prompted a United States–based mega trial, the Global Utilization of Streptokinase and rt-PA for occluded coronary arteries trial (GUSTO), comparing rt-PA to SK and evaluating the role of systemic heparin. However, the message from the current mega trials comparing the different agents and the previous placebo-controlled trials is clear. It does not matter which thrombolytic agent is administered, as long as eligible patients receive a thrombolytic agent as early as possible in the course of their AMI.

Efficacy of Thrombolytic Therapy

Many placebo-controlled trials have documented the efficacy of thrombolytic therapy (Table 2). Compared to standard medical therapy, patients receiving thrombolytic therapy had anywhere from a 15% to 50% reduction in mortality. Although it has not been proven conclusively, it appears that restoration of coronary blood flow is the sine qua non of thrombolytic benefit. What has been well documented is the earlier the therapy is administered the greater the potential benefit. In the Gruppo Italiano Per Lo Studio Della Streptochi-Nasi Nell'Infarcto Miocardico (GISSI-I) trial, patients receiving SK within 1 hour of the onset of their symptoms had a 50% reduction in their mortality compared to control patients.[2] Data from the two largest placebo-controlled trials suggest that a significant reduction in mortality can definitely be achieved with the administration of thrombolytic therapy within 6 hours of infarct onset and perhaps as late as 24 hours.[3,4] Current recommendations support the administration of thrombolytic therapy, in the absence of contraindications, to all patients who present within 6 hours of their infarction. If there is any clinical or electrocardiographic evidence of ongoing ischemia, this window can be extended comfortably to 12 hours.

Unfortunately, despite the clear-cut nature of this recommendation, it is estimated that only 30% to 40% of eligible patients are

Table 2

Early and Late Mortality Trials

| | | | Follow-Up | Mortality | | |
| | | No. of | | Treated | Control | |
Trial	Lytic Agent	Patients	Early/Late	(%)	(%)	p Value
GISSI-1	SK	11,806	3 wks	10.7	13	0.002
			1 yr	17.2	19	0.008
ISIS-2	SK & ASA	8592	5 wks	8.0	13.2	0.0001
			1 yr	13.5	19	0.0001
ISIS-3	SK	41,299	5 wks	10.6	*	p = NS
	APSAC			10.5	*	
	rt-PA			10.3	*	
	SK	41,299	6 mos	14.0	*	p = NS
	APSAC			13.7	*	
	rt-PA			14.5	*	
GISSI-2	SK	12,381	5 wks	9.60		p = NS
	rt-PA			9.20		
	SK	12,381	6 mos	11.80		p = NS
	rt-PA			12.39		
AIMS	APSAC	1258	1 mo	6.4	12.1	p = 0.0006
			1 yr	11.1	17.8	p = 0.0007
ASSET	rt-PA	5011	1 mo	7.2	9.8	26% reduction†

*No placebo control group.
†p value not reported.
GISSI-1 = Gruppo Italiano Per Lo Studio Della; GISSI-2 = Streptochi-Nasi Nell' Infarcto Miocardico, Trials 1 and 2; ISIS-2 = International Study of Infarct Survival; ISIS-3 = Trials 2 and 3; AIMS = APSAC Intervention Mortality Study; ASSET = Anglo-Scandinavian Study of Early Thrombolysis; SK = streptokinase; APSAC = anisoylated plasminogen streptokinase activator; rt-PA = recombinant tissue plasminogen activator.

currently receiving thrombolytic therapy in the United States. The reasons for this are many. The main one is still physician education. Most infarction patients present to community hospitals, not to tertiary centers. An internist, family practitioner, or even an emergency medicine specialist staffing a community hospital emergency room probably is not as experienced as a tertiary care center cardiologist in administering thrombolytic therapy. Lack of experience generates insecurity, especially when the therapy has the potentially serious side effects associated with thrombolytic therapy. However, what all physicians who treat infarction patients have to realize is not administering thrombolytic therapy to an eligible patient can now be viewed as malpractice. They should become familiar with thrombolytic therapy and be comfortable administering it. Understandably, the most frequent concern is the danger of intracranial hemorrhage. However, the physician administering thrombolytic therapy must realize that placebo-controlled trials have demonstrated no difference in the frequency of stroke while documenting a clear mortality benefit, which should alleviate this concern.

Controversial Subgroups

Although some patients might be clear-cut candidates for thrombolytic therapy on presentation, there are subgroups of patients that are still controversial and represent difficult decisions. The subgroups include patients with inferior infarctions, elderly patients, and patients without clear-cut electrocardiogram (ECG) changes. In the case of inferior wall infarction patients, the difficulty lies in the variable risk associated with an inferior wall myocardial infarction. In the case of an uncomplicated inferior infarction the mortality may be as low as 5%, which would be difficult to improve on with any therapy.[32] However, if an inferior infarction is associated with right ventricular involvement, heart block, or precordial ST segment depression, the associated mortality is similar to that of an anterior myocardial infarction.[32,33] In the presence of these complications, the risk-benefit ratio of thrombolytic therapy is clear cut. However, in their absence, one cannot assume a low mortality, especially in the early hours of an infarct when thrombolytic therapy has the most benefit. These complications may not develop for several hours into the infarction, particularly in the case of heart block, when it is too late to administer therapy. Therefore, the data support the administration of thrombolytic therapy to all patients who present with an inferior infarction within 6 hours of the event.[3,5]

Elderly Patients

The early thrombolytic trials excluded elderly patients for the fear of an increased likelihood of serious complications. As experiences increased with thrombolytic therapy, the age restrictions were softened and eventually eliminated, allowing the evaluation of thrombolytic therapy in elderly subgroups. What was already known and reinforced by the placebo arm of these studies was the increased mortality associated with an infarction in elderly patients.[2,4,34,35] Approximately 50% of all deaths in patients hospitalized for AMI occur in patients >75 years of age. What was demonstrated in the treatment arm was that this high mortality rate could be decreased significantly with thrombolytic therapy.[6,7] This was particularly evident in the Anglo-Scandinavian Study of Early Thrombolysis (ASSET) trial, in which the whole population achieved a 27% reduction in mortality, and the patients 65- to 75-years old achieved an even greater 34% reduction.[6] The largest experience comes from the pooled results of GISSI-1 and the Second International Study of Infarct Survival (ISIS-2) with 2678 patients 75 years of age or older.[36] The Collaborative group[37] reported a statistically significant reduction in mortality. Age therefore should never be considered an absolute contraindication to thrombolytic therapy.

Unfortunately, however, elderly patients are more likely to have other contraindications. They are more likely to have had a previous stroke, ulcer disease, or hypertension, which may exclude them from therapy. In the event that they do receive thrombolytic therapy, they are at increased risk of hemorrhagic events including intracranial bleeding.[37,38] Clinical variables such as female gender, diabetes, and hypertension were associated with higher bleeding events in patients ≥75 years old. However, as indicated above, despite these increased risks, the risk-benefit ratio favors administering thrombolytic therapy to the elderly in the absence of absolute contraindications.

Nondiagnostic Electrocardiogram

As was the case with age restrictions, early thrombolytic trials had strict ECG criteria requiring ST segment elevation to exclude questionable infarctions and presumably maximize the risk-benefit ratio. However, the European trials adopted a more clinical approach allowing physicians to enroll any patient suspected of having an AMI regardless of their ECG. This has allowed subgroup analysis of the possible benefits of thrombolytic therapy in patients presenting without classic ST segment elevation.

The results are interesting. In general, patients suspected of having an AMI on clinical grounds but with either a left bundle branch block or nonspecific findings appear to benefit from thrombolytic therapy.[4] One category is particularly perplexing based on available data and needs further investigation before recommendations can be offered. Patients with an AMI presenting with ST segment depression appear to be a particularly high-risk subgroup. Within both the GISSI[3] and ISIS[5] trials, the mortality for this group in the placebo arm was higher than for patients presenting with ST segment elevation. Thrombolytic therapy had no significant effect in the ISIS trial and a disturbing trend toward an increased mortality in the GISSI trial. Smaller studies including angiography suggest that patients presenting with an ST segment depression infarction often have severe three-vessel disease and a large ischemic burden. Perhaps directing therapy only at the culprit lesion is not enough to improve the outcome in these patients. A more aggressive revascularization approach may be necessary. At this time thrombolytic therapy cannot be recommended in patients presenting with the clinical picture of an infarction but with ST segment depression on ECG.

Unstable Angina and Nontransmural Wave Myocardial Infarctions

As discussed above, the pathophysiology of unstable angina and nontransmural (non–Q wave) infarctions involves the development of thrombus at the site of an unstable plaque.[13,14] In contrast to AMI, unstable angina and subendocardial infarctions do not involve complete occlusion of the vessel in most patients. However, since the development of thrombus is associated with a very unstable focus that could progress to complete occlusion, thrombolytic therapy therefore may be effective for the treatment of unstable angina. The risk-benefit ratio is not as favorable as when treating AMI since the mortality associated with unstable angina is substantially less. Also, as already discussed both aspirin and heparin, which have a lower risk profile than thrombolytic therapy, are very effective in treating the unstable angina patient.[18]

Ongoing studies of unstable angina patients involving coronary angiography have documented that when obvious intracoronary thrombus is present, it does appear to resolve more reliably after thrombolytic therapy than with heparin therapy alone. However, clinical endpoints of myocardial infarction and refractory symptoms are similar whether the patients are treated with heparin alone or thrombolytic therapy. The Thrombolysis in Myocardial Infarction

Trial (TIMI III), which is a mortality-based trial of unstable angina patients comparing the efficacy of heparin versus rt-PA, should help to resolve this issue. At present there are not enough data to support the administration of thrombolytic therapy for the syndromes of unstable angina and non–Q wave infarction.

Contraindications and Complications

Based on experience from several randomized trials, 9% to 35% of patients who present early in the course of their acute infarction have contraindications to thrombolytic therapy.[39] This wide range reflects early trials that considered delay time of >6 hours and age >75 as contraindications to lytic therapy. More recent trials have used broader eligibility criteria. Table 3 is a list adapted from a

---

Table 3
Contraindications

Absolute Contraindications
1. Active internal bleeding
2. Suspected aortic dissection
3. Prolonged or traumatic CPR
4. Recent head trauma or known intracranial neoplasm
5. Recorded blood pressure ≥200/120
6. Previous allergy to thrombolytic agent (SK or APSAC)
7. Pregnancy
8. Hx of cerebrovascular accident known to be hemorrhagic
9. Trauma or surgery within 2 weeks, which is a potential source of bleeding

Relative Contraindications
1. Hemorrhagic retinopathy
2. Trauma or surgery >2 weeks
3. Hx of chronic severe HTN (DBP ≥100) with or without drug therapy
4. Active peptic ulcer disease
5. Hx of CVA
6. Known bleeding diathesis or current use of anticoagulants
7. Prior treatment with SK/APSAC, especially if within 6–9 months' time interval; does not apply to rt-PA

Adapted from AHA guidelines. Circulation, 1990; 82(2).
CPR = cardiopulmonary resuscitation; SK = streptokinase; APSAC = anisoylated plasminogen streptokinase activator; Hx = history; HTN = hypertension; DBP = diastolic blood pressure; CVA = cerebrovascular accident; rt-PA = recombinant tissue plasminogen activator.

recent ACC/AHA task force report[40] of the most common absolute and relative contraindications to lytic therapy.

The most serious and common complications of thrombolytic therapy have been broken down into several categories by experienced investigators.[41] These include a) intracranial hemorrhage, b) systemic hemorrhage, c) immunological complications/hypotension, and d) myocardial rupture.

Intracranial Hemorrhage

The most feared complication of thrombolytic therapy is intracranial hemorrhage. It is essentially irreversible and frequently, but not always, associated with significant morbidity or death. Fortunately, it is also a very uncommon complication. The accepted rate for intracranial hemorrhage is approximately 1.0%. This is based on a large number of trials using different agents. The occurrence of hemorrhagic strokes, ischemic strokes, and strokes of undefined cause has been reported recently by GISSI-2/International Study Group investigators.[42] A total of 236 of 20,768 patients suffered strokes in this analysis (1.14%). The breakdown consisted of 36% hemorrhagic strokes, 48% ischemic strokes, and 30% strokes of undefined cause. Patients receiving rt-PA had a small but significant excess of all strokes compared to those receiving SK (1.33% vs. 0.94%). The administration of subcutaneous heparin did not increase stroke risk. However, older age, higher Killip class, and presence of acute anterior wall infarction significantly increased the risk of ischemic stroke, a relationship that has also been described in other trials.[43-45] In addition, female gender, although not significantly correlated with the occurrence of all strokes, was associated with a higher incidence of hemorrhagic strokes. Other risk factors for intracranial hemorrhage and potential contraindications for lytic therapy include known intracranial neoplasm, prior neurosurgery, recent stroke (within 6 months), remote stroke, recent head trauma (within 1 month), and acute, severe hypertension (systolic >180 mm Hg and diastolic blood pressure >120 mm Hg) (Table 3).

Systemic Bleeding

Bleeding frequently has been classified as either major or minor. Major bleeding is defined usually as a significant drop in the hematocrit ($>$15%)[46] or a blood loss associated with hypotension or requiring transfusion. Minor bleeding encompasses all other bleeding. Reported bleeding rates have varied considerably depending on the size and nature of different trials. The risk of major bleeding events reported in large trials not involving cardiac catheterization is $<$1%.[1-8] Understandably, the risk of major bleeding is dramatically higher (12–15%) in study protocols that included cardiac catheterization.[47] In the TIMI-1 trial,[1] major bleeding events occurred in $>$15% of patients, with 27% of all complications occurring at the site of cardiac catheterization in both the rt-PA- and SK-treated patient groups.

In the TIMI-II trial,[48] patients were treated with rt-PA and then assigned to either an invasive or conservative treatment strategy. Of note, initial dosing evaluated 150 mg of rt-PA but this was decreased to 100 mg because of a significantly increased risk of bleeding complications at the higher dose. Patients assigned to the invasive strategy had more frequent and more severe hemorrhagic complications than the conservative group (18.5% vs. 12.8%, $p < 0.001$).

Immunological Complications/Hypotension

Since both SK and APSAC are derived from group C β-hemolytic streptococci, a significant antigenic response may occur in patients treated with these agents. rt-PA is a derivative of human proteins, and thus does not provoke a significant antigenic response.

Acute anaphylaxis is the most serious of all immunological reactions and occurs in $<$0.2% of patients receiving either SK or APSAC.[41] In the setting of AMI, hemodynamic compromise and bronchospasm due to pulmonary edema occur frequently. When these events occur soon after the administration of either SK or APSAC, it is often difficult to distinguish cardiogenic shock secondary to pump failure from an anaphylactic reaction secondary to lytic therapy.

Hypotension unrelated to anaphylaxis occurs in 5% to 10% of patients treated with SK or APSAC.[49] The mechanism is thought to involve activation of the kininogen-kinin system with subsequent vasodilator effects and decreases in systolic blood pressure. Again, it may be difficult to distinguish isolated hypotension related to lytic therapy from hypotension secondary to cardiogenic shock or anaphylaxis. Hypotension due to lytic therapy usually responds quickly to volume repletion and vasopressor support. Other less serious manifestations of SK/APSAC lytic therapy, such as fever, rash, urticaria, arthralgias, or vasculitis, have been reported to occur in 2% to 6% of patients.[49]

Finally, the immunogenic potential of both SK and APSAC is important when considering thrombolytic therapy for the management of either early (<48 hr) or late (>48 hr) reocclusion. A systemic antigenic response with antibody formation is triggered by administration of SK or APSAC. Readministration within a certain time may precipitate an anaphylactic reaction due to a more aggressive amnestic response. Therefore, these agents should not be used for the treatment of reocclusion. Rather, rt-PA is the agent of choice for the treatment of reocclusion after either SK or APSAC therapy. Readministration of these agents 6 to 9 months after initial usage is considered safe for the treatment of subsequent AMI.[50]

Reperfusion Injury and Myocardial Rupture

Late reperfusion is a topic that has created much controversy in thrombolytic research trials. Theoretically, reperfusion by improving blood flow to ischemic myocardium could lead to improved scar formation and preservation of an epicardial rim of viable myocardium. The "rim" could then restrict left ventricular dilatation and aneurysm formation, resulting in improved left ventricular hemodynamics. In contrast, restoration of blood flow also could be detrimental. Reperfusion of ischemic and necrotic myocardium may lead to the release of destructive enzymes, which could enhance necrosis and lead to myocardial rupture. Furthermore, there is some evidence to suggest that thrombolytic therapy promotes hemorrhage into freshly infarcted tissue and can cause dissection of blood through regions of transmural necrosis.[49]

A number of investigators have studied the incidence of myocardial rupture in patients receiving thrombolytic therapy. Honan et al.[51] performed a meta-analysis of four thrombolytic trials involving 1638 patients and 58 episodes of cardiac rupture. He estimated the odds ratio of cardiac rupture or death in both treated and control group patients with respect to time from symptom onset to treatment. Cardiac rupture directly correlated with time to treatment: at 7 hours the odds ratio was 0.4, at 11 hours it was 0.93, and at 17 hours it was 3.21 (with an odds ratio of <1.0 implying reduced risk of an event occurring after therapy, and a ratio of >1.0 implying greater risk).

Currier et al.[52] analyzed the occurrence of cardiac rupture after AMI in patients treated with rt-PA in the TIMI-II study. Thirty-three of the 3501 patients suffered cardiac rupture (0.9%). In contrast to the study by Honan et al., there was no relationship between cardiac rupture and the interval from onset of symptoms to rt-PA infusion. Cardiac rupture accounted for 17.3% of first-day mortality and 18.6% of 30-day mortality in TIMI-II. Female gender and age >65 were both significant risk factors for the development of cardiac rupture. The incidence of cardiac rupture was comparable to historical controls from the prethrombolytic era.

The mechanisms of early death despite thrombolytic therapy was evaluated in the TIMI-II population.[53] Sixty-three patients died (63/3339) within 18 hours of enrollment. Ventricular rupture was the cause of death in 10 of the 63 patients (16%) and occurred in 7 of 43 (16%) patients with anterior wall infarction and 3 of 20 (15%) with nonanterior wall infarction. In a separate, detailed morphological study from the TIMI database, Gertz et al.[54] described the cause of death in 52 patients who died 5 hours to 260 days after treatment with rt-PA. Myocardial rupture occurred in 12 of 52 (23%) patients. Interestingly, in contrast to the hypothesis above, rupture occurred at a similar frequency in both hemorrhagic (6/23, 25%) and nonhemorrhagic infarcts.

The incidence of rupture in a population of patients randomized to thrombolytic therapy versus placebo has not been well studied. In a nonrandomized population, Gertz et al.[55] analyzed the hearts of 61 patients who died 5 hours to 42 days after a fatal, first myocardial infarction. Twenty-three patients had received rt-PA and were compared with 38 who had not. Myocardial rupture occurred in 5 of the 23 (22%) thrombolytic-treated patients, compared to 18 of 38 (47%) of nonlytic-treated patients. In a subset of 29 patients who died within 72 hours of symptom onset, 3 of 15 (20%) lytic therapy patients sustained cardiac rupture, compared with 9 of 14 (64%) nonlytic patients.

In summary, available data suggest that the incidence of myocardial rupture after thrombolytic therapy is similar to the incidence from the prethrombolytic era. Cardiac rupture continues to contribute significantly to first-day and early mortality after AMI. Although there is evidence that thrombolytic therapy causes intramyocardial hemorrhage, data suggest that cardiac rupture occurs equally in both hemorrhagic and nonhemorrhagic infarcts.

Percutaneous Transluminal Coronary Angioplasty

It is clear that thrombolytic therapy offers significant survival benefits to patients who present early in the course of AMI. However, while lytic agents act directly on occlusive intracoronary thrombus, there often are hemodynamically significant stenoses that remain. During the early thrombolytic trials it was hypothesized that thrombolytic therapy would be effective at reperfusing the thrombotic occlusion but that angioplasty would be necessary to reduce the underlying stenosis and prevent reocclusion while maximizing myocardial salvage. Four major trials investigated the use of adjunctive PTCA in combination with lytic therapy.

The four major trials include TIMI-IIA and -IIB, the Thrombolysis and Angioplasty in Myocardial Infarction trial (TAMI-1), and the European Cooperative Study Group (ECSG).[48, 56–58] There are methodological differences between the studies, but taken in total, the data from these trials answer major questions regarding the role of PTCA after thrombolytic therapy. Contrary to the initial hypothesis, routine prophylactic PTCA is not necessary after thrombolytic therapy. The incidence of reocclusion and reinfarction are the same in patients randomized to an invasive strategy of routine prophylactic PTCA, compared to patients randomized to a conservative strategy of PTCA only in the case of spontaneous or exercise-induced ischemia. The mortality and left ventricular function also was comparable in the two groups. Patients who underwent routine PTCA did have less recurrent ischemia. However, the primary objective of acute thrombolytic therapy is to decrease mortality, salvage myocardium, and prevent reocclusion. The conservative strategy is as effective as the invasive strategy in accomplishing these primary objectives. Patients who experience episodes of recurrent ischemia may require revascularization, but they are not placed at increased risk of death or reinfarction by waiting for the ischemia to declare itself either spontaneously or on a discharge low level exercise test.

Interestingly, the underlying lesion responsible for AMI often is only moderately severe in the 50% to 60% range as opposed to a 99% stenosis that conventional wisdom has led us to expect. Furthermore, up to 20% of patients may not even have a hemodynamically significant stenosis. This may explain why prophylactic PTCA with its inherent risk did not improve the results achieved by thrombolytic therapy alone. Therapy to improve on reperfusion rates and patency rates may have to be directed at the hypercoaguable nature of the lesion with more potent antithrombin and antiplatelet therapy as opposed to mechanical manipulation.

It is now established that routine angioplasty after thrombolytic therapy offers no benefits and is associated with greater risk than lytic therapy alone. However, in patients with absolute contraindications to thrombolytic therapy, directed PTCA still remains a potential option for the treatment of AMI. Reperfusion rates are favorable, in the 80% to 90% range, while the risks are somewhat higher than elective angioplasty but acceptable in light of the potential benefit. Although no randomized studies have been completed, comparison of mortality in patients treated with thrombolytic therapy versus primary angioplasty are very similar.

Furthermore, thrombolytic therapy may not be as effective in reducing mortality in patients who present with infarctions that are complicated by congestive heart failure or cardiogenic shock. Approximately 25% of patients participating in large mortality trials have had congestive heart failure.[59] In GISSI-1,[2] 22.7% were in Killip class II and 3.2% were in class III. In-hospital mortality rates were 16.1% and 33%, respectively, compared to 5.9% for those in Killip class I ($p = 0.01$). Similarly, 1-year mortality rates were 26.6% and 50.3%, respectively, compared with 10.6% in Killip I patients. In this trial, 2.5% of patients presented in cardiogenic shock (Killip IV). Despite thrombolytic therapy, hospital and 1-year mortality rates of 69.9% and 76.6% were observed. In contrast, there are data that support a substantial reduction in mortality when either angioplasty alone or in combination with thrombolytic therapy is undertaken in patients with cardiogenic shock.[60] Thus, coronary angioplasty remains an important treatment option for those patients who present with either contraindications to lytic therapy or with associated congestive heart failure or cardiogenic shock.

Coronary Artery Bypass Surgery After Thrombolytic Therapy

Coronary artery bypass grafting (CABG) sometimes is necessary in patients who have received thrombolytic therapy for treatment of AMI. Frequently the decision has to be made during the early hours of the infarction and often in the sickest subgroup of patients. As discussed above, present data would suggest that only patients who have contraindications to thrombolytic therapy, evidence of reocclusion, or hemodynamic compromise warrant evaluation with coronary angiography during the acute event. It is this subgroup of patients undergoing catheterization and possible acute angioplasty that sometimes requires emergent or urgent bypass surgery. If angioplasty fails and there is evidence of myocardial viability or hemodynamic compromise if the culprit vessel is allowed to occlude, then urgent CABG becomes a crucial treatment modality.[61] Coronary angiography in other patients may reveal left main stenosis or severe three-vessel disease not amenable to angioplasty, and these patients also might require bypass surgery.

Petrovich et al.[62] examined both early and late results of CABG after thrombolytic therapy for AMI. One hundred ninety-one patients underwent surgical revascularization 4.1 ± 3.6 days after initial lytic therapy with either intravenous or intracoronary SK. Of these operations, 6.8% occurred after unsuccessful coronary angioplasty. Although 88% of patients were found to have multivessel disease, no information regarding the clinical stability or indications for CABG are provided in this study. Also of note, 67% of patients had inferior wall infarctions. Overall operative mortality was 4.2%, whereas the mortality in patients who had failed PTCA was 15.4%. Most operative mortality was due to left ventricular failure, not bleeding complications. Late mortality defined in a follow-up period of 12 to 48 months (mean 27 ± 8 months) was 1%. Importantly, only nine patients (4.1%) had significant perioperative bleeding necessitating blood transfusions and fresh frozen plasma; an average of 3.8 ± 2.9 units of blood were administered perioperatively. Thus, although clinical indications for CABG were not defined clearly, this study demonstrates that CABG can be performed safely, without excessive bleeding complications, early after thrombolytic therapy.

Kereiakes et al.[63] examined patients requiring emergent CABG in the TAMI trial. In this trial rt-PA was administered 2.6 ± 0.7 hours after onset of AMI in 386 consecutive patients. Emergent CABG was performed 7.3 ± 1.2 hours after onset of symptoms in 24 patients (6.8%). In these patients, indications for surgery were left main or significant three-vessel disease (7 patients), coronary anatomy unsuitable for PTCA (4 patients), and unsuccessful PTCA

(13 patients). Infarct vessel patency was achieved either pharmacologically (rt-PA) or mechanically (PTCA) before surgery in 21 of 24 patients. In contrast to the study by Petrovich et al.,[62] anterior wall infarction occurred more frequently than inferior wall infarction (67% vs. 39%, respectively). Sixteen patients had stable hemodynamics preoperatively and eight patients had cardiogenic shock. Three deaths occurred postoperatively and all of these patients were in the group with preoperative cardiogenic shock (12.5% mortality for CABG group overall, 38% for those patients in cardiogenic shock). Significant bleeding requiring surgical re-exploration occurred in three patients (12.5%) and bleeding attributed to general abnormalities in hemostasis occurred in two patients (8%). Overall, an average of 5.6 units of packed red cells, 4 units of fresh frozen plasma, 3.9 units of cryoprecipitate, and 3 units of platelets were necessary. Of importance was the observation that a significant improvement between pre- and postoperative ejection fraction was noted (pre = $49 \pm 6\%$ compared with $56 \pm 6\%$ postoperatively; $p = 0.008$). Furthermore, patients with multivessel disease had a greater magnitude of preservation of left ventricular function than those with single-vessel disease (multivessel: 46.1% vs. 55.3%; single vessel 53% vs. 57%).

Barner et al.[64] performed an extensive literature review evaluating the use of coronary artery bypass surgery in three patient groups. The groups consisted of a) patients having CABG early after administration of lytic therapy, b) after failed PTCA, and c) as primary management of AMI. Treatment with lytic therapy followed by operation occurred in 143 patients in 11 trials. Intracoronary SK was used in seven trials, intravenous SK in one trial, and a combination of intravenous and intracoronary SK in two trials. Only one trial employed rt-PA (the TAMI trial) and these results already have been described. For the group as a whole, operations were performed within 8 hours and there were four (2.8%) hospital deaths. Specifically, when only intravenous SK (1.5×10^6 units) was used and followed by coronary bypass surgery within 12 hours, there were significant increases in blood loss, transfusion requirements, and a greater need for reoperation for postoperative bleeding compared with nonlytic-treated patients ($p < 0.05$, all groups). Far less morbidity due to excessive bleeding occurred if surgery was delayed (12–72 hours) or late (>72 hours). In summary, current information suggests that CABG can be performed safely after lytic therapy and can lead to overall preservation of left ventricular function. Coagulopathy associated with lytic agents leads to an increase in postoperative bleeding complications. There is evidence to suggest that, when possible, delaying surgery for more than 12 hours may help to minimize hemorrhagic morbidity.

Future Trends

Despite the major advances thrombolytic therapy has made in the treatment of acute myocardial infarction, it is important to realize that this approach is still in its relative infancy. There is room for improvement and a great deal to learn about the optimal regimen that will maximize the benefits of thrombolytic therapy. A great deal of research currently is being done on two important areas of thrombolytic therapy. First, as discussed earlier, reocclusion remains a problem after thrombolytic therapy and is felt to be primarily a thrombin- and platelet-mediated phenomenon. While it is accepted that heparin and aspirin should be standard adjunctive agents used during lytic therapy, several other, more potent, antithrombin and antiplatelet agents currently are being investigated. The second area of intense research involves different dosing regimens for the commonly used agents and different combinations of these agents. Although standard protocols either use 1.5 million units of SK or 100 mg of rt-PA intravenously, ongoing trials are investigating different dosing schedules and combined rt-PA/APSAC and rt-PA/SK regimens.

Adjunctive Therapy

Antithrombin Therapy

Heparin has been shown to be important in helping to prevent reocclusion after therapy with rt-PA.[1,29,65–67] In addition, there is some evidence that heparin, although associated with increased bleeding, may be important when combined with SK[4] in reducing mortality. Other trials, however, have been less clear and indicate that no significant mortality benefits were derived when heparin was administered.[3,68] Controversy exists regarding the route of administration in these trials, which have variably employed either subcutaneous or intravenous heparin therapy. Importantly, both routes of administration will be compared in the ongoing GUSTO trial, which hopefully will resolve the heparin issue. Based on available data, full-dose intravenous heparin should be employed after all thrombolytic agents.

Although the most effective antithrombin agent available is heparin, it does have some deficiencies with respect to the treatment of intracoronary thrombus. Because of the large size of the heparin-antithrombin III moleclue that inactivates circulating thrombin, it cannot act on fibrin-bound thrombin at the surface of a clot. Fibrin-bound thrombin is a potent platelet activator and a potent activator of the clotting cascade. Therefore, even in the presence of heparin, thrombin at the surface of a clot still can stimulate ongoing thrombus formation. These factors have stimulated a search for a more potent antithrombin agent.

Hirudin, a protein derived from Leech saliva, holds much promise as a more potent inhibitor of clot-bound thrombin. Experimental models have shown that hirudin specifically inhibits thrombin and prevents thrombus formation after deep arterial injury.[69] Furthermore, hirudin appears to be more effective than heparin in inhibiting thrombin already bound to fibrin.[70] Several other hirudin-like compounds, as well as synthetic competitive thrombin inhibitors such as argatroban, also display greater antithrombin effects than intravenous heparin in experimental models.[71] Upcoming trials will evaluate the clinical safety and efficacy of recombinant hirudin combined both with rt-PA (TIMI-5) and with SK (TIMI-6). Further clinical trials undoubtedly will incorporate several other antithrombin agents into design protocols.

Antiplatelet Therapy

It is now well known that platelets play a critical role in the balance that exists between the processes of reperfusion and reocclusion.[13,14] ISIS-II demonstrated the beneficial mortality effects of aspirin as an effective antiplatelet drug. Aspirin acts by inhibiting cyclo-oxygenase, which leads to thromboxane A_2 inhibition and at least partial inhibition of platelet aggregation. A new antiplatelet agent, Ridogrel, which is a specific thromboxane A_2 inhibitor, is currently being compared to aspirin in the large multicenter Ridogrel versus Aspirin trial (the RAPT trial). Similar to the heparin-thrombin issue, aspirin is a relatively weak antiplatelet agent. It blocks platelet aggregation via the thromboxane pathway but other factors such as collagen and thrombin can still stimulate platelet aggregation. Therefore, a search for a more potent antiplatelet agent also is underway.

Platelet aggregation requires the interaction of platelet surface receptors glycoproteins IIb/IIIA. Potentially a more potent approach toward inhibiting platelet aggregation involves the blocking of these platelet surface receptors. These receptors mediate platelet aggregation after platelet activation occurs during thrombogenesis. An ongoing trial, TAMI-8, is evaluating the effect of the 7E3 monoclonal antiplatelet glycoprotein IIb/IIIa antibody together with rt-PA on the maintenance of infarct vessel patency. Other naturally occurring and synthetic inhibitors of these platelet receptor sites are currently being developed. These mediators may prove to be important adjunctive agents in thrombolytic therapy.

Future Trials

Neuhaus et al.[72] introduced the concept of "a front-loaded," weight-adjusted, accelerated dosing regimen for rt-PA. These investigators showed that, in contrast to a 100-mg dose of rt-PA infused over 3 hours, a rapid infusion of 100 mg of rt-PA over 90 minutes could be used safely. Furthermore, a higher early patency rate of 92.4% was achieved.

Two trials are currently comparing the accelerated rt-PA dosing regimen to other thrombolytic agents, directly and in combination. TIMI-4 will compare early and sustained patency effects of rt-PA (100 mg over 90 min), with APSAC (30 units over 2–5 min) alone and in combination (65 mg rt-PA over 30 min + 20 units of APSAC).

The GUSTO trial is an ongoing large clinical trial with an expected enrollment of approximately 40,000 patients. This trial is investigating several unresolved issues that have been brought up by previous trials and some that have been discussed above. Patients will be randomized to accelerated intravenous (IV) rt-PA alone, IV SK alone, or a combination of IV rt-PA and SK. All patients will receive IV heparin except a subgroup of patients who will receive IV SK together with subcutaneous heparin. This arm is felt to be necessary to compare directly the effects of subcutaneous heparin with intravenous heparin in the other arms of this study. This comparison may help to clarify previous confusion regarding which route of heparin administration is safest and most efficacious. It also will shed further light on the issue of which thrombolytic agent might be more effective in reducing mortality. Finally, an angiographic arm of the GUSTO trial will attempt to resolve the question of whether or not the timing of vessel patency and vessel patency itself is the sine qua non of thrombolytic benefit.

Summary

It is now well accepted that thrombolytic therapy with any of the commercially available agents affords significant mortality benefits to patients who are treated in the early stages of an AMI. Current and future research will be directed toward expanding existing knowledge regarding mechanisms of action of fibrinolytic agents, improving adjunctive therapy, and refining modes of administration. In addition, increasing physician awareness regarding the use of these agents needs to be a major focus so that the maximum survival benefit in appropriate patients can be achieved.

References

1. Chesebro JH, Knatterud G, Roberts R, Borer J, Cohen LS, et al. Thrombolysis in myocardial infarction (TIMI) trial, phase I: a comparison between intravenous tissue plasminogen activator and intravenous streptokinase. Circulation 1987; 76:142–154.
2. Gruppo Italiano Per Lo Studio Della Streptochinasi nell' Infarto Miocardico (GISSI). Long-term effects of intravenous thrombolysis in acute myocardial infarction: final report of the GISSI study. Lancet 1987; 1:871–874.
3. Gruppo Italiano Per Lo Studio Della Sopravvivenza nell' Infarto Miocardico. GISSI-2: a factorial randomised trial of alteplase versus streptokinase and heparin versus no heparin among 12,490 patients with acute myocardial infarction. Lancet 1990; 336:65–75.
4. ISIS-2 (Second International Study of Infarct Survival) collaborative group. Randomised trial of intravenous streptokinase, oral aspirin, both, or neither among 17,187 cases of suspected acute myocardial infarctions: ISIS-2. Lancet 1988; 2:349–360.
5. ISIS-3 (Third International Study of Infarct Survival) collaborative group. ISIS-3: a randomised comparison of streptokinase vs tissue plasminogen activator vs anistreplase and of aspirin plus heparin vs aspirin alone among 41,299 cases of suspected acute myocardial infarction. Lancet 1992; 339:753–770.
6. Wilcox RG, Olsson CG, Skene AM, Von Der Lippe G, Jensen G,

Hampton J. Trial of tissue plasminogen activator for mortality reduction in acute myocardial infarction. Anglo-Scandinavian Study of Early Thrombolysis (ASSET). Lancet 1988; 2:525–530.

7. AIMS trial study group. Long-term effects of intravenous anistreplase in acute myocardial infarction: final report of the AIM study. Lancet 1990; 335:427–431.

8. The I.S.A.M. study group. A prospective trial of intravenous streptokinase in acute myocardial infarction (I.S.A.M.). Mortality, morbidity, and infarcts size at 21 days. N Engl J Med 1986; 314:1465–1471.

9. DeWood MA, Spores J, Notske R, Mouser LT, Burroughs R, et al. Prevalence of total coronary occlusion during the early hours of transmural myocardial infarction. N Engl J Med 1980; 303:897–901.

10. Herrick JB. Clinical features of sudden obstruction of the coronary arteries. JAMA 1912; 59:2015–2020.

11. Chazov EK, Mateeva LS, Masaev AV, et al. Intracoronary administration of fibrinolysin in acute myocardial infarction. Ter Arkh 1976; 48:8–19.

12. Rentrop KP, Blanke H, Karsh KR, Kreuzer H. Initial experience with transluminal recanalization of the recently occluded infarct-related coronary artery in acute myocardial infarction-comparison with conventionally treated patients. Clin Cardiol 1979; 2:92–105.

13. Fuster V, Badimon L, Badimon JJ, Chesebro JH. The pathogenesis of coronary artery disease and the acute coronary syndromes. N Engl J Med 1992; 326:242–250.

14. Fuster V, Badimon L, Badimon JJ, Chesebro JH. Mechanisms of disease; the pathogenesis of coronary artery disease and the acute coronary syndromes (second of two parts). N Engl J Med 1992; 326:310–318.

15. Folts JD, Crowell EB Jr, Rowe CG. Platelet aggregation in partially obstructed vessels and its elimination by aspirin. Circulation 1976; 54:365–370.

16. Machovich R, ed. Hemostasis in Blood Vessel Wall and Thrombosis, vol 1. Boca Raton, FL: CRC Press. 1988; pp 3–80.

17. Weiss HJ, Baumgartner HR, Turillo VT. Regulation of platelet-fibrin thrombin on subendothelium. Ann NY Acad Sci 1987; 516:380–397.

18. Theroux P, Ouimet H, McCans J, Latour JG, Joly P, et al. Aspirin, heparin, or both to treat acute unstable angina. N Engl J Med 1988; 319:1105–1111.

19. Fuster V, Stein B, Ambrose JA, Badimon L, Badimon JJ, Chesebro JH. Atherosclerotic plaque rupture and thrombosis: evolving concepts. Circulation 1990; 82(Suppl II):II-47–II-59.

20. Barnhart MI, Cress DC, Henry RL, Riddle JM. Influence of fibrinogen split products on platelets. Thromb Diath Haemorrh 1967; 17:78–98.

21. Buluk K, Molefiejew M. The pharmacological properties of fibrinogen degradation products. Br J Pharmacol 1969; 35:79–89.

22. Kopec M. Budzynski A, Stachurska J, Wegrzynowicz Z, Kowalski E. Studies on the mechanism of interference by fibrinogen degradation products (FDP) with the platelet function, role of fibrinogen in the platelet atmosphere. Thromb Diath Haemorrh 1966; 15:476.

23. Thorsen LI, Brosstad F, Gogstad G, Sletten K, Solum NO. Competitions between fibrinogen with its degradation products for interactions with the platelet-fibrinogen receptor. Thromb Res 1986; 44:611–623.
24. Wilson PA, McNicol GP, Douglas AS. Effect of fibrinogen degradation products on platelet aggregation. J Clin Pathol 1968; 21:147–153.
25. Grines CL, Nissen SE, Booth DE, Guley JC, Bennett KA, DeMaria AN. A new thrombolytic regimen for acute myocardial infarction using combination half-dose tissue-type plasminogen activator with full-dose streptokinase: a pilot study. J Am Coll Cardiol 1989; 14:573–580.
26. Zamarron C, Lijnen HR, Collen D. Kinetics of the activation of plasminogen by natural and recombinant tissue type plasminogen activator. J Biochem Chem 1984; 259:2080–2083.
27. Mueller HS, Rao AK, Forman SA, TIMI Investigators: Thrombolysis in myocardial infarction (TIMI). Comparative studies of coronary reperfusion and systemic fibrinogenolysis with two forms of recombinant tissue-type plasminogen activator. J Am Coll Cardiol 1987; 10:479–490.
28. Williams DO, Borer J, Braunwald E, et al. Intravenous recombinant tissue-type plasminogen activator in patients with acute myocardial infarction: a report from the NHLBI Thrombolysis in Myocardial Infarction Trial. Circulation 1986; 73:338–346.
29. Bleich SD, Nichols TC, Schumacher RR, Cooke DH, Tate DA, Teichman SL. Effect of heparin on coronary arterial patency after thrombolysis with tissue plasminogen activator in acute myocardial infarction. Am J Cardiol 1990; 66:1412–1417.
30. Ross AM, Hsia J, Hamilton W, et al. Heparin versus aspirin after recombinant tissue plasminogen activator therapy in myocardial infarction: a randomized trial (abstract). J Am Coll Cardiol 1990; 15:64A.
31. de Bono DP, Simoons ML, Tijssen J, Arnold AE, Betriu A, et al. Effect of early intravenous heparin on coronary patency, infarct size, and bleeding complications after Alteplase thrombolysis: results of a randomized double blind European Cooperative Study Group trial. Br Heart J 1992; 67(2):122–128.
32. Berger PB, Ryan TJ. Inferior myocardial infarction. Circulation 1990; 81:401–411.
33. Berger PB, Ruocco NA, Ryan TJ, Frederick MM, Jacobs AK, Faxon DP, TIMI Investigators. Incidence and prognostic implications of heart block complicating inferior myocardial infarction treated with thrombolytic therapy: results from TIMI II. J Am Coll Cardiol 1992; 20:533–540.
34. Robinson K, Conroy RM, Mulcahy R. Risk factors and in-hospital course of first myocardial infarction in the elderly. Clin Cardiol 1988; 11:519–553.
35. Tofler GH, Muller JE, Stone PH, et al. Factors leading to shorter survival after acute myocardial infarction in patients ages 65 to 75 years compared with younger patients. Am J Cardiol 1988; 62:860–867.
36. Lew AS, Hod H, Cercek B, Shah P, Ganz W. Mortality and morbidity of rates of patients older and younger than 75 years with acute myocardial

infarction treated with intravenous streptokinase. Am J Cardiol 1987; 59:1871:1–5.

37. Collins R. Optimizing thrombolytic therapy of acute myocardial infarction: age is not a contraindication. ISIS Collaborative Group, Radcliffe Infirmiry, Oxford, UK. Circulation 1991; 84(Suppl):II–230.

38. Bovill EG, Terrin ML, Stump DC, Berke AD, Frederick M, et al., for the TIMI Investigators. Hemorrhagic events during therapy with recombinant tissue-type plasminogen activator, heparin, and aspirin for acute myocardial infarction. Ann Intern Med 1991; 115:256–265.

39. Karlson BW, Herlitz J. Can the eligibility criteria for thrombolytic therapy be broadened? Prim Cardiol 1992; 18:39–45.

40. Gunnar RM, Bourdillon PD, Dixon DW, Fuster V, Karp RB, et al. Guidelines for the early management of patients with acute myocardial infarction. A report of the American College of Cardiology/American Heart Association task force on assessment of diagnostic and therapeutic cardiovascular procedures (subcommittee to develop guidelines for the early management of patients with acute myocardial infarction. J Am Coll Cardiol 1990; 16:249–292.

41. Califf RM, Fortin DF, Tenaglia AN, Sane DC. Clinical risks of thrombolytic therapy. Am J Cardiol 1992; 69:12A–20A.

42. Maggioni AP, Franzosi MG, Santoro E, White H, Van deWerf F, et al. The risk of stroke in patients with acute myocardial infarction after thrombolytic and antithrombotic treatment. N Engl J Med 1992; 327:1–6.

43. Maggioni AP, Franzosi MG, Farina ML, et al. Cerebrovascular events after myocardial infarction: analysis of the GISSI Trial. Br Med J 1991; 302:1428–1431.

44. O'Connor CM, Califf RM, Masswy EW, et al. Stroke and acute myocardial infarction in the thrombolytic era: clinical correlates and long-term prognosis. J Am Coll Cardiol 1990; 16:533–540.

45. Thompson PL, Robinson JS. Stroke after acute myocardial infarction: relation to infarct size. Br J Med 1978; 2:457–459.

46. Fennerty AG, Levine MN, Hirsh J. Hemorrhagic complications of thrombolytic therapy in the treatment of myocardial infarction and venous thromboembolism. Chest 1989; 95(Suppl):885–875.

47. Faxon DF. The risk of reperfusion in the treatment of patients with acute myocardial infarction. J Am Coll Cardiol 1988; 12:52A–57A.

48. The TIMI Research Group. Immediate vs delayed catheterization and angioplasty following thrombolytic therapy for acute myocardial infarction. JAMA 1988; 260:2849–2858.

49. Topol EJ. Textbook of interventional cardiology. Philadelphia: Saunders. 1990; pp 77–111.

50. Jalihal S, Morris GK. Anistreptokinase titres after intravenous streptokinase. Lancet 1990; 1:184–185.

51. Honan MB, Harrell FE, Reimer KA, Califf RM, Mark DB, et al. Cardiac rupture, mortality and the timing of thrombolytic therapy: a meta-analysis. J Am Coll Cardiol 1990; 16:359–367.

52. Currier JW, Kalan JM, Ruocco NA Jr, Frederick MM, Faxon DP, et al. Cardiac rupture after myocardial infarction treated with tissue plas-

minogen activator: results from TIMI-II. J Am Coll Cardiol 1991; 17:16A.

53. Kleiman NS, Terrin M, Mueler H, Chaitman B, Roberts R, et al. Mechanism of early death despite thrombolytic therapy: experience from the thrombolysis in myocardial infarction phase II (TIMI) study. J Am Coll Cardiol 1992; 19:1129–1135.

54. Gertz SD, Kalan JM, Kragel AH, Roberts WC, Braunwald E, TIMI Investigators. Cardiac morphologic findings in patients with acute myocardial infarction treated with recombinant tissue plasminogen activator. Am J Cardiol 1990; 65:953–961.

55. Gertz SD, Kragel AH, Kalan JM, Braunwald E, Roberts WC, TIMI Investigators. Comparison of coronary and myocardial morphologic findings in patients with and without thrombolytic therapy during fatal first acute myocardial infarction. Am J Cardiol 1990; 66:904–909.

56. Topol EJ, Califf RM, George BS, Kereiakes DJ, Lee KL, TAMI Study Group. Insights derived from the thrombolysis and angioplasty in myocardial infarction (TAMI) trials. J Am Coll Cardiol 1988; 12:24A–31A.

57. Simons SL, Aer A, Betriu A, et al. Thrombolysis with rt-PA in acute myocardial infarction: no beneficial effects of immediate PTCA. Lancet 1988; 1:197–203.

58. The TIMI Study Group. Comparison of invasive and conservative strategies after treatment with intravenous tissue plasminogen activator in acute myocardial infarction. N Engl J Med 1989; 320:618–627.

59. Bates ER, Topol EJ. Limitations of thrombolytic therapy for acute myocardial infarction complicated by congestive heart failure and cardiogenic shock. J Am Coll Cardiol 1991; 18:1077–1084.

60. Lee L, Bates ER, Pitt B, Walton JA, Laufer N, O'Neil WW. Percutaneous transluminal coronary angioplasty improves survival in acute myocardial infarction complicated by cardiogenic shock. Circulation 1988; 78:1345–1351.

61. Kirklin JW, Akins CW, Blackstone EH, Booth DC, Califf RM, et al. ACC/AHA guidelines and indications for coronary artery bypass graft surgery. A report of the American College of Cardiology/American Heart Association task force on assessment of diagnostic and therapeutic cardiovascular procedures (subcommittee on coronary artery bypass graft surgery). Circulation 1991; 83:1125–1173.

62. Petrovich JA, Schneider JA, Taylor J, Mikell FL, Batchelder E, et al. Early and late results of operation after thrombolytic therapy for acute myocardial infarction. J Thorac Cardiovasc Surg 1986; 92:853–858.

63. Kereiakes DJ, Topol EJ, George BS, Abbottsmith CW, Stack RS, et al. Emergency coronary artery bypass surgery preserves global and regional left ventricular function after intravenous tissue plasminogen activator therapy for acute myocardial infarction. J Am Coll Cardiol 1988; 11:899–907.

64. Barner HB, Lea JW, Naunheim KS, Stoney WS Jr. Emergency coronary bypass not associated with preoperative cardiogenic shock in failed angioplasty, after thrombolysis, and for acute myocardial infarction. Circulation 1989; 79(Suppl I):I-152–I-159.

65. Ohman EM, Califf RM, Topol EJ, Candela R, Abbottsmith C, et al. Consequences of reocclusion after successful reperfusion therapy in acute myocardial infarction. Circulation 1990; 82:781–791.
66. Hsia J, Hamilton WP, Kleiman N, Roberts R, Chaitman BR, Ross AM. A comparison between heparin and low-dose aspirin as adjunctive therapy with tissue plasminogen activator for acute myocardial infarction. The Heparin-Aspirin Reperfusion Trial (HART) Investigations. N Engl J Med 1990; 323:1433–1437.
67. The SCATI (studio sulla calciparina nell'angina e nella thrombosi ventricolare nell' infarto) group. Randomised controlled trial of subcutaneous calcium-heparin after rt-PA for acute myocardial infarction. Lancet 1989; 2:182–186.
68. The International Study Group. In-hospital mortality and clinical course of 20-891 patients with suspected acute myocardial infarction randomised between alteplase and streptokinase with or without heparin. Lancet 1990; 336:71–75.
69. Heras M, Chesebro JH, Penny WJ, Bailey KR, Badimon L, Fuster V. Effects of thrombin inhibition on the development of acute platelet-thrombus deposition during angioplasty in pigs. Heparin versus recombinant hirudin, a specific thrombin inhibitor. Circulation 1989; 79:657–665.
70. Kelly AB, Hanson SR, Marzec U, Harker LA. Recombinant hirudin (r-h) interruption of platelet-dependent thrombus formation (abstract). Circulation 1988; 80(Suppl II):II–311.
71. Jang IK, Gold HK, Ziskind AA, Leinbach RC, Fallon JT, Collen D. Prevention of platelet-rich arterial thrombosis selective thrombin inhibitor. Circulation 1990; 81:219–225.
72. Neuhaus KL, Feuerer W, Jeep-Tebbe S, Niedereer W, Vogt A, Tebbe U. Improved thrombolysis with modified dose regimen of recombinant tissue-type plasminogen activator. J Am Coll Cardiol 1989; 14:1566–1569.

Chapter 3

The Role of Coronary Sinus Interventions to Reduce Myocardial Damage After Acute Coronary Ischemia

Alice K. Jacobs and Harold L. Lazar

Introduction

Coronary artery bypass grafting (CABG) and percutaneous transluminal coronary angioplasty (PTCA) are now established methods for treating both acute and chronic coronary ischemic syndromes. Both modalities restore antegrade blood flow to jeopardized myocardium. It is of interest, however, that the initial attempts to treat myocardial ischemia were directed toward a retrograde approach using the coronary venous system.[1]

There currently is a renewed interest in protecting jeopardized myocardium during regional and global ischemia using coronary sinus venous techniques. Coronary venous retrograde perfusion offers several advantages in comparison to antegrade arterial perfu-

Lazar HL (editor): *Current Therapy for Acute Coronary Ischemia,* © Futura Publishing Co., Inc., Mount Kisco, NY, 1993.

sion during acute coronary ischemia. The venous system is relatively free of atherosclerotic lesions and the coronary sinus can be cannulated relatively quickly. Retrograde perfusion of antiarrhythmic, inotropic, and thrombolytic agents may be more effective in reaching areas of regional ischemia than the intravenous route. In addition, these techniques can provide regional myocardial perfusion during high-risk PTCA. When emergent CABG is required after a failed PTCA, they may also be used for delivering retrograde cardioplegia during aortic cross-clamping. There is experimental evidence to suggest that retrograde cardioplegia may provide superior myocardial protection during the revascularization of an acute coronary occlusion.[2]

Advances in catheter design have made access to the coronary sinus easier and safer. Synchronized retroperfusion (SRP) and pressure-controlled intermittent coronary sinus occlusion (PICSO) have emerged as techniques by which blood can be redirected through the coronary sinus to nourish ischemic myocardium beyond a coronary occlusion. This chapter reviews the current applications of these coronary sinus interventions and the pertinent experimental and clinical studies upon which they are based. The efficacy of these techniques in either reversing or delaying ischemic damage after an episode of acute coronary insufficiency also is discussed.

History of Coronary Sinus Interventions

Gross and his co-workers first documented the feasibility of coronary sinus occlusion in reducing myocardial necrosis in experimental studies in dogs in 1937.[3] When the coronary sinus was ligated, there was a 70% reduction in infarct size and mortality after acute occlusion of the left anterior descending coronary artery (LAD). In 1948, Beck designed a surgical procedure based on the occlusion of the coronary sinus for patients with myocardial ischemia.[1] His operation was performed in two stages. In the first stage, a left thoracotomy was performed to expose the coronary sinus and descending thoracic aorta and a bypass conduit was constructed between the aorta and coronary sinus. Three weeks later, a repeat thoracotomy was performed, and the coronary sinus was ligated just beyond the ostium. The Beck procedure was never accepted because of the difficulty of the operative technique, the need for two operations, and its considerable mortality (18%). Nevertheless, many patients reported dramatic relief of anginal pain. In 1956, Lillehei and colleagues demonstrated that retrograde coronary sinus perfusion could provide effective myocardial protection during cardiac valve surgery.[4] These early studies indicated that coronary sinus retrograde perfusion could minimize the size of an infarct, reduce anginal pain, and protect the myocardium during periods of coronary insufficiency.

The use of retrograde coronary venous perfusion to provide support for patients with acute coronary insufficiency was first suggested by Gensini et al. in the early 1960s after they demonstrated the safety of coronary sinus occlusion and venography.[5,6] Experimental studies by Rassman and co-workers[7] showed that occlusion of the coronary sinus by a balloon catheter could significantly improve survival after circumflex coronary artery ligation. Other investigations showed that arterial perfusion through an occluding coronary sinus balloon catheter further improved myocardial salvage and prevented the development of cardiogenic shock.[8] In addition, studies by Arealis and colleagues demonstrated that nonsynchronized intermittent occlusion of the coronary sinus, without arterial retrograde perfusion, decreased the ischemic response during sequential coronary artery occlusion.[9]

A major modification in coronary venous retrograde perfusion techniques was pioneered by Meerbaum and Corday, who introduced the concept of SRP.[10] In the SRP technique, coronary sinus balloon occlusion occurs during diastole while balloon deflation occurs during systole. This allows for normal venous drainage to occur during systole and thus prevents excessive and prolonged elevation of coronary sinus pressure, which resulted in myocardial edema and hemorrhage in earlier studies. In 1984, based on the work of Arealis, Mohl and his co-workers introduced the concept of PICSO.[11] In this nonsynchronized retrograde technique, a coronary sinus balloon-tipped catheter is inflated and deflated intermittently according to a preset cycle. Coronary sinus occlusion is followed by a rise in the coronary sinus pressure until a plateau is reached when the venous system is filled. This redistribution of flow into the ischemic area is followed by a washout of toxic metabolites and edema after the fall in pressure that accompanies release of the coronary sinus occlusion.[12]

Anatomy of the Coronary Sinus

An understanding of coronary venous anatomy is helpful in determining the efficacy and pathophysiology of coronary sinus interventions. As is the case with most venous anatomy, there is great variation of the venous drainage of the myocardium. In a series of 250 adult heart specimens, in only 21% of the dissections did the coronary sinus collect all the myocardial venous drainage.[13]

The venous outflow from the heart can be divided into three systems: the coronary sinus and its tributaries, the anterior cardiac veins, and the smallest veins of Thebesius.[14] The coronary sinus varies from 4 to 14 mm in diameter and averages approximately 9 to 10 mm.[14] It has been known to dilate significantly in the setting of elevated right atrial pressures that can occur in congestive heart failure. Less than 1% of patients do not have a coronary sinus large enough to permit cannulation. The tributaries of the coronary sinus include the great cardiac vein, the posterior vein of the left ventricle, the oblique vein of Marshall, the posterior interventricular vein, and the small cardiac veins. All five tributaries are present in only 25% of patients. The small cardiac veins, draining the posterior wall of the right ventricle, are the most anomalous tributary; they are absent in 75% of all patients. The anterior cardiac veins drain the anterior surface of the left ventricle directly into the right atrium. The number and course of the anterior cardiac veins are closely connected with the presence of the small cardiac veins. The smallest cardiac veins of Thebesius carry blood from the myocardial wall and drain directly into the atria and ventricles of the heart. The distribution of the Thebesian veins varies, but they are most dense in the right atrium.

In addition to these major systems, there are also venovenous, arteriovenous, and venoluminal anastomoses[15] (Fig. 1). This dense network of alternative venous pathways serves to connect the major tributaries of the coronary sinus with the other venous networks that do not empty directly into the coronary sinus. The success of any method of retrograde perfusion depends on the anatomical variation of the major tributaries of the coronary sinus and the extent of venovenous and arteriovenous anastomoses. Dissections in human hearts with atherosclerotic arterial lesions have shown greater numbers of arteriovenous and venoluminal anastomoses.[16] These interconnections may be of particular importance during retrograde perfusion because they allow perfusion of potentially ischemic areas

Sinus
coronarius

Posterior
interventricular
vein

Left
marginal vein

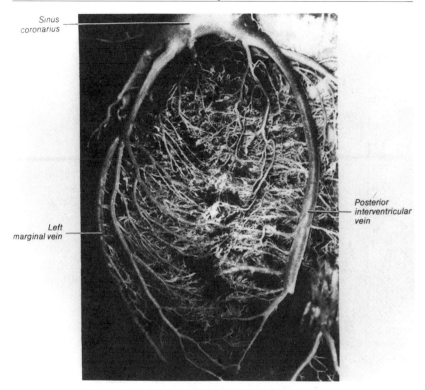

Figure 1: Technovit cast demonstrating the intricate microvasculature and the dense anastomotic network of the cardiac vein. Reprinted with permission of Tschabitscher.[14]

of the myocardium in areas not directly drained by the coronary sinus.

Physiology and Flow Dynamics of the Coronary Sinus

The variations and intricacies of the coronary venous system help to explain its unique physiology and flow dynamics. Normal coronary sinus pressure is similar to right atrial pressure, with discrete "a", "c," and "v" waves. When the coronary sinus is occluded, there is a rise in systolic pressure that reaches a plateau. This plateau of systolic pressure, which usually is 40 to 50 mm Hg,

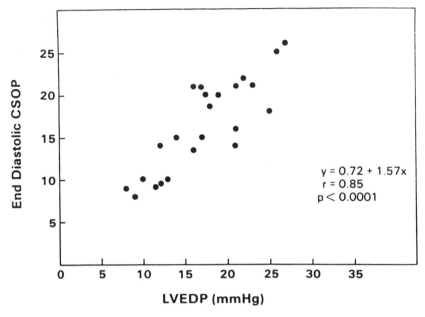

Figure 2: Correlation between the end-diastolic coronary sinus occlusion pressure (CSOP) and left ventricular end-diastolic pressure (LVEDP). Reprinted with permission of Faxon et al.[17]

appears to represent complete filling of the venous circulation. In humans, coronary sinus occlusion pressure (CSOP) correlates with left ventricular end-diastolic pressure (LVEDP) over a wide range of pressures[17] (Fig. 2). In contrast, systolic CSOP is significantly lower than left ventricular systolic pressure. The close relationship between LVEDP and diastolic CSOP is most likely related to the many arteriovenous anastomoses found in the human left ventricle. Due to this rich network of arteriovenous anastomoses, the sudden occlusion of the coronary sinus results in a partial preservation of coronary arterial blood flow.[18]

Technique of Coronary Sinus Catheterization

Cannulation of the coronary sinus is most successful from the right internal jugular vein. Fluoroscopy and pressure-monitoring equipment are essential. The catheter tip is positioned along the lateral wall of the mid-right atrium and rotated counterclockwise and advanced into the right ventricle. It is then withdrawn and rotated slowly so that the tip is posterior and above the tricuspid valve at the entrance of the coronary sinus. The catheter is then advanced into the coronary sinus along the atrioventricular groove into the great cardiac vein. The injection of contrast material may be helpful in visualizing the anatomy and the venous tributaries.

Cannulation of the great cardiac vein via the coronary sinus is successful in 85% of patients within 5 minutes in experienced hands. During coronary angioplasty, access through the femoral vein is more readily available but does make cannulating the coronary sinus more difficult. A standard soft-tipped guidewire placed through the catheter may facilitate the technique. In the operating room, transesophageal 2D echocardiography is helpful in cannulating the coronary sinus for retrograde cardioplegia techniques.

Clinical Applications for Coronary Sinus Interventions

Currently, there are three sinus techniques undergoing clinical evaluation (Table 1). These include (a) retroinfusion of pharmaceutical agents, (b) synchronized retroperfusion, and (c) pressure-controlled intermittent coronary sinus occlusion.

Retroinfusion

Coronary sinus retroinfusion provides an alternative route to deliver pharmacological agents to ischemic myocardium beyond a coronary occlusion. The coronary sinus is catheterized and a pump is used to deliver the drug to the myocardium. This technique usually is combined with a method of coronary sinus occlusion to prevent leakage into the right atrium. The mechanism of retrograde perfusion to ischemic myocardium was defined by Meesmann and his co-workers, who injected monastral blue dye through a catheter in the coronary sinus in dogs with and without LAD occlusions.[19] In the absence of an LAD occlusion with a normal mean aortic pressure, there was no significant perfusion of myocardial tissue. However, in the presence of an LAD occlusion, the distal myocardium beyond the

Table 1

Clinical Applications for Coronary Sinus Interventions

Modality	Methods	Advantages	Disadvantages
All modalities		CS catheterization simple to accomplish	Potential risk of damage to venous system
		Avoid coronary artery manipulation and potential trauma	Additional time and equipment needed to establish technique
		No evidence of vascular damage in published clinical reports	SRP and PICSO provide only temporary support of ischemic myocardium
Retroinfusion	Transvenous cannulation of CS and delivery of pharmacological agents	No arterial access Uniform delivery of cardioplegia (useful with severe proximal coronary artery stenosis, aortic valve surgery)	Potential inadequate RV protection Myocardial edema and hemorrhage when CS occluded During cardiac surgery, longer time to diastolic arrest and RA incision required
SRP	Blood from femoral artery pumped during diastole into CS catheter; CS balloon occlusion occurs during diastole	Normal venous drainage Delivery of pharmacological agents to ischemic myocardium	Arterial access required Potential for hemolysis with gated pumping
PICSO	Intermittent balloon occlusion of CS maintained until CS pressure reaches a plateau and the obstruction is released	No arterial access Simple system Facilitates washout of ischemic myocardium Continuous monitoring of LVEDP	Not effective during brief ischemia

CS = coronary sinus; LVEDP = left ventricular end-diastolic pressure; PICSO = pressure-controlled intermittent coronary sinus occlusion; RA = right atrium; SRP = synchronized retroperfusion; RV = right ventricle.

occlusion was selectively perfused. Furthermore, during systemic hypotension (systolic BP <55 mm Hg), retrograde perfusion occurred in both the myocardium beyond the LAD occlusion as well as in unobstructed areas. There have been several experimental studies showing the efficacy of retroinfusion of cardioprotective drugs. In pigs with LAD occlusions, Ryder et al. showed that retroinfusion of metoprolol resulted in higher drug concentrations in the area of ischemic myocardium than in nonischemic areas.[20] Furthermore, the drug concentrations of metoprolol infused retrogradely were similar to those obtained when the drug was given antegradely beyond the coronary occlusion. In a similar model, Miyazaki and his co-workers found that the retrograde administration of recombinant tissue-type plasminogen activator resulted in more rapid clot lysis, better recovery of regional wall motion, and decreased infarct size than when the drug was systemically administered.[21] Similar results have been reported with the retroinfusion of streptokinase.[22] Kobayashi et al., using the iron chelator deferoxamine, found that the retroinfusion of deferoxamine resulted in a significant decrease in infarct size after LAD occlusion whereas the systemic infusion of the same drug failed to reduce infarct size.[23] Similar experimental models of coronary occlusion also have shown enhanced antiarrhythmic effects by retroinfusion of lidocaine[24] and procainamide,[25] and decreased infarct size using oxygen free radical scavengers.[26]

There are several reasons to explain the improved drug delivery to ischemic areas of the myocardium using the retrograde technique. The decrease in antegrade flow beyond the coronary occlusion results in lower capillary pressures, thus reversing the arteriovenous gradient and resulting in increased flow to low pressure areas of the myocardium. Since there is less antegrade flow to the ischemic myocardium, there is less washout of tissues and, therefore, the retrograde-delivered drug has a better chance to accumulate at the microvascular level. These experimental studies suggest that clinical retroinfusion techniques will further protect jeopardized ischemic myocardium if pharmacological agents are added to the retroperfusate.

Synchronized Retroperfusion

Since its introduction by Meerbaum and his colleagues in 1976,[10] SRP techniques have undergone extensive experimental and clinical evaluation. The current SRP system consists of an electronic pumping console, a specially designed retroperfusion catheter, and an arterial catheter (Fig. 3). Arterial blood is withdrawn from an 8F arterial catheter placed percutaneously in the femoral artery. The catheter is equipped with both a distal end hole and side holes to provide adequate arterial supply and to prevent intimal damage. The coronary sinus retroperfusion catheter is an 8.5F triple lumen catheter that features an inflatable balloon located 1 cm from the distal end of the catheter (Fig. 4). At full inflation, the balloon is oval shaped, with a 10-mm diameter. Carbon dioxide gas is delivered via a second lumen to inflate the balloon during diastole. The third

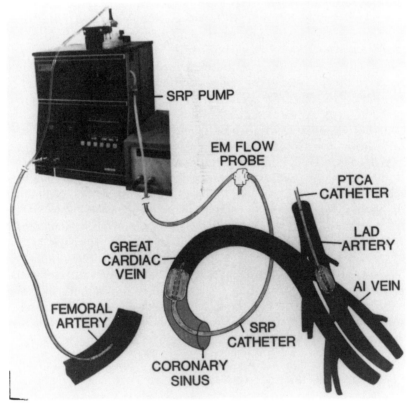

Figure 3: Schematic representation of the retroperfusion system. AI = anterior interventricular; EM = electromagnetic; LAD = left anterior descending coronary artery; PTCA = percutaneous transluminal coronary angioplasty; SRP = synchronized retroperfusion. Reprinted with permission of Kar et al.[35]

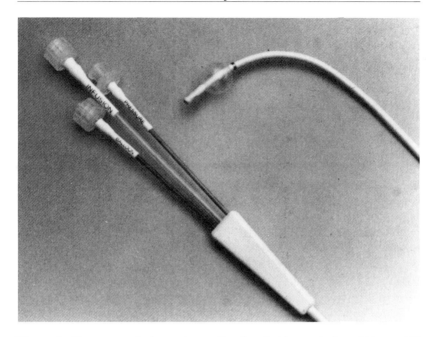

Figure 4: The retroperfusion catheter. Reprinted with permission of Kar et al.[35]

lumen is used to monitor coronary venous pressure continuously so as not to exceed 60 mm Hg, which may damage the venules. A radiopaque band proximal to the balloon aids in fluoroscopic placement. The arterial blood supply catheter is connected to the pumping console, which pumps blood during diastole by means of a piston whose motion is triggered by the R wave of the monitored electrocardiogram. This is in turn connected to the blood infusion lumen of the coronary sinus retroperfusion catheter. Arterial flow is initiated at 50 ml/min and is increased until a maximum flow of 250 ml/min is achieved or the peak coronary sinus pressure exceeds 60 mm Hg. The pump is equipped with a safety mechanism that terminates retroperfusion if these coronary venous pressures are exceeded.

Microsphere studies in experimental preparations with acute LAD occlusion indicate that SRP provides increased blood flow to the acutely ischemic myocardium.[27] Furthermore, these studies indicate that initiation of SRP soon after LAD occlusion results in significant improvement in regional ventricular function and decreased infarct size.[27,28]

In preparation for clinical use, Gore and his co-workers studied the effects of SRP in animals for up to 24 hours.[29] Gross and microscopic examination of the coronary sinus, coronary veins, and right atrium did not reveal any evidence of major damage from prolonged retroperfusion. Based on these studies, a protocol to evaluate the clinical feasibility and safety of SRP was initiated.[30] Patients with unstable angina unresponsive to maximal medical management were selected. Retroperfusion was initiated at a flow rate of 0.5 ml/kg of body weight per minute and increased every 10 minutes until there was relief of symptoms of ischemia or until the maximum output of the system was achieved. SRP was performed at the bedside and took an average of 30 minutes from the preparation of the patient to the institution of therapy. In most patients, the coronary sinus was cannulated in less than 1 minute. There were no adverse effects on red cell or platelet counts. In the five patients studied, the frequency of anginal attacks and incidence of electrocardiographic changes indicated a major clinical improvement during SRP therapy. In four of five patients, there was normalization of the ischemic electrocardiographic changes within 10 minutes of instituting retroperfusion. After medical stabilization on SRP, all patients underwent coronary angiography, at which time a decision was made as to whether a PTCA or CABG was required. Barnett and Touchon reported the effects of retroperfusion in eight patients with unstable angina and myocardial infarction, of whom two were in cardiogenic shock.[31] During retroperfusion, there was reduction in the degree of ST segment elevation, with a corresponding improvement noted in the wall motion of the infarct zone seen on 2D echocardiography. Both these studies demonstrated the feasibility and safety of retroperfusion in patients with unstable angina and an evolving myocardial infarction. These encouraging results prompted the initiation of clinical protocols to determine whether SRP had a role in protecting jeopardized myocardium during LAD angioplasty.

Weiner and her co-workers first employed SRP during angioplasty of the LAD in three patients.[32] Each patient underwent four angioplasty balloon dilatations, two with and two without retroperfusion (Fig. 5). SRP resulted in a significant delay in the onset of angina (100 vs. 28 sec) and the time to ST segment change (137 vs. 60 sec) compared to inflations where SRP was not used. In a similar group of LAD angioplasty patients, Constantini and co-workers showed better preservation of cardiac and stroke work indices in patients receiving SRP.[33] Berland and co-workers studied

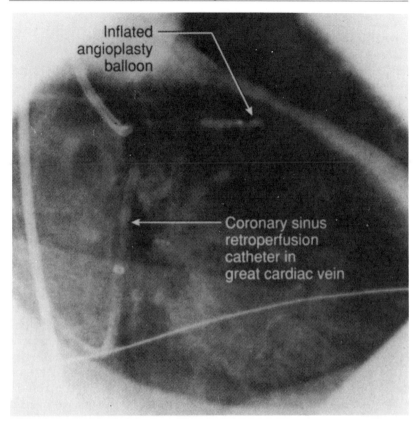

Figure 5: Single-frame cineangiogram in a patient undergoing left anterior descending coronary artery angioplasty during synchronized retroperfusion. Reprinted with permission of Lincoff et al.[44]

16 patients undergoing SRP during angioplasty of the LAD.[34] Forty-eight PTCA balloon inflations were evaluated: 16 during retroperfusion and 32 without SRP. Thirty-one percent of the SRP inflations resulted in angina as opposed to 72% of the untreated inflations. The average ST segment elevation in leads V_1 through V_4 was significantly lower with SRP. There also was better preservation of ejection fraction as determined by 2D echocardiography with SRP. These studies demonstrated that SRP was a safe technique that reduced ischemia and preserved both regional and global myocardial function during PTCA.

To evaluate the feasibility, safety, and efficacy of SRP during

PTCA, a multicenter trial was initiated in 1987.[35] SRP was performed during alternate PTCA balloon inflations such that untreated inflations served as controls. Data were pooled from 164 patients undergoing LAD angioplasty. A total of 499 PTCA inflations were reported: 198 with SRP and 301 without. Angina occurred in 43% of the SRP inflations as compared to 58% of the untreated controls ($p<0.01$). The average time to the onset of angina was significantly prolonged in the SRP group (48 vs. 38 sec; $p<0.01$). The average ST segment change also was lower in the SRP group (2.4 vs. 3.3 mV, $p<0.01$). Regional wall motion analysis showed significantly fewer segmental changes during SRP. The global ejection fraction also was significantly higher in the SRP group (44 vs. 36%, $p<0.01$). There was no evidence of hemolysis or any other major adverse effects associated with SRP in these patients.

Although these initial clinical studies indicate that SRP is beneficial in decreasing acute ischemia, it is important to note that the ischemic response is delayed or decreased but not totally prevented or abolished. The position of the coronary sinus catheter tip is crucial and should be in as close proximity as possible to the myocardium distal to the coronary artery occlusion. The flow rate is important and variable in a given patient. The pressure gradient between the coronary veins and the zone distal to the coronary artery occlusion is also important. Most studies have been performed during LAD occlusions while the effects of SRP on right coronary and circumflex coronary artery occlusions are not as well documented.

Currently, clinical indications for the initiation of SRP exist in those patients undergoing LAD angioplasty who are at high risk for ischemic complications. These include patients with unstable angina, low output syndrome, or an evolving myocardial infarction in whom thrombolytic therapy is contraindicated. Ongoing clinical trials will determine the efficacy of new catheter designs, the role of SRP combined with pharmaceutical therapy, and effects of retroperfusion during right coronary and left circumflex angioplasty.

Pressure-Controlled Intermittent Coronary Sinus Occlusion

In the PICSO technique, a 7 to 9F balloon-tipped catheter is positioned in the orifice of the coronary sinus and is connected to a pneumatic pump. The pump automatically inflates and deflates the

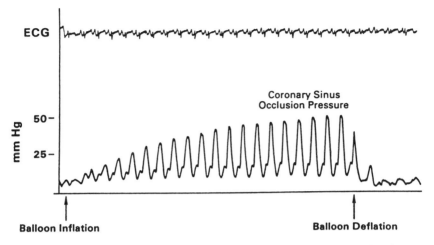

Figure 6: Coronary sinus pressure. After inflation of a balloon-tipped catheter positioned in the coronary sinus, the coronary sinus pressure rises until the coronary sinus occlusion pressure reaches a plateau. Balloon deflation is followed by a rapid return to baseline pressure. Reprinted with permission of Faxon DP, Jacobs AK.[45]

balloon according to a preset cycle of 10 seconds of inflation and 4 seconds of deflation.[11] During the occlusion phase, there is a slow increase in coronary sinus pressure until a plateau is reached (Fig. 6). After this plateau phase, the pneumatic pump automatically deflates the balloon, thereby resulting in an abrupt decrease in coronary sinus pressure and allowing drainage of the coronary venous system. When the coronary sinus pressure returns to baseline, the balloon is automatically inflated and the PICSO cycle is repeated. The timing of the inflation-deflation cycle is critical since prolonged occlusion of the coronary sinus can cause hemorrhage, edema, thrombosis, arrhythmias, and conduction disturbances. The intermittent nature of the inflation-deflation process avoids these complications despite peak coronary sinus pressures as high as 50 mm Hg. The inflation-deflation cycle also promotes washout of toxic metabolites formed during ischemia that results in tissue acidosis impairing regional function. Experimental studies have shown enhanced lactate washout and changes in purine nucleotides after PICSO treatment.[36]

As noted in Chapter 7, experimental studies have shown that after an acute coronary occlusion subjected to surgical revasculariztion, PICSO improves the distribution of antegrade cardioplegia, increases myocardial tissue pH, improves regional and global ventricular function, and decreases tissue necrosis.[37–39] These studies correlate with previous experimental studies involving coronary occlusions without cardiopulmonary bypass, which have shown that PICSO increases blood flow to ischemic and border zones, preserves regional wall motion, and decreases infarct size.[11,40,41] The above studies were performed in animals with prolonged (≥15 min) periods of LAD occlusion. However, PICSO is less effective during brief periods of ischemia. In a canine model of 3-minute LAD occlusions, PICSO did not prevent, reduce, or shorten the transient period of left ventricular dysfunction that occurred.[42] This suggests that PICSO may not be as useful in reducing ischemia after brief periods of ischemia such as that caused by uncomplicated angioplasty inflations. Clinically, PICSO has been limited to intraoperative use. In 30 patients undergoing CABG surgery, PICSO was performed for 1 hour during reperfusion.[43] Using 2D echo criteria, it appeared that segments with preoperative dysfunction had better preservation after surgery when PICSO was used. There were no complications using the PICSO technique.

Unlike SRP, PICSO does not require catheterization of the femoral artery. This makes it more applicable to patients with severe peripheral vascular disease. Since PICSO works on a preset cycle, the constant monitoring and manipulation necessary for SRP is not required. Experimental studies appear to indicate that unlike SRP, PICSO offers limited benefits for short periods (<15 min) of coronary ischemia and is more beneficial after prolonged periods of coronary occlusion. This may make it a suitable technique for PTCA when complicated by prolonged ischemia followed by abrupt closure of the coronary artery, especially with those patients who require urgent surgical revascularization. The PICSO catheter also can be used to deliver retrograde cardioplegia, which may be the technique of choice for myocardial protection in the face of an acute coronary occlusion.[2]

Clinical Applications for Coronary Sinus Techniques After Acute Coronary Insufficiency

The role of coronary sinus techniques in the treatment of acute coronary insufficiency continues to evolve. Unlike the intra-aortic balloon and percutaneous bypass, SRP and PICSO cannot indepen-dently support the failing heart during the low cardiac output syndrome.[44] However, there are numerous clinical applications for these techniques. Coronary sinus interventions can help to avoid ischemic injury in the setting of high-risk PTCA. This would include patients with unstable angina with large territories at risk as well as those patients who are evolving a myocardial infarction at the time of their PTCA. Both SRP and PICSO may be of benefit in patients with an acute myocardial infarction. These techniques may be initiated at local community hospitals that do not have catheteri-zation laboratories but have access to fluoroscopy. Inotropic, anti-arrhythmic, lytic, substrate, and free radical scavenger agents can be delivered as the patient is transported to a tertiary care center for catheterization. This helps to expand the time window in which it is necessary to perform cardiac catheterization to determine what type of revascularization procedure (PTCA vs CABG) will be required. As noted in Chapter 7, PICSO can be especially helpful for patients with a failed PTCA requiring urgent surgical revascularization when a bailout or autoperfusion catheter cannot be used due to loss of antegrade access to the vessel. The initiation of PICSO may limit infarct size during the time of transport to the operating room. The catheter also can be used to measure LVEDP providing a useful guide to left ventricular function without the need for a Swan-Ganz catheter. In addition to delivering pharmacological agents, the PICSO catheter also can be used to deliver retrograde cardioplegia in the operating room. After aortic unclamping, PICSO can be reinsti-tuted during the reperfusion period and left in place in the intensive care unit for monitoring purposes. Finally, the use of coronary sinus techniques appears to enhance support devices such as the intra-aortic balloon and percutaneous bypass by increasing myocardial blood supply.

Future Directions

Both PICSO and SRP have been shown to be safe techniques with minimal morbidity. While initial experimental and clinical studies are encouraging, carefully matched randomized studies involving patients with evolving myocardial infarctions and unsta-ble angina will be necessary to define their roles further in clinical practice. Sophisticated diagnostic techniques such as 2D echocardiography and positron emission tomography scanning may be needed to quantify wall motion changes and infarct size in the area at risk. Nevertheless, as the practice of cardiovascular medicine changes to include more patients who present with acute coronary insufficiency, coronary sinus interventions have the potential to play an important role in limiting infarct size and decreasing morbidity and mortality in patients requiring urgent revascularization.

References

1. Beck CS. Revascularization of the heart. Ann Surg 1948; 128:854–864.
2. Haan C, Lazar HL, Bernard S, Rivers S, Zallnick J, Shemin RJ. Superiority of retrograde cardioplegia after acute coronary occlusion. Ann Thorac Surg 1991; 51:408–412.
3. Gross L, Blum L, Silverman G. Experimental attempts to increase the blood supply to the dog's heart by means of coronary sinus occlusion. J Exp Med 1937; 65:91–108.
4. Lillehei CW, Dewal RA, Gott VL, Varco RL. The direct vision correction of calcific aortic stenosis by means of a pump-oxygenator and retrograde coronary sinus perfusion. Dis Chest 1956; 30:123–132.
5. Gensini GG, DiGiorgi S, Murad-Netto S. Coronary venous occluded pressure. Arch Surgery 1963; 86:72–80.
6. Gensini GG, DiGiorgi S, Coskun O, Palacio A, Kelly AE. Anatomy of the coronary circulation in living man: coronary venography. Circulation 1965; 31:778–784.
7. Rassman WR, Tanaka S, Fleming R, Lillehei LW. Acute revascularization of the heart by coronary sinus occlusion without thoracotomy. Circulation 1968; 161:37–38.
8. Carabello BA, Lemoie GM, Lee KW, Spann JF. Retrograde coronary capillary perfusion for prevention and reversal of cardiogenic shock in experimental myocardial infarction. Ann Thorac Surg 1976; 21:405–411.
9. Arealis EG, Moulopoulos SD, Kolff WJ. Attempts to increase blood supply to an acutely ischemic area of the myocardium by intermittent occlusion of the coronary sinus (preliminary results). Med Res Eng 1977; 12:4–7.
10. Meerbaum S, Lang TW, Osher JV, et al. Diastolic retroperfusion of acutely ischemic myocardium. Am J Cardiol 1976; 37:588–598.
11. Mohl W, Glogar D, Mayr H, et al. Reduction of infarct size induced by intermittent coronary sinus occlusion. Am J Cardiol 1984; 53:923–928.
12. Moser M, Mohl W, Gallasch E, Kenner T. Optimization of pressure-controlled intermittent coronary sinus occlusion intervals by density measurements. In: Mohl W, Werner E, Glogan D, eds. The Coronary Sinus. Steinkopff Verlag, Darmstadt: Springer-Verlag. 1984; pp 529–536.
13. Ludinghausen M. Anatomy of the coronary arteries and veins. In: Mohl

W, Wolner E. Glogar D, eds. The Coronary Sinus. Steinkopff Verlag, Darmstadt: Springer-Verlag. 1984; pp 5–7.

14. Tschabitscher M. Anatomy of coronary veins. In: Mohl W, Wolner E, Glogar D, eds. The Coronary Sinus. Steinkopff Verlag, Darmstadt: Springer-Verlag. 1984; pp 8–25.

15. Ratajczyk-Pakalska E, Kolff WJ. Anatomical basis for the coronary venous outflow. In: Mohl W, Wolner E, Glogar D, eds. The Coronary Sinus. Steinkopff Verlag, Darmstadt: Springer-Verlag. 1984; pp 40–46.

16. Ratajczyk-Pakalska E. Thebesian veins in the human hearts with atherosclerotic lesions in the coronary arteries. In: Mohl W, Faxon D, Wolner E, eds. Clinics of CSI. Steinkopff Verlag, Darmstadt: Springer-Verlag. 1986: pp 141–145.

17. Faxon DP, Jacobs AK, Kellett MA, McSweeney SM, Coats WD, Ryan TJ. Coronary sinus occlusion pressure and its relation to intracardiac pressure. Am J Cardiol 1985; 56:457–460.

18. Jacobs AK, Faxon DP, Apstein CS, et al. The hemodynamic consequences of coronary sinus occlusion. In: Mohl W, Wolner E, Glogar D, eds. The Coronary Sinus, Steinkopff Verlag, Darmstadt: Springer-Verlag. 1984; pp 430–435.

19. Meesmann M, Karagueuzian HS, Takashi I, et al. Selective perfusion of ischemic myocardium during coronary venous retroinjection: a study of the causative role of venoarterial and venoventricular pressure gradients. J Am Coll Cardiol 1987; 10:887–897.

20. Ryder L, Tadokoro H, Sjoquist PO, et al. Pharmacokinetic analysis of coronary venous retroinfusion: a comparison with antegrade coronary artery drug administration using metoprolol as a tracer. J Am Coll Cardiol 1991; 18:603–612.

21. Miyazaki A, Tadokoro H, Drury JK, Ryder L, Haendchen RV, Corday E. Retrograde coronary venous administration of recombinant tissue-type plasminogen activator: a unique and effective approach to coronary artery thrombolysis. J Am Coll Cardiol 1991; 18:613–620.

22. Meerbaum S, Lang TW, Povzhitkov M, et al. Retrograde lysis of coronary artery thrombosis by coronary venous streptokinase administration. J Am Coll Cardiol 1983; 1:1262–1267.

23. Kobayashi S, Tadokoro H, Wakida Y, et al. Coronary venous retroinfusion of deferoxamine reduces infarct size in pigs. J Am Coll Cardiol 1991; 18:621–627.

24. Otsu F, Carew TE, Maroka PR. Myocardial concentration and antiarrhythmic effect of lidocaine via coronary veins. J Am Coll Cardiol 1985; 5:467A.

25. Karagueuzian HS, Ohta M, Drury JK, et al. Coronary venous retroperfusion of procainamide: a new approach for the management of spontaneous and inducible sustained ventricular tachycardia during myocardial infarction. J Am Coll Cardiol 1986; 7:551–563.

26. Hatori N, Miyazaki A, Tadokoro H, et al. Beneficial effects of coronary venous retroinfusion of superoxide dismutase and catalase on reperfusion arrhythmias, myocardial function, and infarct size in dogs. J Cardiovasc Pharmacol 1989; 14:396–404.

27. Farcot JC, Meerbaum S, Lang TW, et al. Synchronized retroperfusion of

coronary veins for circulatory support of jeopardized ischemic myocardium. Am J Cardiol 1978; 21:1191–1201.

28. Yamazaki S, Drury JK, Meerbaum S, Corday E. Synchronized coronary venous retroperfusion: prompt improvement of left ventricular function in experimental myocardial ischemia. J Am Coll Cardiol 1985; 5:655–663.

29. Gore JM, Weiner BH, Sloan KM, Cuenoud HF. The safety of synchronized coronary sinus retroperfusion (SCSR) for up to 24 hours. Chest 1985; 88:73–80.

30. Gore JM, Weiner BH, Benotti JR, et al. Preliminary experience with synchronized coronary sinus retroperfusion in humans. Circulation 1986; 74:381–388.

31. Barnett CR, Touchon CT. Use of coronary venous retroperfusion in acute myocardial ischemia. Cardiovasc Rev Rep 1990; 10:64–65.

32. Weiner BH, Gore JM, Sloan KM, et al. Synchronized coronary sinus retroperfusion during LAD angioplasty. J Am Coll Cardiol 1986; 7:64A.

33. Constantini C, Sampaolesi A, Pieroni M, et al. Coronary venous retroperfusion support during high risk coronary angioplasty in patients with acute ischemic syndromes. J Am Coll Cardiol 1989; II–625A.

34. Berland J, Farcot JC, Barrier A, Dellac A, Gamra H, Letac B. Coronary venous synchronized retroperfusion during percutaneous transluminal angioplasty of left anterior descending coronary artery. Circulation 1990; 81:35–42.

35. Kar S, Jacobs AR, Faxon DP. Synchronized coronary venous retroperfusion during coronary angioplasty. In: Shawe F, ed. Supported Complex and High Risk Coronary Angioplasty. Boston: Kluwer Academic Publishers. 1991; pp 215–230.

36. Schopf G, Mohl W, Schuster M, Mullen M. Effects of PICSO on purine nucleotides in ischemic canine and reperfused human hearts. In: Mohl W, Wolner E, Glogar D, eds. The Coronary Sinus. Steinkopff Verlag, Darmstadt: Springer-Verlag. 1984; pp 508–515.

37. Lazar HL, Khoury T, Rivers S. Improved distribution of cardioplegia with pressure controlled intermittent coronary sinus occlusion. Ann Thorac Surg 1988; 46:202–207.

38. Lazar HL, Rajai A, Roberts AJ. Reversal of reperfusion injury following ischemic arrest with pressure-controlled intermittent coronary sinus occlusion. J Thorac Cardiovasc Surg 1988; 95:637–642.

39. Lazar HL, Haan C, Bernard S, Rivers S, Shemin RJ. Reduction of infarct size following revascularization of an acute coronary occlusion with pressure-controlled intermittent occlusion (PICSO). J Mol Cell Cardiol 1990; 22:515.

40. Mohl W, Pruzengruber C, Moser M, et al. Effects of pressure controlled intermittent coronary sinus occlusion on regional ischemic myocardial function. J Am Coll Cardiol 1985; 5:939–943.

41. Guerci AD, Diuffo AA, DiPaula AF, Weisfeldt ML. Intermittent coronary sinus occlusion in dogs: reduction of infarct size 10 days after reperfusion. J Am Coll Cardiol 1987; 9:1075–1081.

42. Jacobs AK, Faxon DP, Coats WD, Vogel WM, Ryan TJ. Coronary sinus

occlusion: effect on ischemic left ventricular dysfunction and reactive hyperemia. Am Heart J 1991; 121:442–449.

43. Mohl W, Simon P, Neumann F, Schreiner W, Punzengruber C. Clinical evaluation of pressure-controlled intermittent coronary sinus occlusion: randomized trial during coronary artery surgery. Ann Thorac Surg 1988; 46:192–201.

44. Lincoff AM, Popma JJ, Ellis SG, Vogel RA, Topol EJ. Percutaneous support devices for high risk or complicated coronary angioplasty. J Am Coll Cardiol 1991; 17:770–780.

45. Faxon DP, Jacobs AK. Coronary sinus retroperfusion and intermittent occlusion. In: Topal J, ed. Acute Coronary Intervention. New York: Alan R. Liss. 1988; pp 255–269.

Chapter 4

The Current Role of Percutaneous Transluminal Coronary Angioplasty for Acute Coronary Ischemic Syndromes

Jeffrey N. Berman and David P. Faxon

Introduction

Unstable angina and myocardial infarction, the acute coronary syndromes, are caused by an abrupt reduction in myocardial oxygen supply. This is in contrast to stable angina pectoris in which symptoms of ischemia are caused by an excess in myocardial oxygen demand that outstrips the supply provided by a stenosed coronary artery. Three mechanisms are felt to cause the abrupt reduction in oxygen supply: plaque disruption, thrombus formation, and vasoconstriction.[1] These three mechanisms can occur in varying degrees, which results in a continuum of the severity of the resultant clinical

Lazar HL (editor): *Current Therapy for Acute Coronary Ischemia,* © Futura Publishing Co., Inc., Mount Kisco, NY, 1993.

syndrome. In unstable angina, the plaque disruption may be relatively minor and the thrombus may be labile and not completely occlusive. This may result in an accelerating pattern of angina or rest symptoms, but myocardial necrosis does not occur. In acute Q-wave myocardial infarction, total coronary occlusion frequently is found.[2] This may result from a more severe plaque rupture with a subsequent fixed thrombus. Non–Q-wave myocardial infarction is intermediate in severity between unstable angina and Q-wave myocardial infarction. The ischemia is severe enough in non–Q-wave myocardial infarction to cause myocardial necrosis, but generally not to the same extent as is found in Q-wave myocardial infarction. Total coronary occlusion is found infrequently early in the course of non–Q-wave myocardial infarction,[3] and when present, collateral vessels frequently are visible (Fig. 1).

The improved understanding of the pathogenesis of the acute coronary syndromes has resulted in specifically targeted therapy. Nitrates and calcium blockers help prevent vasoconstriction. Aspirin and heparin exert antiplatelet and antithrombotic effects. Thrombolytic therapy and percutaneous transluminal coronary angioplasty (PTCA) represent the most profound changes in therapy for the acute coronary syndromes that have occurred in the recent past.

The role of PTCA in both unstable angina and myocardial infarction is discussed in this chapter. Despite the fact that unstable angina, non–Q-wave myocardial infarction, and Q-wave myocardial infarction are felt to represent a continuum, there are important differences between these syndromes that result in differences in the use of PTCA. Most notably is the role of thrombolytic therapy in their respective treatments. DeWood et al. showed in 1980 that acute myocardial infarction (AMI) is caused most commonly by acute thrombosis and total occlusion of a coronary artery.[2] This demonstration led rapidly to trials of intracoronary and, subsequently, intravenous thrombolytic therapy. A number of very large, well designed, randomized trials have proven that thrombolytic therapy reduces mortality in AMI that presents with ST segment elevation.[4–7] A mortality benefit has not been found, however, in patients with ST depression and myocardial infarction,[6] nor in patients with unstable angina,[4] although large scale trials are still ongoing (e.g., TIMI II and IV). Thus, despite the similar pathogenetic mechanisms in the acute coronary syndromes, to date, thrombolysis has been found to be of benefit only in AMI accompanied by ST

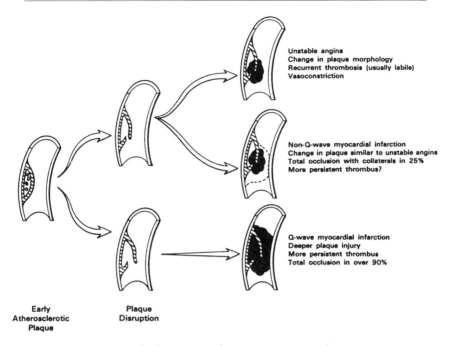

Unstable angina
Change in plaque morphology
Recurrent thrombosis (usually labile)
Vasoconstriction

Non-Q-wave myocardial infarction
Change in plaque similar to unstable angina
Total occlusion with collaterals in 25%
More persistent thrombus?

Q-wave myocardial infarction
Deeper plaque injury
More persistent thrombus
Total occlusion in over 90%

Early
Atherosclerotic
Plaque

Plaque
Disruption

Figure 1: Pathogenesis of acute coronary syndromes.

elevation. This is of importance in the discussion that follows, since PTCA for AMI must be considered in relation to thrombolytic therapy.

PTCA was first performed in a human coronary artery by Gruntzig et al. in 1977.[8] This therapy was first used for the treatment of patients with stable angina pectoris. Within a few years, however, it was used increasingly in patients with unstable angina and with AMI. The necessity of catheterization for the administration of intracoronary thrombolytic therapy made acute PTCA a logical step in AMI. Although thrombolysis currently is considered first-line therapy for AMI in most centers, there are a number of centers in which PTCA is the primary intervention, and the reported results are impressive. With improvements in equipment and adjunctive therapy, the success rate for PTCA in patients with acute coronary syndromes is high and the complication rates are relatively low. The utilization of PTCA must be viewed in the context of other available therapies, including thrombolysis and coronary artery bypass grafting (CABG), which have similarly been shown to be highly effective in the appropriate settings. Unfortunately, at present there is a paucity of data directly comparing these different therapies, although a number of studies are ongoing.

PTCA in Unstable Angina

PTCA has become a frequently utilized therapy in the management of patients with unstable angina. Although angioplasty originally was conceived as management for chronic stable angina, in the 1985–1986 National Heart Lung and Blood Institute Registry, 49% of new patients undergoing PTCA were diagnosed as having unstable angina.[9] Concerns over safety of the procedure in unstable patients were resolved in several studies in the early 1980s.[10,11] Understanding the role of thrombus in abrupt closure and the now universal usage of aspirin and heparin has resulted in decreases in the rate of complications to a level that is almost as low as the complications of PTCA in stable patients. Improvements in techniques and equipment have resulted in a very high success rate.

Efficacy of PTCA in Unstable Angina

A number of recent series of PTCA in patients with unstable angina have been published. All are series of consecutive patients who have had rest pain accompanied by electrocardiogram (ECG) changes, including a substantial number of patients who are refractory to medical therapy. The recently published series with more than 100 patients is shown in Table 1. Success is categorized as either angiographic or clinical. Angiographic success is defined as the reduction of the stenosis by more than 20% with a residual stenosis of less than 50%. Clinical success is defined as angiographic success without the occurrence of death, myocardial infarction, or emergency coronary artery bypass surgery. In general, angiographic success is 5% to 10% greater than clinical success. The initial clinical success rates in these studies vary from 84% to 94%.[12–16] Analysis of the causes of failure in one study[12] indicate that approximately half of the failures resulted from inability to cross totally occluded stenoses. The other half of the failures (5% of patients in this study) were due to abrupt vessel closure, which necessitated emergency coronary artery bypass surgery.

The long-term results also have been good (Table 2). In the study

Table 1

PTCA in Unstable Angina: Success and Complications

Study	No. of Pts	Clinical Success (%)	In-Hospital Mortality (%)	MI (%)	EMCABG (%)
deFeyter et al.[12]	200	90	0.5	8.0	9.0
Myler et al.[13]	807	84	0.2	3.6	5.1
Bentivoglio et al.[15]	952	84	1.3	3.3	4.4
Plokker et al.[14]	469	88	1.0	4.9	6.0
Suryapranata et al.[16]	200	90	0.5	3.0	3.0

Pts = patients; MI = myocardial infarction; EMCABG = emergency coronary artery bypass surgery; success = all lesions dilated with a >20% change, and a residual stenosis <50% without in-hospital mortality, MI, or emergency CABG.

Table 2

PTCA in Unstable Angina: Long-Term Results

Study	No. of Pts	F/U (mos)	Death (%)	MI (%)	CABG (%)	rePTCA (%)	Class 1 or 2 (%)	ASX (%)
deFeyter et al.[12]	200	24	3	12	15	11.5	95	74
Myler et al.[13]	807	37	3.2	8.4	11.7	31.2	—	—
Bentivoglio et al.[15]	952	24	5	9	15	22	89	71

Pts = patients; F/U = follow-up; MI = myocardial infarction; CABG = coronary artery bypass grafting; rePTCA = second percutaneous transluminal coronary angioplasty; class = Canadian Heart Association class of angina; ASX = asymptomatic.

of deFeyter et al.,[12] complete 2-year follow-up data was obtained in all patients, including those in whom the PTCA was unsuccessful. The 2-year incidences of mortality, nonfatal myocardial infarction and CABG were 3%, 12%, and 15%, respectively. This includes the periprocedural complications. Additionally, 12% of patients underwent repeat PTCA. The angiographic restenosis rate was 32%. At 2 years, 82% of the patients who had undergone PTCA were asymptomatic. This includes those who had subsequent CABG or PTCA.

Plokker et al. reported 5-year actuarial results on the 411 of 469 patients who had a successful angioplasty. The survival rate was 94%, and 79% were free of events (recurrent angina, myocardial infarction, repeat PTCA, CABG, or death).[14] In this latter study, all patients treated with PTCA had unstable angina refractory to medical therapy.

Complications of PTCA in Unstable Angina

Early concern over the potential risks of PTCA in patients with unstable angina prompted a number of studies. Faxon and co-workers compared patients with stable angina (SAP) with patients with unstable angina (UAP) who underwent PTCA in the NHLBI registry between September 1979 and October 1981.[11] The success rates were similar in the two groups (63% in UAP vs. 61% in SAP). The low success rates in this study reflect the relatively crude equipment used in the early days of PTCA. The in-hospital mortality was low in both groups (0.9% in UAP vs. 0.4% in SAP) and the rate of in-hospital myocardial infarction also was similar (9.5% in UAP vs. 8.0% in SAP). These results also were comparable to those obtained with bypass surgery in patients with unstable angina who underwent single-vessel CABG in the CASS registry. In these patients, the mortality was 0.9% and the rate of myocardial infarction was 7.0%. It should be pointed out that these results were obtained despite the fact that 29% of the patients undergoing PTCA for unstable angina had bypass surgery because of an unsuccessful procedure, again a reflection of the techniques and equipment of the early days of PTCA.

The complication rate of PTCA has improved dramatically in recent years so that the rate of emergency CABG has decreased from 29% in the NHLBI registry study[11] to rates of 2.6% to 9.0% in more recent studies.[12–16] Despite these improvements, the incidence of abrupt closure and subsequent myocardial infarction or need for CABG remains higher in patients with unstable angina than in those with stable angina. In a retrospective review of 1423 consecutive patients undergoing PTCA, deFeyter and co-workers found that abrupt vessel closure occurred in 104 patients (7.3%).[17] Abrupt closure was defined as clinical or ECG evidence of myocardial ischemia and a complete or critical reduction in coronary flow in the vessel previously dilated, leading to either emergency repeat PTCA, emergency bypass surgery, or myocardial infarction during or after PTCA. Most of these patients were treated with immediate redilation and 42 of the patients had successful procedures. In 58 patients (56% of those with abrupt closure), a major complication (death, myocardial infarction, or emergency surgery) resulted with a mortality rate of 6% of the patients who had abrupt closure. On multivariate analysis, unstable angina was found to be one of the three independent predictive variables, the others being multivessel disease and complex lesions. In this study, 63% of the patients who had acute coronary artery occlusion had unstable angina versus 34% of patients in the comparison group without abrupt closure.[17] Thus, although PTCA in patients with unstable angina has been found to have an acceptably low complication rate, there is a higher risk of abrupt vessel closure in this group.

Coronary Artery Thrombus in Unstable Angina

Coronary artery thrombus is most likely the reason for the increased risk of abrupt closure. Thrombus is felt to be part of the pathogenesis of unstable angina, although the detection rate of thrombus on angiography in patients with unstable angina has ranged from 35% to 85% in various studies.[18-20] This variable presence of thrombus may be explained by different definitions of thrombus on angiography, different subgroups of patients with unstable angina, differences in the timing of angiography, and the inherent insensitivity of angiography in the detection of thrombus. An angioscopic study reported thrombus in 7 of 10 patients with unstable angina and in all 7 patients with angina at rest. Only one of the seven thrombi was detected on angiography.[21] In another angioscopic study involving 15 consecutive patients with rest angina, intracoronary thrombus was identified in 14 of the patients.[22]

Several studies have demonstrated that thrombus is a potent risk factor for abrupt closure. Mabin et al. found that acute vessel closure occurred in 11 of 15 patients (73%) who had thrombus identified on angiography compared to an 8% risk of abrupt closure in the 223 patients who did not have thrombus.[23] This dramatic incidence of abrupt closure has been reduced by the use of periprocedure heparin. After adding heparin for 24 hours after the procedure, the same group that reported the 73% abrupt closure rate found that only 8 of 34 (24%) patients with intracoronary thrombus on angiography had abrupt closure.[24] Pretreatment with heparin may further reduce the risk. Pow and associates showed that pretreatment with heparin for 3 days reduced the abrupt closure rate from 9% to 0%.[25] Three other studies have documented similar reductions.[26–28]

"Culprit Lesion" PTCA

Although many patients with unstable angina have multivessel coronary artery disease, a single lesion, the "culprit lesion," often is responsible for the patient's symptoms. This concept of the culprit lesion was introduced by Wohlgelernter and colleagues, who reported on 27 patients with multivessel disease and unstable angina refractory to medical therapy.[29] The lesion responsible for the patients' symptoms was identified angiographically (stenosis greater than 75% with irregular borders or an intraluminal filling defect consistent with thrombus, or a 99% stenosis with delayed flow). In 78% of the cases, spontaneous ECG changes occurred in the distribution of the culprit. PTCA of the culprit lesion was successful in 89% (24/27) without complications. The remaining three patients underwent uncomplicated CABG within 24 hours. During 26 months of follow-up, only 17% of the patients had recurrent angina. Subsequent studies in patients with multivessel disease have confirmed that culprit lesion PTCA in appropriate patients is a successful strategy with a high primary success rate and a good long-term outcome. In the study of deFeyter and co-workers cited earlier,[12] 65 patients had multivessel disease and underwent culprit lesion angioplasty. The success rate was 91% and there was a 9% complication rate. They did report a significantly higher rate of persistent or recurrent angina and more frequent exercise-induced ischemia than in the group of patients with single-vessel disease. In the 59 patients who had successful culprit lesion PTCA, 23 of 59 (39%) patients had recurrent angina at 1 year. The incidence of death and myocardial infarction at 1 year in this group was 2 of 59 (3%).

This relatively high rate of recurrent angina points out one of the major concerns in the use of angioplasty in patients with multivessel disease: the potential advantage of complete revascularization. The surgical literature indicated that incomplete revascularization resulted in a less favorable long-term survival rate and a higher incidence of subsequent symptoms.[30] It is impossible to apply these data to angioplasty, because noninvasive testing has enabled therapy to be directed to the culprit vessel. Seven studies have examined the influence of incomplete revascularization on long-term outcome (Table 3).[31-37] Three showed a greater need for a second revascularization in the incompletely revascularized group, while the other four showed no significant difference. Faxon and colleagues[37] demonstrated that functional significance is perhaps the most important factor in determining immediate and long-term outcome. Patients with incomplete revascularization were divided retrospectively into an incompletely but adequately revascularized group and an incompletely and inadequately revascularized group. The incompletely and inadequately revascularized patients had lesions that could be bypassed in vessels serving viable myocardium remaining after angioplasty, whereas adequately revascularized patients had lesions that served infarcted territory or that were considered not to be possible to bypass. When these two groups were compared, the incompletely and inadequately revascularized group had a higher incidence of bypass surgery during follow-up over a 1-year period. Incompletely but adequately revascularized patients had an outcome that was similar to that of the completely revascularized patients with multivessel disease. The relative roles of

Table 3

Completeness of Revascularization and Outcome

Study	No. of Pts	FU (yr)	CABG (%)		rePTCA (%)		ASX (%)	
			C	IC	C	IC	C	IC
Mabin et al.[31]	66	1.0	13.0	23.0*	6	6	87	63
Vandormael et al.[32]	117	0.5	3.0	16.0*	3	16	63	63
Reeder et al.[33]	286	2.0	33.0	35.0	20	8	69	67
Faxon et al.[37]	139	1.0	15.0	18.0	30	19	78	67
Deligonul et al.[35]	397	2.0	7.0	16.0*	14	13	80	78
Thomas et al.[36]	92	0.5	1.0	5.0	11	12	63	63
Bourassa et al.[34]	1553	1.0	1.5	10.7	19	17	—	—

*$p < 0.005$.
Pts = patients; C = complete; IC = incomplete; FU = follow-up; CABG = coronary artery bypass grafting; rePTCA = second percutaneous transluminal coronary angioplasty; ASX = asymptomatic.
Reprinted with permission of Faxon.[40]

angioplasty and bypass surgery in patients with unstable angina and multivessel disease remains a controversial question. The Bypass Angioplasty Revascularization Investigation, which randomized 1800 patients with multivessel disease, was designed to address these issues. Several smaller trials also are ongoing.

Restenosis

Restenosis continues to be a major unsolved problem in the use of PTCA. In the studies discussed in the previous sections, restenosis rates varied from 28% to 37% with angiographic follow-up in 54% to 79% of patients.[12,13,15,16] In a recent meta-analysis, unstable angina was found to be a risk factor for restenosis with a relative risk 1.2 to 1.7 times higher in patients with unstable angina than for patients with stable symptoms.[38] As yet, there is no method by which one can identify a patient who is at very high risk for restenosis. A recent study reported that in patients with unstable angina, hyperventilation-induced abnormal coronary vasoconstriction may be a useful discriminator.[39] Abnormal vasoconstriction was observed in 48 patients, and 29 of these patients (73%) had restenosis. In contrast, the restenosis rate in the 58 patients with a normal response was only 25%. The usefulness of this marker for restenosis needs further testing, but markers for restenosis risk would be of great benefit.

Selection of Patients

The decision to perform PTCA in unstable angina is based on a number of factors both clinical and angiographic. Careful consideration of the risks and benefits of PTCA in the individual patient must be attempted along with a consideration of the alternatives, bypass surgery and medical therapy. Clinical factors influencing success and complications of angioplasty include age greater than 70 [relative risk (RR) = 2.0], female gender (RR = 3.1), congestive heart failure (RR = 5), and the extent of coronary artery disease (for three-vessel, RR = 3.0).[40]

The ACC/AHA combined task force has published guidelines for the selection of patients for coronary angioplasty.[41] In addition to clinical indications, angiographic criteria have been identified in attempts to predict the likelihood of success as well as the risk of complications. The angiographic criteria divide coronary lesions into three categories: types A, B, and C.

Type A lesions are lesions that are associated with a high success rate and low complication rate. Angiographic characteristics in this group include single, discrete, accessible, nonangulated lesions that are not totally occluded and are concentric. These characteristics were considered ideal for angioplasty when it was first introduced and were adopted by the initial NHLBI PTCA registry. In this setting, angiographic success is expected to be more than 85%, with an abrupt closure rate of less than 1%.

Type B lesions are associated with a lower success rate but still could be dilated if clinically justified. Characteristics of this type of lesion include eccentric or calcified lesions, lesions on bends of less than 90° but greater than 45°, lesions distal to tortuous proximal vessels, bifurcation lesions, totally occluded vessels of less than 3 months' duration, and lesions with evidence of thrombus.

Type C lesions are lesions associated with a poor success or high complication rate. Examples include chronic total occlusions, of greater than 3 months' duration, diffuse disease greater than 2 cm in length, excessive tortuousity, and lesion angulation. In general, angioplasty of these lesions is not recommended.

Ellis and co-workers prospectively evaluated these criteria and substantiated their clinical utility.[42] They also suggested that improved discrimination could be obtained in type B lesions when they were categorized into type B1 and B2, whereas the presence of one type B characteristic would be categorized as B1 and two or more as B2. In addition, the current improvement in equipment and introduction of new interventional devices has further improved the success in unfavorable anatomy such that many type B lesions have success comparable to type A lesions.

Although the guidelines are helpful in the selection of patients, they are operator-dependent and are influenced by the clinical situation. In addition, other issues, particularly incomplete revascularization, were not considered in this classification. Patients who are not ideal candidates for angioplasty often are poor surgical candidates as well, and they represent a group that is at high risk on medical therapy. Colle and Delarche studied a group of patients with unstable angina that included a substantial number of patients who had been refused for bypass surgery who underwent angioplasty for unstable angina.[67] Their population of 277 patients included 36.4% with occluded vessels, 24.9% with three-vessel disease, 5.7% in whom the target lesion was in the only patent vessel, and 3.6% who were in cardiogenic shock. Overall they had an 85% success rate, a 6.8% incidence of AMI, and a mortality of 3.2%. Risk factors for failure, infarction, and mortality included emergency procedure, multivessel disease, and prior complete obstructions. All but one of the deaths in this study occurred in patients who had at least one occluded vessel and five of the nine deaths occurred in patients in whom the single patent vessel was dilated. The mortality in this group was 33%. The mortality in patients with cardiogenic shock was 33% also. These data point out the importance of patient selection in the success and complication rates. It may be appropriate in certain clinical settings to accept high-risk patients when there are no other good alternatives.

Conclusions

Coronary angioplasty has assumed an important role in the management of patients with unstable angina, which currently is the most common clinical indication for PTCA. It can be performed safely with acceptable risks of myocardial infarction and emergency coronary bypass, although these risks are higher than in patients with stable angina. In patients with refractory symptoms and single-vessel disease, PTCA is the procedure of choice. Patients with unstable angina refractory to medical therapy and multivessel disease who have a clearly identifiable culprit lesion or in whom adequate revascularization is possible may benefit from PTCA, although the relative merits of PTCA and bypass surgery remain to be determined. Currently, patients with multivessel disease who have no clear culprit lesion or who would be revascularized inadequately by PTCA should undergo CABG. In patients with unstable angina who stabilize on medical therapy, PTCA is an appealing option, although the long-term benefits of PTCA over medical therapy in this subgroup have not been proven. Ongoing clinical trials are addressing these issues.

PTCA in Acute Myocardial Infarction

The use of PTCA in AMI is inextricably connected to the use of thrombolytic therapy. In the early 1980s, intracoronary streptokinase (SK) was the first thrombolytic regimen utilized. It was recognized that PTCA could be performed in patients receiving intracoronary therapy, and the initial results were excellent. O'Neill and colleagues completed a randomized trial that showed that PTCA had some advantages over intracoronary thrombolysis.[43] In this study, the success rates of the two approaches were similar (83% for PTCA vs. 85% for SK), but patients treated with PTCA had less severe residual stenoses and a greater improvement in left ventricular function. By the time of publication of this trial, however, it was clear that intravenous thrombolytic therapy had significant advantages over the intracoronary route, and several large studies confirmed the lifesaving advantages of thrombolysis. Patients no longer were required to be in the catheterization laboratory for the administration of thrombolysis and it became a therapy that could be administered in the community hospital. In several centers, however, direct (i.e., as primary therapy instead of thrombolysis) angioplasty continued to be utilized and its role remains controversial. It became apparent that the rate of recurrent angina and reinfarction after thrombolysis was approximately 20%.[44] Also, it was known that most patients were left with significant (i.e., >70%) stenoses after successful thrombolysis.[45] Furthermore, in a number of patients, thrombolysis is unsuccessful. Angioplasty has been utilized in various strategies in attempts to address these problems.

The use of angioplasty in AMI can be divided into five approaches: a) direct PTCA, i.e., PTCA used as primary therapy for AMI without thrombolysis, b) immediate PTCA, i.e., PTCA performed within hours of PTCA as a routine adjunct to open residual stenoses, c) rescue PTCA, i.e., PTCA performed immediately after thrombolysis in those who have not had reperfusion, d) deferred PTCA, i.e., PTCA performed routinely several days after thrombolysis to dilate residual stenoses, and e) elective PTCA, i.e., PTCA utilized only as needed to treat recurrent or provocable ischemia.[44] Much has been learned about these various strategies through published series and most importantly in randomized trials. It is of interest that in some of these studies, the anticipated "logical" result was disproven.

Direct Coronary Angioplasty

The current status of direct coronary angioplasty for AMI is best illustrated by the opposing views taken in two editorials. In an editorial entitled "Because We Can, Should We?," Brundage concludes that "conservative medical management of single vessel disease is recommended," and he states that "at this juncture it is even difficult to recommend a randomized controlled study of the two forms of therapy."[46] In contrast, Meier in an editorial entitled "Balloon Angioplasty for Acute Myocardial Infarction: Was It Buried Alive?" states that angioplasty is "preferable in cases of large infarctions and in those having access to a well-staffed angioplasty laboratory within 30 minutes." He commends the practitioners of direct angioplasty "for persevering in a stressful and time-consuming mode of therapy" and he accuses those who abandoned angioplasty of a lack of dedication and lethargy.[47] The truth, of course, lies somewhere in between these two views. The ongoing Primary Angioplasty in Myocardial Infarction study, a large randomized trial of thrombolysis and infarct PTCA, hopefully will resolve the issue and define more clearly the role of direct angioplasty. The data accumulated thus far, summarized in the following paragraphs, indicate that this form of therapy is highly effective with high success rates and a low short- and long-term morbidity and mortality, similar to the claims that can be made for intravenous thrombolysis.

There are some advantages of direct angioplasty over thrombolytic therapy, including a) the avoidance of thrombolytics and the attendant risk of bleeding complications, plaque hemorrhage, and intramyocardial hemorrhage, b) a higher initial patency rate, and c) possible improvement in left ventricular function, coronary blood flow, and a reduction of recurrent ischemic events. There are some problems as well. There appear to be more arrhythmias with the sudden reperfusion achieved with angioplasty than with the more gradual reperfusion of thrombolysis.[48] There also is a significant incidence of reocclusion of the dilated vessel before hospital discharge. There are logistic and cost issues as well. Only 12% of hospitals in the United States have the facilities for angioplasty.[49] Direct angioplasty requires an additional commitment of resources to maintain rapid response when the situation arises. Thrombolytic therapy, which can be administered in the community hospital and even in the prehospital setting, has advantages in terms of widespread applicability.

Much of the data on direct angioplasty in AMI comes from Geoffrey Hartzler and co-workers at the Mid America Heart Institute. O'Keefe et al. summarized their 8-year experience during which 500 patients were treated, including 85 who were greater than 70 years of age, 39 who were in cardiogenic shock, and 49 with prior CABG.[50] Successful PTCA of the infarct artery was achieved in 94%

of patients. Overall mortality was 7.2% and they point out that in the 222 patients who were eligible for the contemporaneous thrombolytic trials, the mortality was 1.8%. Vascular complications occurred in 3% of patients and urgent bypass surgery was required in 2%. There were no strokes and no cardiac ruptures. The reocclusion rate before discharge was 15%. Actuarial survival at 1 year was 95% and at 5 years, 84%. The subsets of patients with single-vessel disease and multivessel disease were analyzed separately. In the 215 patients with single-vessel disease, the success rate was 99%, with one urgent bypass and no procedure-related deaths.[51] The in-hospital mortality was 1%. Eight patients (4%) had recurrent ischemia. Long-term follow-up (mean 34 months), revealed an actuarial event-free survival of 84% at 3 years, with 9 nonfatal myocardial infarctions, 11 patients undergoing coronary artery bypass surgery, and 17 deaths, 5 of which were noncardiac. Repeat angioplasty was required in 52 patients (24%).

The 285 patients with multivessel disease represented a sicker population with an anterior myocardial infarction in 123 (43%), cardiogenic shock in 33 (12%), and age greater than 70 in 59 (21%).[52] Two-vessel disease was present in 163 patients (57%) and three-vessel disease in 122 (43%). Angioplasty of the infarct-related artery was successful in 256 patients (90%), with a slightly higher success rate in those with two-vessel disease than the ones with three-vessel disease. The in-hospital mortality was 12% (33 patients), 45% in the patients in cardiogenic shock, and 7% in those without shock. There were no strokes and no myocardial rupture. Reocclusion of the infarct-related artery during hospitalization occurred in 33 patients (18%). Follow-up at a mean of 35 months found 31 deaths. The actuarial 1- and 3-year event-free survival rates were 80% and 71% overall, 88% and 82% in those with two-vessel disease, and 68% and 55% in those with three-vessel disease. Repeat angioplasty was performed in 59 patients (23%).

To address the question of safety, Kahn and co-workers described the results in 250 patients treated between 1987 and 1989.[53] Forty-nine patients were at least 70 years of age (20%), multivessel disease was present in 142 patients (57%), and cardiogenic shock was present in 16 patients (6%). Major events (defined as cardioversion, cardiopulmonary resuscitation, dopamine or intra-aortic balloon pump for hypotension, and urgent surgery) occurred in 22 patients, all 16 patients with cardiogenic shock and only 6 of the 234 patients without shock. There was one cath lab death, in a patient with left anterior descending coronary artery occlusion and shock, and 14 in-hospital deaths (6.4%). The procedural success rate was 96%. The survival in patients not in cardiogenic shock was 97.5%.

Thus, Hartzler and his co-workers have demonstrated the feasibility, the high success rate, and the relative safety of direct angioplasty. They have not, however, demonstrated its superiority or even equivalence to thrombolytic therapy as an initial strategy. This question remains to be answered in a randomized trial. The role of direct angioplasty is clearer in certain patient subgroups including those in whom thrombolytic therapy is contraindicated and patients with cardiogenic shock.

Direct PTCA in Noncandidates for Thrombolysis

Thrombolytic therapy has been clearly documented to reduce mortality in AMI, yet it has been shown in numerous studies that only about 33% of patients presenting with a myocardial infarction are eligible for this therapy. Cragg and co-workers reported that of 1471 patients presenting with a myocardial infarction at a large community-based hospital, 1144 patients did not receive reperfusion therapy because of contraindications, which included age greater than 76, stroke or bleeding risk, delayed presentation, ineligible ECG, and miscellaneous exclusions.[54] The mortality rate among the ineligible patients was fivefold higher (19%) than among the patients who received thrombolysis according to a protocol (4%). Continuing investigation of the exclusions for thrombolysis may expand the use of these agents; however, probably fewer than 50% of patients will be eligible for thrombolysis. When one considers the relatively high mortality in patients not eligible for thrombolysis, these patients may derive great benefit from direct angioplasty.

Brodie and co-workers examined the use of direct angioplasty in patients who were candidates and noncandidates for thrombolysis.[55] The noncandidates were older (mean age 65 vs. 57), were more often female (39% vs. 24%), had a lower ejection fraction on presentation (48% vs. 54%), had more multivessel disease (62% vs. 50%), and had a longer time to reperfusion (6.4 vs. 3.2 hr). Twenty-two percent of the noncandidates were in cardiogenic shock on presentation. The success rates were similar (88% vs. 92%), but the in-hospital mortality was significantly higher in the noncandidates (24% vs. 3.9%). These data confirm the high mortality in noncandidates of thrombolytic therapy. It is difficult to determine how great an impact angioplasty would make in this group, but clearly there are some patients who would benefit.

Direct PTCA in Patients with Cardiogenic Shock

Cardiogenic shock in the setting of AMI carries with it a very high mortality that has changed little in the past 15 years. Goldberg and co-workers in a recent study reported that the incidence of cardiogenic shock had remained constant at about 7.5%, as has the mortality associated with it.[56] In 1975, the mortality in this study was 74%, and in 1988, it was 82%. Thrombolytic therapy has not been shown to be effective in improving survival in this group of patients,[4,57] and it has been suggested that thrombolytic therapy may be more useful in preventing the development of shock rather than in reversing it once shock has occurred. Bates and Topol suggest that the low output state associated with cardiogenic shock may result in less effective thrombolysis.[58]

There have been numerous studies of direct PTCA in the management of patients with myocardial infarction shock. Bates and Topol summarized the results of 14 studies published between 1985 and 1991. There were 386 patients treated in these studies. The reperfusion rate was 73% and the overall mortality was 44%. Of the 243 patients with successful PTCA, the mortality rate was 30% compared to an 80% mortality in the PTCA failures.[58] A recent multicenter trial yielded similar results and showed that the survival benefit of PTCA was maintained at long-term follow-up.[59] Thus, a substantial body of data suggests that emergent PTCA may be very helpful in patients with AMI and cardiogenic shock.

Immediate Angioplasty

In the immediate angioplasty strategy, PTCA is performed as soon as possible after the administration of thrombolytic therapy. The rationale for this approach is that some patients, approximately 20% to 30%, will have had unsuccessful reperfusion while another 50% will have significant residual stenosis. It was hypothesized that angioplasty in these patients would confer a significant survival benefit. In a pilot study, an improvement in infarct-zone regional wall motion was noted in the patients who underwent PTCA after thrombolysis.[60] Three well designed, relatively large randomized trials were subsequently conducted, and all three yielded surprisingly similar results despite some differences in patient selection, randomization, and PTCA strategy.[61–63] In the European Cooperative Study Group trial, a significantly higher mortality was noted in the patients who underwent immediate angioplasty. In the other studies, a trend toward increased mortality was found. In addition, the patients who underwent emergency angioplasty had a higher transfusion requirement and a higher rate of need for urgent coronary bypass surgery. The results of these three trials are summarized in Figure 2.

There are some data to suggest that the thrombolytic agent used may be important in determining the results of immediate angioplasty. In the three studies described above, tissue plasminogen activator (t-PA) was the thrombolytic agent used. t-PA has been shown to be associated with a high rate of reocclusion. SK has been found to be associated with a reduced reocclusion rate.[64] Despite the fact that improved results may have been obtained with a non–

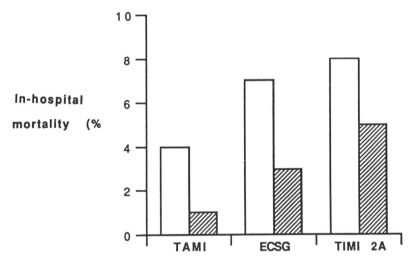

Figure 2: Mortality in the immediate coronary angioplasty trials. The mortality in the patients undergoing immediate PTCA (solid white) was higher than in those treated with deferred or no PTCA (striped bars). Statistical significance was present only in the ECSG trial. TAMI = Thrombolysis and Angioplasty in Myocardial Infarction Study Group; ECSG = European Cooperative Study Group; TIMI 2A = Thrombolysis in Myocardial Infarction Study Group. Data adapted from Topol et al.,[45] Simoons et al.,[63] and the TIMI Research Group.[62]

fibrin-specific agent, the three studies cited above provided rather convincing evidence that immediate angioplasty as a matter of routine is not likely to be a fruitful strategy.

Rescue Angioplasty

Rescue angioplasty is defined as angioplasty after thrombolysis for failed reperfusion. The major problem with this strategy is that there are as yet no noninvasive markers with sufficient specificity and sensitivity to identify reliably those in whom thrombolysis has been unsuccessful. Thus, to perform rescue angioplasty, many patients with successful reperfusion would need to be studied to find those in whom thrombolysis has not been successful. The recently reported TAMI-5 trial provides suggestive evidence that rescue angioplasty may be beneficial.[65] In this study, 575 patients were randomized to either emergency coronary angiography with rescue coronary angioplasty, if necessary, or to routine predischarge cardiac catheterization. The initial patency rate for the infarct-related vessel 90 minutes after thrombolysis was 76% and improved to 96% with the use of rescue PTCA. At the time of discharge the patency rate was 94% in the emergency catheterization group versus 90% in the delayed catheterization group. There was an improvement in regional wall motion among the patients who had undergone PTCA. It is important to note that this study does not provide a true evaluation of rescue angioplasty because the control group did not undergo angiography. The Randomized Evaluation of Salvage Angioplasty with Combined Utilization of Endpoints (RESCUE), which is now in progress, is designed to determine the role of this strategy by randomizing patients with occluded left anterior descending arteries after thrombolysis to either PTCA or medical therapy.

Deferred versus Elective PTCA

In the "deferred angioplasty" strategy, patients are routinely catheterized and undergo PTCA within several days after thrombolysis if there is a residual stenosis. The premise of this approach is that the underlying stenosis must be treated to prevent subsequent events. In the elective approach, patients undergo revascularization only if they demonstrate either spontaneous or induced reversible ischemia. The TIMI II B trial was designed to compare these two strategies.[66] In this study, 3262 patients who had been treated with t-PA were randomized to an invasive strategy consisting of coronary arteriography 18 to 48 hours after the administration of recombinant t-PA (rt-PA) followed by prophylactic PTCA if anatomy was suitable or to a conservative strategy in which patients underwent arteriography and PTCA only if they demonstrated spontaneous or reversible ischemia. In the group assigned to the invasive strategy, 928 of 1636 patients (56.7%) underwent PTCA with a 93.3% success rate. In the conservative group, 262 patients (16.1%) underwent PTCA within 14 days for clinical indications. In the invasive group, 195 patients underwent CABG within 42 days, and 50 patients had this procedure after PTCA. In the conservative group, 170 patients underwent bypass surgery, 21 after PTCA. The patients assigned to the invasive strategy were found to have a slightly higher, but statistically nonsignificant, incidence of death or reinfarction (10.9% vs. 9.7%; Fig. 3). There was no difference in left ventricular ejection

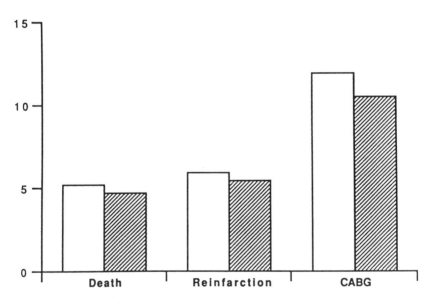

Figure 3: Adverse outcomes in the TIMI II-B trial. Patients were randomized to an invasive strategy (n = 1636, solid white bars) or a conservative strategy (n = 1626, striped bars). There was a slightly higher, but not significant, incidence of death, reinfarction, and coronary artery bypass surgery in the patients randomized to the invasive strategy. There was no difference in left ventricular function. Data adapted from the TIMI Study Group.[56]

fraction. The authors of this study concluded that a strategy of "watchful waiting" after thrombolytic therapy represents the most prudent course.[66]

Conclusions

The use of PTCA in AMI is inextricably linked to the use of thrombolytic therapy. While direct PTCA has been shown to be an effective approach to opening acutely obstructed coronary arteries, there are as yet no randomized clinical trials to support its use over thrombolytic therapy in patients who are candidates for thrombolytic therapy. Noncandidates for thrombolytic therapy may benefit by direct PTCA, but again there are no randomized trials to support this. Direct PTCA may have a role in patients who present in cardiogenic shock in whom thrombolytic therapy has not been found to improve outcome.

After thrombolytic therapy has been given, patients with spontaneous or provocable ischemia are known to be at high risk for reinfarction or infarct extension. These patients form a subgroup with unstable angina and if anatomy is appropriate, they are candidates for revascularization. In single-vessel disease, PTCA is the procedure of choice. In patients with multivessel disease, the same considerations as discussed in the unstable angina patients apply. Culprit lesion angioplasty may be an effective approach. Additionally, in patients who can be completely or adequately revascularized, PTCA is an acceptable option. The final word on multivessel PTCA in patients with unstable angina, including post–myocardial infarction angina, awaits the results of several large ongoing clinical trials. The largest trial, sponsored by the NHLBI, is the Bypass, Angioplasty Revascularization Investigation (BARI) trial. Conducted in 18 clinical centers, it has randomized 1800 patients with multivessel disease to PTCA or CABG. A sizable proportion of these patients have unstable or postinfarction angina. Only when the results of the BARI and other randomized trials are reported will the optimum roles of PTCA and CABG in these patients be determined.

The strategies of rescue angioplasty and routine angioplasty immediately after thrombolysis have not been shown to be advantageous over the conservative approach of catheterization and revascularization only for provocable or spontaneous ischemia.

Summary

Coronary angioplasty has become an important therapeutic technique in patients with acute coronary syndromes. The procedure has been demonstrated to be highly efficacious and relatively safe in appropriately selected patients. There remain important questions regarding the role of angioplasty in comparison to medical therapy and coronary artery bypass surgery, many of which will be answered in ongoing clinical trials.

The technique of angioplasty is constantly being improved. The marked improvement in the success rates in patients with unstable angina in the past 10 years highlights this improvement. New devices including directional coronary atherectomy, rotational atherectomy, stents, and the excimer laser may improve the success or reduce the complications further and may expand the use of angioplasty. Specifically targeted therapies may reduce the complications of abrupt vessel closure and restenosis.

References

1. Fuster V, Badimon L, Badimon JJ, Chesebro JH. The pathogenesis of coronary artery disease and the acute coronary syndromes. N Engl J Med 1992; 326:242–250, 310–318.
2. DeWood MA, Spores J, Notske R, et al. Prevalence of total coronary occlusion during the early hours of transmural myocardial infarction. N Engl J Med 1980; 303:897–902.
3. DeWood MA, Stifter WF, Simpson CS, et al. Coronary arteriographic findings soon after non–Q-wave myocardial infarction. N Engl J Med 1986; 315:417–423.
4. Gruppo Italiano per lo Studio della Streptochinasi nell'Infarcto Miocardico (GISSI). Effectiveness of intravenous thrombolytic treatment in acute myocardial infarction. Lancet 1986; 1:397–401.
5. The AIMS Trial Study Group. Effect of intravenous APSAC on mortality after acute myocardial infarction: preliminary report of a placebo-controlled clinical trial. Lancet 1988; 1:545–549.
6. ISIS-2 Collaborative Group. Randomised trial of intravenous streptokinase, oral aspirin, both, or neither among 17,187 cases of suspected acute myocardial infarction: ISIS-2. Lancet 1988; 2:349–360.
7. Wilcox RG, von der Lippe G, Olsson CG, Jensen G, Skene AM, Hampton JR. Trial of tissue plasminogen activator for mortality reduction in acute myocardial infarction. Anglo-Scandinavian Study of Early Thrombolysis (ASSET). Lancet 1988; 2:525–530.
8. Gruntzig AR, Myler RK, Hanna ES, Turina MI. Transluminal angioplasty of coronary artery stenosis. Circulation 1977; 56:84.

9. Detre K, Holubkov R, Kelsey S. Percutaneous transluminal coronary angioplasty registry: percutaneous transluminal coronary angioplasty in 1985-1986 and 1977-1981. The National Heart Lung and Blood Institute Registry. N Engl J Med 1988; 318:265–270.

10. Williams DO, Riley RS, Singh AK, Gewirtz H, Most AS. Evaluation of the role of coronary angioplasty in patients with unstable angina pectoris. Am Heart J 1981; 102:1–9.

11. Faxon DP, Detre KM, McCabe CH, et al. Role of percutaneous transluminal coronary angioplasty in the treatment of unstable angina: report from the NHLBI PTCA and CASS registries. Am J Cardiol 1984; 53:131C–135C.

12. deFeyter PJ, Suryapranta H, Serruys PW, et al. Coronary angioplasty for unstable angina: immediate and late results in 200 consecutive patients with identification of risk factors for unfavorable early and late outcome. J Am Coll Cardiol 1988; 12:324–333.

13. Myler RK, Shaw RE, Stertzer SH, et al. Unstable angina and coronary angioplasty. Circulation 1990; 82(Suppl II):82–95.

14. Plokker HWT, Ernst SMPG, Bal ET, et al. Percutaneous transluminal coronary angioplasty in patients with unstable angina pectoris refractory to medical therapy: long-term clinical and angiographic results. Cathet Cardiovasc Diagn 1988; 14:15–18.

15. Bentivoglio LG, Holubkov R, Kelsey SF, et al. Short and long term outcome of percutaneous transluminal coronary angioplasty in unstable versus stable angina pectoris: a report of the 1985-1986 NHLBI PTCA registry. Cathet Cardiovasc Diagn 1991; 23:227–238.

16. Suryapranata H, deFeyter PJ, Serruys PW. Coronary angioplasty in patients with unstable angina pectoris: is there a role for thrombolysis. J Am Coll Cardiol 1988; 12:69A–77A.

17. deFeyter PJ, van den Brand M, Jaarman G, Van Domburg R, Werruys PW, Suryapranata H. Acute coronary artery occlusion during and after percutaneous transluminal coronary angioplasty: frequency, prediction, clinical course, management and follow-up. Circulation 1991; 83:927–936.

18. Vetrovec GW, Leinbach RC, Gold HK, Cowley MJ. Intracoronary thrombolysis in syndromes of unstable ischemia: angiographic and clinical results. Am Heart J 1982; 104:946–952.

19. Capone G, Wolf NM, Meyer B, Meister SG. Frequency of intracoronary filling defects by angiography in angina pectoris at rest. Am J Cardiol 1985; 56:403–406.

20. Bresnahan DR, Davis JL, Holmes DR, Smith HC. Angiographic occurrence and clinical correlates of intraluminal coronary artery thrombus: role of unstable angina. J Am Coll Cardiol 1985; 6:285–289.

21. Sherman CT, Litvack F, Grundfest W, et al. Coronary angioscopy in patients with unstable angina pectoris. N Engl J Med 1986; 315:913–919.

22. Mizuno K, Satomura K, Miyamoto A, et al. Angioscopic evaluation of coronary artery thrombi in acute coronary syndromes. N Engl J Med 1992; 326:287–291.

23. Mabin TA, Holmes DR, Smith HC, et al. Intracoronary thrombus: role

in coronary occlusion complicating percutaneous transluminal coronary angioplasty. J Am Coll Cardiol 1985; 5:198–202.

24. Sugrue DD, Holmes DR, Smith HC, et al. Coronary artery thrombus as a risk factor for acute vessel occlusion during percutaneous transluminal coronary angioplasty: improving results. Br Heart J 1986; 56:62–66.

25. Pow TK, Varricchione TR, Jacobs AK, et al. Does heparin alter coronary stenosis in unstable angina? Circulation 1988; 78:II–421.

26. Hettleman BD, Aplin RA, Sullivan PR, Lemal H, O'Connor GT. Three days of heparin pretreatment reduces major complications of coronary angioplasty in patients with unstable angina pectoris. J Am Coll Cardiol 1990; 15:154A.

27. Laskey MAL, Deutsch E, Barnathan E, Laskey WK. Influence of heparin therapy on percutaneous transluminal coronary angioplasty outcome in unstable angina pectoris. Am J Cardiol 1990; 65:1425–1429.

28. Lukas MA, Deutsch E, Jr Hirshfeld JW, Kussmaul WG, Barnathan E, Laskey WK. Influence of heparin therapy on percutaneous transluminal coronary angioplasty outcome in patients with coronary arterial thrombus. Am J Cardiol 1990; 65:179–182.

29. Wohlgelernter D, Cleman M, Highman HA, Zaret BL. Percutaneous transluminal coronary angioplasty of the "culprit lesion" for management of unstable angina pectoris in patients with multivessel coronary artery disease. Am J Cardiol 1986; 58:460–464.

30. Jones EL, Craver JM, Guyton RA. Importance of complete revascularization and performance of bypass operation. J Am Coll Cardiol 1983; 51:7–12.

31. Mabin TA, Holmes DR, Smith HC, et al. Follow up clinical results of inpatients undergoing percutaneous transluminal coronary angioplasty. Circulation 1985; 71:754–760.

32. Vandormael MG, Chaitman BR, Ischinger T, et al. Immediate and short-term benefit of multilesion coronary angioplasty: influence of degree of revascularization. J Am Coll Cardiol 1985; 6:983–991.

33. Reeder GS, Holmes DR, Detre K, et al. Degree of revascularization in patients with multivessel coronary disease: a report from the National Heart, Lung and Blood Institute Percutaneous Transluminal Coronary Angioplasty registry. Circulation 1988; 77:638–644.

34. Bourassa MG, David PR, Costigan, et al. Completeness of revascularization early after coronary angioplasty (PTCA in the NHLBI PTCA Registry). J Am Coll Cardiol 1987; 9:19A.

35. Deligonul U, Vandormael MG, Kern MJ, et al. The therapeutic option for symptomatic patients with two- and three- vessel coronary artery disease. J Am Coll Cardiol 1988; 11:1173–1179.

36. Thomas ES, Most AS, Williams DO. Coronary angioplasty for patients with multivessel coronary artery disease: follow-up clinical studies. Am Heart J 1988; 115:8–13.

37. Faxon DP, Ghalili K, Jacobs AK, et al. The degree of revascularization and outcome after multivessel coronary angioplasty. Am Heart J 1992; 123:854–859.

38. Califf R. Restenosis after coronary angioplasty: an overview. J Am Coll Cardiol 1991; 17:2B–13B.

39. Ardissino D, Barberis P, DeServi S, et al. Abnormal coronary vasoconstriction as a predictor of restenosis after successful coronary angioplasty in patients with unstable angina pectoris. N Engl J Med 1991; 325:1035–1037.
40. Faxon DP. Percutaneous coronary angioplasty in stable and unstable angina. Cardiol Clin 1991; 9:99–113.
41. Ryan TJ, Faxon DP, Gunnar RM, et al. Guidelines for percutaneous transluminal coronary angioplasty: a report of the American College of Cardiology/American Heart Association Task Force on assessment of diagnositic and therapeutic cardiovascular procedures (subcommittee on percutaneous transluminal coronary angioplasty). J Am Coll Cardiol 1988; 12:529–545.
42. Ellis S, Cowley M, Vandormael M, et al. Risk of coronary angioplasty in multivessel disease: improved assessment with modified ACC/AHA score. Circulation 1989; :II–372.
43. O'Neill W, Timmis GC, Bourdillon P, et al. A prospective randomized clinical trial of intracoronary streptokinase versus coronary angioplasty therapy of acute myocardial infarction. N Engl J Med 1986; 314:812–828.
44. Topol EJ. Coronary angioplasty for acute myocardial infarction. Ann Intern Med 1988; 109:970–980.
45. Topol EJ, Holmes DR, Rogers WJ. Coronary angiography after thrombolytic therapy for acute myocardial infarction. Ann Intern Med 1991; 114:885–887.
46. Brundage BH. Because we can, should we? J Am Coll Cardiol 1990; 15:544–545.
47. Meier B. Balloon angioplasty for acute myocardial infarction: was it buried alive? Circulation 1990; 82:2243–2245.
48. Ramos RG, Patel C, Gangadharan V, Gordon S, Timmis GC. Outcome of coronary angioplasty (PTCA) following thrombolytic therapy in acute myocardial infarction. Circulation 1986; 74(Suppl II):II–124.
49. Topol EJ, Bates ER, Walton JA Jr, et al. Community hospital administration of intravenous tissue plasminogen activator in acute myocardial infarction: improved timing, thrombolytic efficacy and ventricular function. J Am Coll Cardiol 1987; 10:1173–1177.
50. O'Keefe JH Jr, Rutherford BD, McConahay DR. Early and late results of coronary angioplasty without antecedent thrombolytic therapy for acute myocardial infarction. Am J Cardiol 1989; 64:1221–1230.
51. Stone GW, Rutherford BD, McConahay DR, et al. Direct coronary angioplasty in acute myocardial infarction: outcome in patients with single vessel disease. J Am Coll Cardiol 1990; 15:534–543.
52. Kahn JK, Rutherford BD, McConahay DR, et al. Results of primary angioplasty for acute myocardial infarction in patients with multivessel coronary artery disease. J Am Coll Cardiol 1990; 16:1089–1096.
53. Kahn JK, Rutherford BD, McConahay DR, et al. Catheterization laboratory events and hospital outcome with direct angioplasty for acute myocardial infarction. Circulation 1990; 82:1910–1915.
54. Cragg DR, Friedman HZ, Bonema JD, et al. Outcome of patients with

acute myocardial infarction who are ineligible for thrombolytic therapy. Ann Intern Med 1991; 115:173–177.

55. Brodie BR, Weintraub RA, Stuckey RD, et al. Outcomes of direct coronary angioplasty for acute myocardial infarction in candidates and non-candidates for thrombolytic therapy. Am J Cardiol 1991; 67:7–12.

56. Goldberg RJ, Gore JM, Alpert JS, et al. Cardiogenic shock after acute myocardial infarction: incidence and mortality from a community-wide perspective, 1975 to 1988. N Engl J Med 1991; 325:1117–1122.

57. Kennedy JW, Gensine GG, Timmis GC, Maynard C. Acute myocardial infarction treated with intracoronary streptokinase: a report of the Society for Coronary Angiography. Am J Cardiol 1985; 55:871–887.

58. Bates ER, Topol EJ. Limitations of thrombolytic therapy for acute myocardial infarction complicated by congestive heart failure and cardiogenic shock. J Am Coll Cardiol 1991; 18:1077–1084.

59. Lee L, Erbel R, Brown TM, Laufer N, Meyer J, O'Neill WW. Multicenter registry of angioplasty therapy of cardiogenic shock: initial and long-term survival. J Am Coll Cardiol 1991; 17:599–603.

60. Topol EJ, O'Neill WW, Langburd AB, et al. A randomized, placebo-controlled trial of intravenous recombinant tissue-type plasminogen activator and emergency coronary angioplasty in patients with acute myocardial infarction. Circulation 1987; 75:420–428.

61. Topol EJ, Califf RM, George BS, et al. A randomized trial of immediate versus delayed elective angioplasty after intravenous tissue plasminogen activator in acute myocardial infarction. N Engl J Med 1987; 317:581–588.

62. The TIMI Research Group. Immediate vs delayed catheterization and angioplasty following thrombolytic therapy for acute myocardial infarction. JAMA 1988; 260:2849–2858.

63. Simoons ML, Arnold AE, Betriu A, et al. Thrombolysis with tissue plasminogen activator in acute myocardial infarction: no additional benefit from immediate percutaneous coronary angioplasty. Lancet 1988; 1:197–203.

64. Stack RS, O'Connor CM, Mark DB, et al. Coronary perfusion during acute myocardial infarction with a combined therapy of coronary angioplasty and high-dose intravenous streptokinase. Circulation 1988; 77:151–161.

65. Califf RM, Topol EJ, Stack RS. Evaluation of combination thrombolytic therapy and timing of cardiac catheterization in acute myocardial infarction: results of thrombolysis and angioplasty in myocardial infarction-phase 5 randomized trial. Circulation 1991; 83:1543–1556.

66. The TIMI Study Group. Comparison of invasive and conservative strategies after treatment with intravenous tissue plasminogen activator in acute myocardial infarction: results of the thrombolysis in myocardial infarction (TIMI) phase II trial. N Engl J Med 1989; 320:618–627.

67. Colle JP, Delarche M. Clinical factors affecting PTCA for patients with unstable angina. Cath CV Diagn 1991; 23(3):155–163.

Chapter 5

Principles of Myocardial Protection During Acute Coronary Ischemia and Reperfusion

Friedhelm Beyersdorf and Gerald D. Buckberg

Introduction

Acute myocardial infarction (AMI) is caused by acute coronary occlusion and is the major cause of death in Europe and in the United States. In-hospital mortality is due principally to cardiogenic shock because of extensive ischemic muscle damage. Previous surgical results of coronary artery bypass grafting (CABG) for left ventricular (LV) power failure have been disappointing,[1-5] as intraoperative ischemic injury is superimposed on severely damaged myocardium. Surgical revascularization has, in general, been restricted to patients with acute occlusion after elective percutaneous transluminal coronary angioplasty (PTCA), because the rapidity of reperfusion has been considered the principal determinant of muscle salvage,

Lazar HL (editor): *Current Therapy for Acute Coronary Ischemia,* © Futura Publishing Co., Inc., Mount Kisco, NY, 1993.

and this can be done more quickly in naturally occurring occlusion by thrombolysis and/or PTCA. Successful medical reperfusion is possible in 70% to 90% by pharmacological or mechanical medical interventions,[6,7] but mortality remains between 9% and 13% in larger unselected series[7,8] and early recovery of contractile function and/or avoidance of electrocardiographic (ECG) infarction are rare, and revascularization is restricted to the infarct related artery. Conversely, surgical reperfusion allows more complete revascularization since many patients have multivessel disease. Hospital mortality is low in larger surgical series,[5,9,10] especially when cardiogenic shock patients are excluded, but logistical constraints delay most surgical interventions beyond the time limits conventionally thought reasonable to avoid irreversible damage. This communication includes experimental and clinical data that may provide a basis for a reappraisal of conventional approaches to patients with AMI.

Acute coronary artery occlusion causes the ischemic muscle segment to stop beating immediately, inasmuch as anaerobic adenosine triphosphate (ATP) production is insufficient to support mechanical function.[11] Systolic shortening is replaced by passive bulging (dyskinesia), because the noncontracting ischemic region is stretched during systole by remote contracting muscle. The magnitude of passive lengthening is dependent on the systolic pressure, ventricular volume, and ventricular compliance. To maintain a sufficient cardiac output to sustain life, remote noninfarcting myocardium must hypercontract to compensate for dissipation of energy during passive stretching of the ischemic segment. Loss of more than 40% of contracting LV muscle results in cardiogenic shock,[12,13] and this can occur with very proximal acute coronary occlusions. Survival after an acute coronary occlusion that renders less than 40% of the LV nonfunctional depends on the compensatory capacity of the remote, "nonischemic" myocardium[14–17]; this can be assessed by analysis of regional wall motion (e.g., by echocardiography, ventriculography, or radionuclide ventriculography). LV power failure will develop if the mass of the remaining myocardium is reduced by a previous myocardial infarction; "normal" contractility (normokinesis) or even reduced contractility (hypokinesis) in viable remote muscle has severe prognostic implications.[18]

Our observations on the pathophysiology of ischemic *and* remote myocardium[11,14,15,19,20] prompted us to develop operative strategies intended to a) restore early segmental contractility in the previously ischemic area despite prolonged (> 6 hr) ischemic periods, and b) restore or maintain hypercontractility in remote myocardium. These strategies involve the use of mechanical cardiac decompression on total vented bypass and the use of warm, substrate-enriched blood cardioplegia to resuscitate *both* acute ischemic muscle and metabolically depleted remote muscle.

This chapter summarizes a) our current understanding of the pathophysiology of acute coronary occlusion on ischemic and nonischemic (remote) myocardium, b) the pathophysiology of LV power failure after acute coronary occlusion, c) the effect of the method of reperfusion on muscle salvage after prolonged temporary regional ischemia, d) the technical details of controlled regional blood cardioplegic reperfusion and maximal protection of remote myocardium, and e) our clinical results after controlled reperfusion in the ischemic segment in patients with acute evolving infarction and in patients in cardiogenic shock secondary to acute coronary occlusion.

Experimental Background

Our studies over the last several years of the natural history of acute regional ischemia and controlled reperfusion after coronary occlusion[21] have shown that acute occlusion of a coronary artery not only affects the ischemic myocardium, but also causes structural, functional, and metabolic alterations in the remote and adjacent myocardium.[14,15,20] These changes in the remote myocardium are even more severe if the remote myocardium is supplied by a stenotic coronary artery.[14]

Myocardial Changes During Acute Coronary Artery Occlusion

Acute coronary occlusion results in immediate systolic bulging (dyskinesia) of the ischemic muscle segment.[14,15,19,22–25] This can be quantified by placing ultrasonic crystals on the ischemic region,[19,26] or observed clinically by echocardiography or ventriculography[27,28] and electrocardiographic changes. These regional wall motion abnormalities are accompanied by progressive ultrastructural[29,30] and biochemical sequences, which include a) depletion of high energy phosphates leading to inactivation of the Na^+/K^+ pump and the Ca^{2+} pump and to an accumulation of inosine and hypoxanthine,[19,31-36] b) anaerobic glycolysis leading to intracellular acidosis and an increase in intracellular osmolarity,[32,33,37,38] c) catabolism of amino acids (Table 1), intermediate products of the Krebs' cycle,[19,35,39] and d) depletion of endogenous oxygen free radical scavengers.[40,41]

Despite these alterations, the myocardial cell remains structurally intact even after 6 hours of ischemia,[19] as long as the damaged tissue is not exposed to a sudden reperfusion with normal blood. Our data (Table 1) as well as those of others show that prolonged ischemia (without reperfusion) cause only a) mild mitochondrial ultrastructural changes (low protein denaturation embedding technique),[19,35,42] b) a mild decrease in mitochondrial function,[19] and c) slight calcium accumulation and edema formation.[19,43] These observations are at variance with previous conclusions that 6 hours of regional ischemia produce irreversible damage[44-47]; prior conclusions were, however, based on the assumption that the method of reperfusion per se does not affect the fate of previously ischemic tissue.

Table 1

Biochemical and Ultrastructural Data after 6 hr of Regional Ischemia (LAD Ligation) in the Anterior Wall of the LV

| | Control | | 6 hr Ischemia‡ | |
	Epicardium	Endocardium	Epicardium	Endocardium
Ultrastructural mitochondrial score	0.5 ± 0.2	0.8 ± 0.1	1.2 ± 0.1	2.0 ± 0.3
Glutamate*	14.1 ± 1.1	14.7 ± 1.1	5.9 ± 0.6	4.9 ± 0.5
Alpha-ketoglutarate†	96.2 ± 17.3	132.0 ± 22.5	20.6 ± 6.6	23.4 ± 7.8
Oxaloacetic acid†	18.7 ± 2.5	19.2 ± 1.8	6.1 ± 2.8	3.5 ± 3.5
RCI	7.61 ± 0.93	7.21 ± 0.37	6.49 ± 0.52	4.85 ± 0.47
ST_3	362.2 ± 22.5	397.4 ± 23.3	295.0 ± 31.6	208.4 ± 22.0
% H_2O content	77.4 ± 0.3	77.6 ± 0.7	78.5 ± 0.4	80.4 ± 0.3

Data are mean ± SEM.
*μmol/g dry weight.
†nmol/g dry weight.
‡$p < 0.05$ vs. control.
ST_3 = state 3 respiration (nanoatoms of O_2/mg of protein); RCI = respiratory control index; LV = left ventricle; LAD = left anterior descending coronary artery.

Effect of the Type of Reperfusion on the Viability After Prolonged Temporary Ischemia

Studies by Jennings et al.[31] suggest that the damage imposed by a 15-minute coronary occlusion can be reversed successfully by normal blood reperfusion. However, after 40 minutes of regional ischemia, massive structural, biochemical, and functional changes occur in the subendocardial muscle after reperfusion with normal blood in the working heart that were not present before the onset of reflow.[29,46,48] These alterations include further calcium accumulation, increase in water content, low- or no-reflow phenomenon, and severe histochemical and ultrastructural damage that result in persistent wall motion abnormalities [either bulging (dyskinesia) or no movement at all (akinesia)].[21,25,29,35,43,49,50] Normal blood reperfusion after longer periods of regional ischemia (6 hr) produces such extensive transmural necrosis that muscle salvage is unlikely.[44-47]

The mechanisms responsible for the additional damage caused by unmodified (normal blood) reperfusion after prolonged severe ischemia include:

1. Malfunctioning ATP-dependent enzymes (e.g., Na^+/K^+-ATPase, Ca^{2+}-ATPase) leading to an impairment of cell volume and calcium regulation with accumulation of calcium and sodium and loss of potassium and magnesium,[36,48,51,52] which in turn causes arrhythmias,[53,54] marked increase in water content,[55] no- or low-reflow phenomenon,[55] reduced oxygen consumption,[56] myocardial fiber necrosis,[57] and severe mitochondrial damage.[42,58]

2. High intracellular osmolar load[37] leads to further cell swelling.

3. Tissue acidosis inhibits optimal enzyme function.[59]

4. Loss of Krebs' cycle intermediates and their precursors (e.g., glutamate and aspartate)[19,39,60] may be a cause for the reduced myocardial oxygen extraction.[61] After temporary global ischemia, uptake of glutamate and aspartate correlate with myocardial oxygen consumption and glutamate uptake seems to be limited by substrate availability.[62]

5. High levels of hypoxanthine and loss of endogenous free radical scavengers[40,41] allow the production of oxygen free radicals[63-67] when blood supply is restored.

6. Neutrophil plugging of capillaries[68] and generation of reactive oxygen intermediates also may contribute to the low-reflow phenomenon.

The occurrence of this myocardial reperfusion injury after normal blood reperfusion is related to the severity of ischemia.[69,70] Short ischemic periods or high collateral blood flow[71] might preserve cellular regulatory mechanisms and this might prevent reperfusion injury, whereas normal blood reperfusion after prolonged severe ischemia always leads to the above-mentioned alterations.

These experimental data are supported by clinical evidence where follow-up ventriculograms 1 year after normal blood reperfusion by coronary artery bypass grafting (CABG) reveals failure to recover regional muscle function[27] in segments revascularized after 6 hours of coronary occlusion and >10% hospital mortality despite thrombolysis after 3 hours of ischemia or more.[8] Furthermore, unmodified blood reperfusion after 2 to 3 hours of occlusion or more leads to electrocardiographic evolution of infarction and provides marginal recovery of regional contractility.[6] One or 2 hours are the upper limit for intravenous thrombolysis therapy to result in myocardial salvage[72] sufficient to restore immediate return of contractile function after PTCA.[73]

We do not believe that normal blood reperfusion extends the infarct process beyond the confines of the area at risk. *Normal blood reperfusion* may a) salvage those myocardial cells that are not severely ischemic (e.g., in the borderzone of the area at risk), and b) seal the fate of severely ischemic cells that are not able to compensate the sudden reintroduction of normal blood. Our data have shown that "treatment" of severely injured cells during the initial reperfusion phase will result in a gradual recovery from the ischemic insult and some regulatory mechanisms will be restored before the onset of normal blood reperfusion.

Studies using our surgical strategy of controlled regional reperfusion as an initial treatment for the jeopardized cells suggest that the duration of ischemia causing irreversible damage may be longer than 6 hours, and that the fate of heart muscle subjected to temporary ischemia may be determined in large part by "how" the muscle is reperfused, rather than "how quickly" blood supply is restored.[14,15,19,21,35,74-81] Conversely, normal blood reperfusion preceding controlled reperfusion may nullify immediate functional recovery.[82]

Our current strategy for controlled reperfusion incorporates *each* of the principles of modification of the conditions of reperfusion and the composition of the reperfusate that evolved from our previous studies.[20,21,50,60,76,83-91]

Conditions of Reperfusion

The conditions of reperfusion that were modified included a) *total heart decompression* by vented bypass to prevent the damaged muscle from developing wall tension during reperfusion and thereby increasing its oxygen demands,[84] b) *gentle reperfusion pressure* (i.e., 50 mm Hg) to limit postischemic edema produced by sudden reperfusion[89]; this also may decrease shear stress and minimize endothelial dysfunction[92] and reduce postreperfusion arrhythmias, c) *regional cardioplegia* to keep energy demands as low as possible during temporarily controlled reperfusion,[87] d) *normothermia* to optimize the rate of cellular repair,[90,93] and e) *prolonged reperfusion duration* (i.e., 20 min) to maximize oxygen uptake relative to demands and avoid premature imposition of high-energy demands that divert the limited oxygen utilization capacity to unnecessary electromechanical work.[94]

Composition of the Reperfusate

The reperfusate composition was modified to allow incorporation of the following principles: a) *oxygenation* with blood to provide substrate (O_2) to generate energy for repair of cellular processes,[94] b) *cardioplegia* (K^+) to keep the heart from resuming electromechanical activity and raising O_2 demand,[87] c) *replenishing of amino acid precursors* of Krebs' cycle intermediates (i.e., glutamate, aspartate) needed to ensure more effective oxidative metabolism to produce energy for cell repair and subsequent mechanical function,[81,95] d) *limitation of calcium influx* by reperfusate hypocalcemia (150–250 μmol/l) with citrate-phosphate-dextrose to reduce calcium load and addition of a calcium channel blocking drug (i.e., diltiazem) that could continue to retard calcium cell entry after normocalcemic reperfusion is started,[77,85] e) *reversal of acidosis* with a buffer to provide an optimal intracellular milieu for effective resumption of metabolic function,[78] f) *hyperosmolarity* (i.e., glucose) to minimize postischemic edema and allow cell volume regulation to occur gradually when normothermic blood flow is restored,[88] g) *counteracting* of oxygen free radicals with *oxygen free radical scavenger* (i.e., coenzyme Q_{10}) to limit cytotoxic effects of these compounds,[96] h) *hyperglycemia* to enhance osmotic effects and perhaps initiate compartmental anaerobic energy production at the start of reperfusion,[88,97] and i) *leukopenia* to reduce the number of white blood cells that can become activated to generate toxic oxygen species, and plug capillaries to contribute to the low-reflow phenomenon.[68,91]

Our experimental studies have shown that controlled reperfusion is followed by immediate recovery of systolic shortening after 2, 4, and 6 hours of ischemia (Fig. 1), whereas normal blood reperfusion in the working heart even after only 2 hours of acute coronary occlusion does not result in an immediate recovery of contractile function (Fig. 1). Furthermore, in contrast to the low-reflow rate after uncontrolled reperfusion after 2 hours of ischemia, there is a marked hyperemic response even after 6 hours of ischemia if controlled reperfusion is used (Fig. 2) and significantly less histochemical injury is seen after 4 hours of regional ischemia when

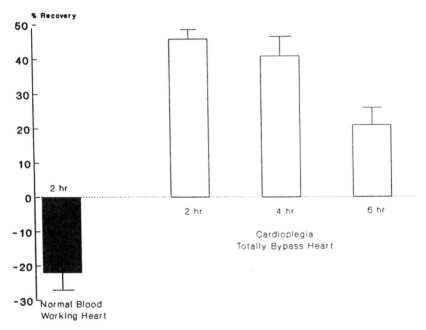

Figure 1: Segmental shortening after reperfusion expressed as percent recovery of systolic shortening, in comparison with control value, after normal blood reperfusion in working heart (solid bar) and substrate enriched blood cardioplegic reperfusion during total vented bypass (stippled bars). Note a) failure to recover systolic shortening after uncontrolled reperfusion at 2 hr (solid bar), and b) immediate recovery of systolic shortening after 2, 4, and 6 hr of ischemia after controlled reperfusion.

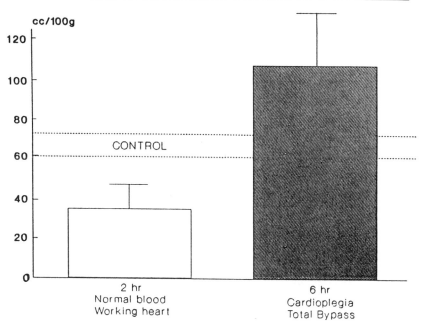

Figure 2: LV transmural blood flow (microspheres) after reperfusion with normal blood in working heart (open bar) and substrate-enriched blood cardioplegic solution during total bypass (hatched bar). Control values are seen in stippled bar. Note low-reflow rate after uncontrolled reperfusion after 2 hr of ischemia and hyperemic flow rates after 6 hr of ischemia and controlled reperfusion.

controlled reperfusion is used in comparison to normal blood reperfusion (Fig. 3).

The superiority of modifying the initial reperfusion phase is confirmed by the work of other investigators, in terms of controlled reflow,[54,92,98,99] reduced calcium reperfusion,[100–103] addition of diltiazem,[104] substrate enhancement,[105–107] ventricular unloading,[108] addition of oxygen free radical scavengers,[109,110] and electromechanical quiescence and initially reduced reperfusion pressure.[111–114] Confirmation of the superiority of our concept of controlling the conditions of reperfusion and the composition of the reperfusate is reported by other authors in the experimental setting[115–118] as well as in the clinical arena (with shorter intervals of controlled reperfusion) in patients with AMI[119] and after global ischemia.[120] Furthermore, Cheung and co-workers[117] showed in a

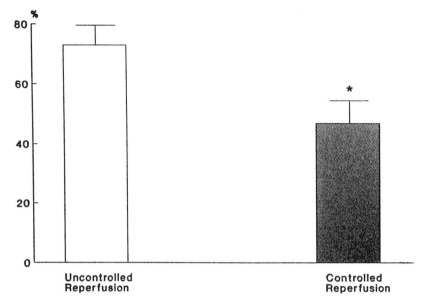

Figure 3: Histochemical myocardial cell damage after 4 hr of regional ischemia followed by uncontrolled (left bar) and controlled (right bar) reperfusion. Note significantly less histochemical injury after controlled reperfusion. Values are mean ± standard error of the mean.* $p<0.05$.

model of 2-hour coronary occlusion that the immediate benefits of controlled reperfusion (30 min after reperfusion) in terms of regional function and myocardial salvage were found to have improved further 1 week post reperfusion.

Remote Myocardium During Acute Coronary Occlusion

The function of remote muscle is the principle determinant of early survival after an otherwise nonlethal coronary occlusion (i.e., 30% of LV at risk).[14] Survival after acute coronary occlusion is determined by a) the infarct size[121–123] and b) the capacity of remote, nonischemic myocardium to support the systemic circulation.[14,18,124] Cardiogenic shock or LV power failure occurs if >40% of the LV muscle mass acutely loses its contractile properties[12,13] or if there is insufficient remote myocardium to compensate for the acute loss of <40% of contractile mass. Failure of remote muscle to hypercontract may be caused by one or more of the following factors:

1. A previous myocardial infarction that reduces the available muscle mass in the remote myocardium; that is, a patient with an acute left anterior descending artery (LAD) occlusion and a previous inferior infarction secondary to prior occlusion of the right coronary artery has only a limited capacity to develop hypercontractility in the now "nonischemic myocardium" and might develop cardiogenic shock after a short time interval after the acute coronary occlusion.

2. Remote muscle hypercontractility that might be present during the initial few hours after the acute coronary occlusion may decrease progressively to normokinesis and finally to hypokinesis.[14,125] Our experimental studies have shown that despite maintenance of normal or increased blood flow, mild energy and substrate depletion and evidence of anaerobic metabolism in the remote muscle occurs several hours after the acute coronary occlusion (Table 2): ATP, creatine phosphate (CP), glycogen, and glutamate become depleted in the remote muscle with only LAD occlusion.[14,25] Glutamate is an amino acid precursor that is essential for aerobic ATP generation by the Krebs' cycle. In another study[15] we found that intravenous metabolic support solutions that replenish depleted substrates can restore and temporarily maintain compensatory

Table 2

Biochemical Data in the Remote Myocardium after Acute LAD Occlusion for 6 hr

	Control	LAD Ligation	LAD Ligation + LCX Stenosis
ATP			
Epicardium	19.0 ± 0.9	20.4 ± 2.5	11.9 ± 2.9
Endocardium	17.7 ± 1.3	25.1 ± 1.8	11.3 ± 3.4
CP			
Epicardium	42.5 ± 3.1	27.9 ± 5.2	15.7 ± 5.6
Endocardium	37.2 ± 2.2	30.7 ± 4.0	18.9 ± 6.1
G-6-P			
Epicardium	0.72 ± 0.19	0.93 ± 0.24	2.51 ± 0.98
Endocardium	0.62 ± 0.10	1.66 ± 0.36	2.50 ± 1.01

Data are mean ± SEM.
*$p<0.05$ vs. LAD ligation.
ATP = adenosine triphosphate; CP = creatine phosphate; G-6-P = glucose-6-phosphate; LAD = left anterior descending coronary artery; LCX = left circumflex coronary artery.

hypercontractility in energy and substrate-depleted remote muscle before definite treatment (i.e., CABG).

3. Remote myocardium may become relatively ischemic if it is supplied by stenotic coronary arteries when called on to increase contractile function, and compensatory hypercontractility either may not occur or be sustained and lead to cardiogenic shock and/or intractable ventricular fibrillation. We found remote muscle to become progressively hypocontractile with resultant reduction in stroke work index when it was supplied by a noncritically stenotic coronary artery[14]; the functional deterioration was accompanied by moderate substrate and energy depletion and more pronounced evidence of anaerobic metabolism despite normal blood flow. Functional impairment despite normal blood flow to remote muscle suggests either autoregulatory failure or substrate depletion as the cause of hypocontractility.

The critical importance of remote muscle in determining the natural history of patients having AMI is reinforced by a recent report by Jaarsma and associates[18] showing a 69% mortality rate (usually from LV power failure) in such patients who did not have remote hypercontractility. Schuster and Buckley[124] report a 72% late mortality rate in patients with "ischemia at a distance" and suggest that prognosis appears related more to ischemic events in remote muscle than to the quantity of myocardium lost during the acute infarction.

These experimental and clinical observations indicate that unimpaired blood supply to remote muscle should be provided by revascularization in patients with multivessel disease if the normal hypercontractile state is not present. Extrapolation of our experimental data suggests that remote muscle normokinesia or hypokinesia should be viewed as a warning sign of impending cardiogenic shock, because wall motion abnormalities precede changes in systemic hemodynamics.

These observations and studies form the basis for the strategy directed at maximizing of myocardial protection of ischemic *and* remote myocardium during operation for acute coronary occlusion. We believe the surgical mortality in patients with evolving myocardial infarction, especially in those with cardiogenic shock, occurs because intraoperative damage is superimposed on a heart whose functioning muscle has limited ischemic tolerance.[95] Consequently, successful revascularization may not restore satisfactory contractility to either ischemic or remote myocardium, and the preoperative low-output state remains uncorrected and causes death from multi-system organ failure and arrhythmias.

Clinical Studies

Myocardial Protection Strategy for Patients with Acute Myocardial Infarction

Our myocardial protection strategy for patients with acute evolving myocardial infarction is designed to a) avoid reperfusion injury after temporary ischemia and "treat" the area damaged by ischemia with the goal to immediately restore segmental contractility and b) provide maximal myocardial protection to remote muscle to avoid additional damage to a segment that already has a limited ischemic tolerance.

Cardiopulmonary bypass is established as quickly as possible by means of single venous and aortic cannulation technique. For patients who need preoperative cardiopulmonary resuscitation, the femoral vein is cannulated with a catheter passed into the right atrium and the femoral artery is cannulated in the usual fashion. The LV is vented routinely by a catheter passed through the right pulmonary vein.

As bypass conduits, we use only vein grafts into the infarcting segment because the controlled reperfusate has to be administered through them. Internal thoracic artery grafts are feasible if they are placed in conjunction with vein grafts into the ischemic region, or if the remote segment is not large, since they will not immediately accommodate the high flows that are conducted through vein grafts and that may be needed to supply remote segments containing a large volume muscle mass.

The strategies for blood cardioplegia may be separated into the phases of a) induction, b) maintenance and distribution, and c) reperfusion. Combined antegrade/retrograde delivery of cardioplegia is used for all patients to ensure optimal distribution beyond the occlusion and stenosis. Antegrade cardioplegia is given in the usual manner through the aortic root. For retrograde delivery of blood cardioplegia, transatrial cannulation of the coronary sinus with the Retroplegia cannula (Research Medical, Inc., Salt Lake City, UT) is performed and the coronary sinus pressure is always measured. Antegrade cardioplegia is always delivered first.

The total blood cardioplegic dose is divided relatively equally between antegrade and retrograde delivery for induction, maintenance, and reperfusion. The doses are never given simultaneously by the two routes. All patients receive substrate-enriched blood cardioplegia diluted at a ratio of 4:1 (blood to cardioplegia) during controlled reperfusion. The desired solution temperature is achieved by circulating either warm or cold water through the heat exchanger (BCD Plus, Shiley Inc., Anaheim, CA) used for cardioplegic delivery.

Blood Cardioplegic Induction

Cardioplegia may be induced immediately after extracorporeal circulation has begun and the pulmonary artery is collapsed. Starting the antegrade infusion before aortic clamping ensures aortic valve competence. The blood cardioplegic induction may be given cold or warm.

Cold Blood Cardioplegic Induction

Patients who are hemodynamically stable receive cold blood cardioplegic induction with a 4° to 8°C cardioplegic solution infused at 250 to 300 ml/min. The 5-minute period for cold cardioplegic induction is divided into 2.5 minutes given antegrade and 2.5 minutes given retrograde. During the retrograde administration flow is reduced to 200 ml/min, and the pressure in the coronary sinus should never exceed 50 mm Hg.

Warm Blood Cardioplegic Induction

Patients in cardiogenic shock or otherwise depleted energy stores are placed on normothermic bypass and receive warm cardioplegic induction over 5 minutes with a 37°C substrate-enriched (glutamate/aspartate) cardioplegic solution containing 20 to 25 mEq/L potassium chloride.[90,95,126] Normothermic blood cardioplegic infusion is started at 250 to 300 ml/min and causes arrest within 1 to 2 minutes. The infusion rate is then reduced to 150 ml/min and the cardioplegic bag is exchanged for one that contains the same constituents but in which the delivered potassium is reduced to 8 to 10 mEq/L. Immediately after the 5-minute warm induction the perfusionist switches the heater-cooler to the maximum cooling mode, circulates cold water (4–6°C) through the disposable heat exchanger (BCD Plus, Shiley Inc., Anaheim, CA), increases the flow rate to 250 to 300 ml/min, and continues the cold low potassium substrate-enriched blood cardioplegic infusion at a rate of 250 to 300 ml/min for 3 to 4 minutes.

Order of Grafting

The first vein graft is always placed into the vessel involved in the acute coronary occlusion. Construction of proximal LAD and/or right coronary anastomoses are begun during retrograde cardioplegic induction if local vessel occlusion with snares controls bleeding sufficiently to permit precise suture placement.

Maintenance of Cardioplegia

Multidose cold blood cardioplegic solution is delivered through the coronary cardioplegic adapter into the aorta and into each graft at 200 ml/min over 2 minutes after completion of each distal anastomosis. Furthermore, blood cardioplegia is delivered retrograde through the coronary sinus for an additional minute. Systemic rewarming is begun after the last distal anastomosis is started.

Controlled Regional Reperfusion

After completion of the last distal anastomosis, warm (37°C) diltiazem-containing, substrate-enriched blood cardioplegia is given into the aorta and all grafts for 2 minutes at 150 ml/min (Table 3). Thereafter the aortic clamp is removed and the controlled blood cardioplegic solution is given at a flow rate of 50 ml/min for an additional 18 minutes only into the graft supplying the region revascularized for acute coronary occlusion. In patients with acute occlusion of the left main coronary artery or with acute occlusion of two coronary arteries, flow is increased to 100 ml/min and given into both vein grafts. Normal blood is delivered into the remainder of the heart via aortic segment not included in this tangential clamp. Cannulation of a side branch of the vein graft may allow delivery of the controlled blood cardioplegic reperfusate while the proximal anastomosis is performed so that no additional ischemic time is imposed on the previously ischemic region. The heart is kept in the

Table 3

Regional Controlled Blood Cardioplegic Reperfusate

Cardioplegic Additive	Volume Added (ml)	Component Modified	Concentration Delivered
KCl (2 mEq/ml)	15	K^+	8–10 mEq/L
THAM (0.3 M)	225	pH	pH 7.5–7.6
CPD	225	Ca^{2+}	0.15–0.25 mM/L Ca^{2+}
Diltiazem	300 μg/kg bw	Ca^{2+}	
Aspartate/ glutamate	250	Substrate	13 mM each
D50W	40	Glucose	400 mg%
D5W	200	Osmolarity	380–400 mosmol

bw = body weight; CPD = citrate-phosphate-dextrose; D50W = dextrose 50% in water; D5W = dextrose 5% in water.

beating empty state for 30 more minutes after completion of the regional cardioplegic infusion, with extracorporeal circulation discontinued immediately thereafter. Additional bypass is used if cardiac output is not satisfactory.

Results After Controlled Regional Reperfusion in Patients with Acute Evolving Infarction

Until 1991, 74 patients with acute coronary occlusion at the Johann Wolfgang Goethe-University Medical Center in Frankfurt/ M. and the University of California at Los Angeles Medical Center underwent emergency surgical revascularization followed by controlled reperfusion. In patients with naturally occurring occlusions, the onset of coronary occlusion was defined as the time of origin of chest pain and was always corroborated by angiographic evidence of coronary occlusion. In elective or emergency PTCA patients (n = 39) with previously patent but stenotic arteries, the onset of acute coronary occlusion was defined as the time of acute vessel closure. In both subsets, electrocardiographic evidence of hyperacute ST elevation with or without Q waves or loss of R-wave progression was present. The duration of ischemia was defined as the period of time until the start of reperfusion, and averaged 4.6 ± 3.0 hours (range 1.5–23 hr). Cardiogenic shock was present preoperatively in 28 patients. Regional contractility was assessed in all patients during the immediate postoperative period by echocardiography and/or radionuclide ventriculography. The wall motion score was graded from 0 = normal to 4 = dyskinesia.

Early recovery of substantial regional contractility occurred in 66 of 74 patients treated by controlled reperfusion; *89% of patients showed either normokinesis or only mild to moderate hypokinesis on the 7th postoperative day* (Fig. 4). Reperfusion arrhythmias were infrequent, hemodynamic instability, present preoperatively in 43 of 74 patients (58%), usually was reversed 18 to 24 hours postoperatively, and hospitalization averaged only 9 days despite delay of treatment for up to 23 hours. Hospital mortality was 5% (4/74).

These clinical results together with our recent reports[74,75]

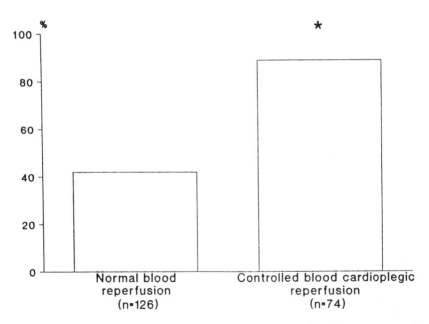

Figure 4: Combined results from UCLA and Frankfurt/M. after emergency CABG in patients with acute coronary occlusion. The ordinate shows the percentage of patients having either normo- or slight hypokinesis in the previously ischemic area after normal blood reperfusion (left bar) or regional controlled blood cardioplegic reperfusion (right bar) 7–14 days postoperatively. Note significantly more patients show substantial recovery of regional wall motion after controlled regional reperfusion as compared to normal blood reperfusion. $^*p<0.05$.

provide confirmation of our belief that the fate of jeopardized myocardium is determined by how the reperfusion strategy is managed, rather than by how quickly the blood supply is restored. In contrast, a consecutive series between 1977 and 1989 at the University of Frankfurt of 126 patients with acute coronary occlusion after PTCA failure who underwent uncontrolled reperfusion (i.e., normal blood) showed that after only 3.5 hours of ischemia recovery of regional wall motion was incomplete (mean wall motion score 1.8) and hospital mortality was 10.3%. Furthermore, a recent review of PTCA for AMI in five series in the medical literature containing 1203 patients showed overall mortality of 9.2% despite successful PTCA in 93% of patients after only 3.6 hours of ischemia.[7,127–130] In these PTCA series, subgroup mortality was highest if there was LAD occlusion, multivessel disease, age >70 years, cardiogenic shock, or unsuccessful PTCA. Additionally, mortality in the GISSI[8] trial was 9% in unselected patients treated by thrombolysis within 2 hours of chest pain and increased to 13% in patients treated after a longer time interval. We presume a >70% success rate of reperfusion in these patients. In the recent ISIS-III study, the preliminary results presented at the American College of Cardiology showed 35-day mortality rates in the groups receiving streptokinase (SK), anisoylated plasminogen streptokinase activator (APSAC), and tissue plasminogen activator (t-PA) were approximately 10.5%.[131] These clinical results of reperfusion of unmodified blood in beating, working, or bypassed hearts suggest that the value of these methods of reperfusion must be reassessed, since early return of contractile function is marginal; these clinical findings are consistent with the experimental studies on unmodified reperfusion.[26,44,46,132]

Reperfusion damage may be reversible, and delayed recovery of contractile function (i.e., "stunned myocardium") may occur in the weeks or months after normal blood reperfusion.[26,132,133] Such delayed recovery is of no functional benefit in the immediate postinfarction interval, and occurs inconsistently in patients undergoing SK thrombolysis after 4 hours of ischemia,[134–138] and therefore will not avert LV power failure, which remains the most common cause of death after AMI. Consequently, successful reperfusion and biochemical evidence of salvage (i.e., thallium uptake)[139,140] in a previously ischemic muscle that cannot regain consistent contractile function may not alter the natural course of acute infarction substantially, as reported by Rentrop and associates[141] and the GISSI trial,[8] where mortality of nonselected patients was reduced from 13% (untreated) to 11% with an anticipated success rate of 74% by thrombolysis.

Our clinical observation that controlled reperfusion produces early functional recovery after ischemic periods up to >6 hours is inconsistent with previous surgical reports suggesting that mechanical recovery occurs rarely if revascularization is delayed for 6 or more hours.[142,143] We suspect that the prior unavailability and application of information concerning the possible benefits of a controlled reperfusion strategy may have limited the previous success of surgical revascularization. We hope that further testing of the controlled reperfusion strategies that yielded the encouraging preliminary results will be tested by others, since confirmation of our findings will offer the potential of extending the time window for salvaging myocardium in patients with prolonged ischemia.

Cardiogenic Shock Secondary to LV Power Failure

Cardiogenic shock secondary to LV power failure is the most frequent complication leading to death in the intensive care unit,[1,144] since in-hospital peri-infarction arrhythmias usually are treated promptly and successfully. Cardiogenic shock occurs in 10% to 20% of patients after acute myocardial infarction[144] and is associated with an in-hospital mortality of 80% to 95% when treated pharmacologically.[144–146] Previous reports after surgical revascularization in patients with LV power failure have been disappointing, with mortality rates ranging from 30% to 63%[1–3,126,147] unless there is a mechanical cause of power failure (i.e., ventricular septal defect or rupture of papillary muscle).

The interval from acute coronary occlusion to the onset of shock is variable, with less than 10% of patients developing this complication in the first hour after myocardial infarction[144] despite maximal dysfunction of infarcting muscle immediately after coronary occlusion.[11] Cardiogenic shock after AMI develops when more than 40% of the LV is nonfunctional[12,13] and is thought to be caused by an extension of the infarct process, especially if associated with continued chest pain.[144,145] An imbalance between oxygen supply and demand in the ischemic zone of the myocardium is thought to be the pathogenetic mechanism in infarct extension.[148] Consistently, the major therapeutic approach to reduce infarct mortality was directed toward limiting the infarct size (i.e., early reperfusion, vasodilators, beta blockade, afterload reduction).[149]

The most favorable results of nonsurgical treatment for LV power failure occur after PTCA, where overall mortality approximates 50%, increasing to 80% if PTCA is unsuccessful.[150] Survival reportedly improves to 54%[150] if angioplasty is successful, especially if there is only single-vessel disease. Nonsurgical results are disappointing in multivessel disease patients, averaging 62% mortality, with 66% of deaths in patients with successful PTCA having multivessel disease.[150] The favorable results after successful PTCA must reflect some improvement in function of the peri-infarction zone, whereas failure to correct remote muscle ischemia is a plausible explanation of the increased death rate in this multivessel disease cohort.

Previous surgical approaches to acute coronary occlusion rarely restored function to the infarcted muscle, and we ascribe the increased perioperative mortality in previous surgical series of revascularization of cardiogenic shock[1–5,151,152] to inadequate protection of the remote muscle, which is vital for survival. Failure of remote muscle to compensate adequately[14] is associated with energy depletion and loss of substrate.[17,153] The substrate-enriched blood cardioplegic solution delivered during warm induction is distributed to remote muscle and replenishes its substrate stores, resuscitates it, and increases its tolerance to ischemia,[95] and the subsequent cold blood cardioplegic solutions reduce metabolic demand while anastomoses are performed during intervals of ischemia used to provide a quiet bloodless field. The first grafts are placed into the largest area of functioning remote muscle to maximize protection of the LV mass responsible for maintaining cardiac output even in patients with evolving infarction, since immediate substantial contractile recovery of the infarct zone is inconsistent immediately after extracorporeal circulation. Vein grafts are used exclusively for the remote and ischemic area because the magnitude of blood flow to muscle supplied by the internal mammary artery currently is not predictable. Furthermore, intraoperative myocardial protection by antegrade delivery of blood cardioplegia may be insufficient if the internal mammary artery is used. Retrograde techniques may circumvent these limitations,[154–157] but will not ensure that the internal mammary artery will carry sufficient flow to support early cardiac function, especially if it supplies substantial remote muscle mass.

We consider the infarct zone the "least important" region for revascularization during operation for cardiogenic shock after an established infarction (i.e. >18 hr of ischemia) and graft into that region last. Although early recovery of ischemic muscle is unlikely after normal blood reperfusion,[134,135,137,138,158] controlled blood cardioplegic reperfusion results in progressively increasing recovery of early contractile function after 6 hours of ischemia or more;[21,35,74,75] early multiple-gated acquisition scans, however, showed only minimal recovery of revascularized ischemic muscle at 24 hours, with more complete recovery delayed until 1 week.[74] Our policy to revascularize remote muscle first during operation for cardiogenic shock is based on the idea that the infarct zone will sustain only minimal added ischemic muscle damage in the decompressed cold heart,[86,159] compared with that occurring during the prolonged preoperative normothermic ischemia while wall tension is high.[84]

The technical considerations for myocardial protection during revascularization in patients with cardiogenic shock include a) warm cardioplegic induction, b) viable areas are grafted first to ensure cardioplegic distribution, c) controlled regional blood cardioplegic reperfusion for the ischemic area, and d) additional 30-minute interval of keeping the heart in the beating, empty state.

These operative strategies were employed in 112 patients admitted to the University of California at Los Angeles Medical Center and to the Johann Wolfgang Goethe-University in Frankfurt/M. with myocardial infarction who underwent emergency coronary revascularization for cardiogenic shock caused by LV power failure. All patients were dependent on inotropic drugs and/or intra-aortic balloon counterpulsation for circulatory support at the time of operation. Mechanical causes of shock, including rupture of the LV septum, free wall, or papillary muscle were excluded. Perioperative 30-day mortality was 19% (21/112 patients). The major cause of early death was multisystem organ failure (10/21 patients) and was present preoperatively in seven patients. Seven patients (6%) died of LV power failure in the immediate postoperative period and three patients died suddenly, presumably of arrhythmia. One patient succumbed due to ventricular rupture. LV power failure was reversed by operation in 94% of patients (105/112 patients) and hemodynamic improvement was evident in the early postoperative period.

Analysis of our data suggests that early and late mortality for patients in LV power failure is related to four factors: a) time from infarct to operation, b) time from shock to operation, c) preoperative organ failure, and d) history of previous infarction.[160]

Time from Infarct to Operation

The best results occurred after operation for acute evolving infarction (Fig. 5), as reported by others.[2,5,9] Hospitalization averaged only 9 days in the patients with AMI, and radionuclide ventriculography before discharge showed only mild to moderate residual hypocontractility in the revascularized zone. We ascribe this recovery to provision of a prolonged controlled regional reperfusion[35,74,75] and the recovery of remote muscle to "active resuscitation" by the warm substrate-enriched cardioplegic solution.[74,95,126]

Time from Shock to Operation

Conventional treatment of cardiogenic shock includes maximum pharmacological and mechanical support and progress to CABG only in balloon-dependent patients or in those whose condition improves sufficiently to allow semielective revascularization. The concept of "stabilization to buy time" is not borne out by the

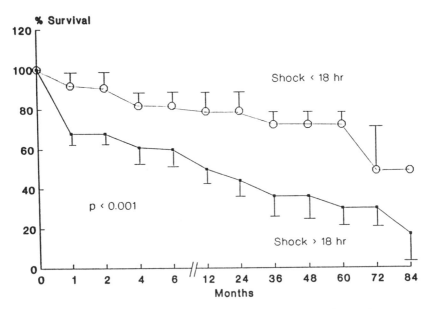

Figure 5: CABG after cardiogenic shock: influence of time of operation. *p* = Wilcoxon, mean ± standard error.

results. Early operation (<18 hr) allowed a 91% early survival rate (9% mortality), avoided preoperative organ failure, and resulted in 70% survival at 5 years. Conversely, delay of operation (>18 hr) prolonged the need for inotropic support, caused more leg complications from the intra-aortic balloon, allowed organ failure to develop, prolonged hospitalization, and increased early and late mortality rates to 33% and 67%, respectively. We suspect that progressive remote muscle necrosis occurred while circulatory support was prolonged and impaired subsequent functional recovery. The overall early and late (follow-up to 5 yr) mortality rate after delayed operation was 67%, which is comparable with the 72% overall mortality of nonsurgical patients reported on by Schuster and Buckley,[161] who have "ischemia at a distance" after AMI.

Preoperative Organ Failure

Cardiac indices before operation were impaired comparably in patients operated on less than and more than 18 hours after shock, but low output state persisted longer in patients undergoing delayed operation and allowed combinations of sepsis, renal failure, and mental obtundation to develop (Fig. 6). Delay of operation until it became clear that "stabilization" was unsuccessful did not reverse organ failure in 6 of 10 patients who died despite reasonable hemodynamic recovery; the other 4 died within 1 year after operation. We currently consider preoperative organ failure after LV failure for more than 18 hours as an avoidable complication of shock that is a contraindication to operation.

Previous Infarction

Previous infarction (Fig. 7) is a common risk factor in patients with cardiogenic shock,[12,13,144,162,163] since it reduces the remote muscle mass responsible for supporting cardiac output during an AMI. The influence of prior infarction on early death was most apparent if operation was delayed, since most early deaths after operations performed more than 18 hours after shock (12/16, 75%) occurred in patients with previous infarction. The influence of prior muscle damage on late results is most evident regarding the timing of operation relative to infarction, since all late deaths in patients

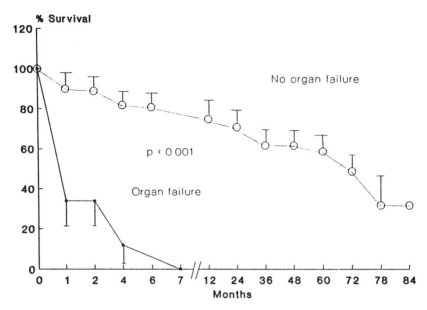

Figure 6: Influence of preoperative organ failure on CABG after cardiogenic shock. p = Wilcoxon, mean ± standard error.

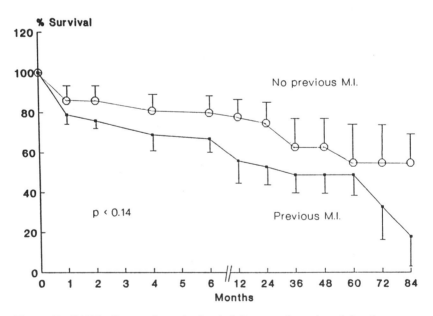

Figure 7: CABG after cardiogenic shock: influence of previous infarction. p = Wilcoxon, mean ± standard error; M.I. = myocardial infarction.

having a previous infarction were restricted to those whose new infarct was allowed to become established before the operation was performed. Conversely, no late deaths occurred in patients with a previous infarction who were undergoing operation for an evolving infarction.

A broader testing of these surgical principles for revascularization in patients with acute coronary occlusion with or without cardiogenic shock might improve the prognosis of patients with severely restricted cardiac function after AMI and might avoid a large transmural myocardial infarction.

Conclusions

Our recent experimental and clinical studies suggest that myocardial salvage with early recovery of contractile function after acute coronary occlusion is possible beyond the generally accepted 2 hours, provided that the initial reperfusion is controlled carefully. Overall in-hospital survival depends on the function of the remote, nonischemic myocardium as failure of remote muscle compensation may cause cardiogenic shock. Surgical revascularization has to restore and maintain significant hypercontractility in the remote area to allow the generation of a sufficient cardiac output in patients with LV power failure. Myocardial protection techniques are described for improving salvage and restoring contractile function in the ischemic area, and to restore successfully hypercontractility in the remote myocardium. Hopefully, subsequent clinical studies will test these approaches, and if confirmatory, reduce the mortality of acute coronary occlusion.

References

1. DeWood MA, Spores J, Notske R, et al. Medical and surgical management of myocardial infarction. Am J Cardiol 1979; 44:1356–1364.
2. DeWood MA, Notske RN, Hensley GR, et al. Intraaortic balloon counterpulsation with and without reperfusion for myocardial infarction shock. Circulation 1980; 61:1105–1112.
3. Subramanian VA, Roberts AJ, Zema JM, et al. Cardiogenic shock following acute myocardial infarction. NY State J Med 1980; 80:947–952.
4. Sanders CA, Bulkley MJ, Leinbach RL, Mundth ED, Austen WG. Mechanical circulatory assistance: current status and experience com-

bining circulatory assistance, emergency coronary angiography, and acute myocardial revascularization. Circulation 1972; 45:1292–1313.

5. Berg RJ, Selinger SL, Leonard JL, Grunwald RP, O'Grady WP. Immediate coronary artery bypass for acute evolving myocardial infarction. J Thorac Cardiovasc Surg 1981; 81:493–497.

6. Topol EJ, Califf RM, George BS, et al. A randomized trial of immediate versus delayed elective angioplasty after intravenous tissue plasminogen activator in acute myocardial infarction. N Engl J Med 1987; 317:581–588.

7. O'Keefe JH, Rutherford BD, McConahay DR, et al. Early and late results of coronary angioplasty without antecedent thrombolytic therapy for acute myocardial infarction. Am J Cardiol 1989; 64:1221–1223.

8. Gruppo Italiano per lo Studio della Streptochinasi nell'Infarto Miocardico (GISSI). Effectiveness of intravenous thrombolytic treatment in acute myocardial infarction. Lancet 1986; 1:397–402.

9. Phillips SJ, Kongtahworn C, Skinner JR, Zeff RH. Emergency coronary artery reperfusion: a choice therapy for evolving myocardial infarction. Results in 339 patients. J Thorac Cardiovasc Surg 1983; 86:679–688.

10. Phillips SJ, Zeff RH, Skinner JR, Toon RS, Grignon A, Kongtahworn C. Reperfusion protocol and results in 738 patients with evolving myocardial infarction. Ann Thorac Surg 1986; 41:119–125.

11. Beyersdorf F, Okamoto F, Buckberg GD, et al. Studies on prolonged acute regional ischemia. II. Implications of progression from dyskinesia to akinesia in the ischemic segment. J Thorac Cardiovasc Surg 1989; 98:224–233.

12. Page DL, Caulfield JB, Kastor JA, DeSanctis R, Sanders CA. Myocardial changes associated with cardiogenic shock. N Engl J Med 1971; 285:133–137.

13. Alonso DR, Scheidt S, Post M, Killip T. Pathophysiology of cardiogenic shock: quantification of myocardial necrosis, clinical, pathologic and electrocardiographic correlations. Circulation 1973; 48:588–596.

14. Beyersdorf F, Acar C, Buckberg GD, et al. Studies of prolonged acute regional ischemia. III. Early national history of simulated single and multivessel disease with emphasis on remote myocardium. J Thorac Cardiovasc Surg 1989; 98:368–380.

15. Beyersdorf F, Acar C, Buckberg GD, et al. Studies on prolonged acute regional ischemia. V. Metabolic support of remote myocardium during left ventricular power failure. J Thorac Cardiovasc Surg 1989; 98:567–579.

16. Naccarella FF, Weintraub WS, Agarwal JB, Helfant RH. Evaluation of "ischemia of a distance": effects of coronary occlusion on a remote area of the left ventricle. Am J Cardiol 1984; 54:869–874.

17. Corday E, Kaplan L, Meerbaum S, et al. Consequences of coronary arterial occlusion on remote myocardium: effects of occlusion and reperfusion. Am J Cardiol 1975; 36:385–394.

18. Jaarsma W, Visser CA, Van Einige JM, et al. Prognostic implication of regional hyperkinesia and remote asynergy of noninfarcted myocardium. Am J Cardiol 1986; 58:394–398.

19. Beyersdorf F, Allen BS, Buckberg GD, et al. Studies of prolonged acute

regional ischemia. I. Evidence of preserved cellular viability after 6 hours of coronary occlusion. J Thorac Cardiovasc Surg 1989; 98:112–126.

20. Beyersdorf F, Acar C, Buckberg GD, et al. Studies on prolonged acute regional ischemia. IV. Aggressive surgical treatment for intractable ventricular fibrillation after acute myocardial infarction. J Thorac Cardiovasc Surg 1989; 98:557–566.

21. Buckberg GD. Studies of controlled reperfusion after ischemia. J Thorac Cardiovasc Surg 1986; 92:483–448.

22. Banka VS, Helfant RH. Temporal sequence of dynamic contractile characteristics in ischemic and nonischemic myocardium after acute coronary ligation. Am J Cardiol 1974; 34:158–163.

23. Guth BD, White FC, Gallagher KP, Bloor CM. Decreased systolic wall thickening in myocardium adjacent to ischemic zones in conscious swine during brief coronary artery occlusion. Am Heart J 1984; 107:458–464.

24. Kerber RE, Marcus ML, Ehrhardt J, Wilson R, Abbour FM. Correlation between echocardiographically demonstrated segmental dyskinesis and regional myocardial perfusion. Circulation 1975; 52:1097–1104.

25. Puri PS. Contractile and biochemical effects of coronary reperfusion after extended periods of coronary occlusion. Am J Cardiol 1975; 36:244–251.

26. Lavallee M, Cox D, Patrick TA, Vatner SF. Salvage of myocardial function by coronary artery reperfusion 1, 2, and 3 hours after occlusion in conscious dogs. Circ Res 1983; 53:235–247.

27. Selinger SL, Berg R Jr, Leonard JJ, Coleman WS, DeWood MA. Surgical intervention in acute myocardial infarction. Texas Heart Inst J 1984; 11:44–51.

28. Stamm RB, Gibson RS, Bishop HL, Carabello BA, Beller GA, Martin RP. Echocardiographic detection of infarct-localized asynergy and remote asynergy during acute myocardial infarction: correlation with the extent of angiographic coronary disease. Circulation 1983; 67:233–244.

29. Jennings RB, Ganote CE. Structural changes in myocardium during acute ischemia. Circ Res 1974; 34/35(Suppl III):156–168.

30. Schaper J. Ultrastructure of the myocardium in acute ischemia. In: Schaper W, ed. The Pathophysiology of Myocardial Perfusion. Amsterdam: Elsevier/North-Holland Biomedical Press. 1979; pp 581–673.

31. Jennings RB, Schaper J, Hill ML, Steenbergen C, Reimer KA. Effect of reperfusion late in the phase reversible ischemic injury. Circ Res 1985; 56:262–278.

32. Jennings RB, Reimer KA, Steenbergen C Jr. Acute regional ischemia. In: Schettler G, Jennings RB, Rapaport E, Wenger NK, Bernhardt R, eds. Reperfusion and Revascularization in Acute Myocardial Infarction. Berlin, Heidelberg, New York, London, Paris, Tokyo: Springer. 1988; pp 3–9.

33. Jennings RB, Reimer KA. Lethal myocardial ischemic injury. Am J Pathol 1981; 102:241–255.

34. Levitzky S, Feinberg H. Biochemical changes of ischemia. Ann Thorac Surg 1975; 20:21–29.

35. Allen BS, Okamoto F, Buckberg GD, et al. Studies of controlled reperfusion after ischemia. XV. Immediate functional recovery after 6 hours of regional ischemia by careful control of conditions of reperfusion and composition of reperfusate. J Thorac Cardiovasc Surg 1986; 92(Suppl):621–635.

36. Shen AC, Jennings RB. Kinetics of calcium accumulation in acute myocardial ischemic injury. Am J Pathol 1972; 67:441–452.

37. Jennings RB, Reimer KA, Steenbergen C Jr. Myocardial ischemia revisited. The osmolar load, membrane damage, and reperfusion (editorial). J Mol Cell Cardiol 1986; 18:769–780.

38. Kübler W, Spieckermann PG. Regulation of glycolysis in the ischemic and anoxic myocardium. J Mol Cell Cardiol 1970; 1:351–359.

39. Tixier D, Matheis G, Buckberg GD, Young HH. Donor hearts with imparied hemodynamics. J Thorac Cardiovasc Surg 1991; 102:207–214.

40. Ferrari R, Ceconi C, Cureelo S, Cargnoni A, Medici D. Oxygen free radicals and reperfusion injury: the effect of ischemia and reperfusion on the cellular ability to neutralize oxygen toxicity. J Mol Cell Cardiol 1986; 18:67–69.

41. Meerson FZ, Kagan VE, Kozlov YP, Belkina LM, Arkhipenko YV. The role of lipid peroxidation in pathogenesis of ischemic damage and the antioxidant protection of the heart. Basic Res Cardiol 1982; 77:465–485.

42. Sjöstrand F, Allen BS, Buckberg GD, Okamoto F, Young H, et al. Studies of controlled reperfusion after ischemia. IV. Electron microscopic studies. Importance of embedding techniques in quantitative evaluation of cardiac mitochondrial structure during regional ischemia and reperfusion. J Thorac Cardiovasc Surg 1986; 92(Suppl):512–524.

43. Whalen DA, Hamilton DG, Ganote CE, Jennings RB. Effect of a transient period of ischemia on mitochondrial cells. I. Effects of cell volume regulation. Am J Pathol 1974; 74:381–397.

44. Kloner RA, Ellis SG, Carlson NV, Braunwald E. Coronary reperfusion for the treatment of acute myocardial infarction: post-ischemic ventricular dysfunction. Cardiology 1983; 70:233–246.

45. Kloner RA, Ellis SG, Lange R, Braunwald E. Studies of experimental coronary artery reperfusion. Effects on infarct size, myocardial function, biochemistry, ultrastructure and microvascular damage. Circulation 1983; 68(Suppl I):8–15.

46. Jennings RB, Reimer KA. Factors involved in salvaging ischemic myocardium: effect of reperfusion of arterial blood. Circulation 1983; 68(Suppl I):25–36.

47. Reimer KA, Jennings RB. The "wavefront phenomenon" of myocardial ischemic cell death. II. Transmural progression of necrosis within the framework of ischemic bed (myocardium at risk) and collateral flow. Lab Invest 1979; 40:633–644.

48. Jennings RB, Sommers HM, Kaltenbach JP, West JJ. Electrolyte alterations in myocardial ischemic injury. Circ Res 1964; 14:260–269.

49. Kloner RA, Przklenk K, Lange R, Ellis S. Reperfusion pathophysiology. In: Roberts AJ, ed. Myocardial Protection in Cardiac Surgery. New York: Marcel Dekker. 1987; pp 29–52.

50. Vinten-Johansen J, Buckberg GD, Okamoto F, Rosenkranz ER, Bugyi H, Leaf J. Studies of controlled reperfusion after ischemia. V. Superiority of surgical versus medical reperfusion after regional ischemia. J Thorac Cardiovasc Surg 1986; 92:525–534.

51. Poole-Wilson PA. Effect of hypoxia and ischemia on calcium fluxes in rabbit myocardium. In: Caldarera CM, Harris P, eds. Advances in Studies on Heart Metabolism. Bologna, Italy: CLUEB. 1982; pp 185–192.

52. Ferrari R, Williams A, DiLisa F. The role of mitochondrial function in the ischemic and reperfused myocardium. In: Caldarera CM, Harris P, eds. Advances in Studies on Heart Metabolism. Bologna, Italy: CLUEB. 1982; pp 254–255.

53. Opie LH. Reperfusion injury and its pharmacologic modification. Circulation 1989; 80:1049–1062.

54. Yamazaki S, Fujibayashi Y, Rajagopalan RE, et al. Effects of staged versus sudden reperfusion after acute coronary occlusion in the dog. J Am Coll Cardiol 1986; 7:564–572.

55. Kloner RA, Ganote CE, Jennings RB. The "no reflow" phenomenon after temporary coronary occlusion in the dog. J Clin Invest 1975; 54:1496–1508.

56. Braun E, Rohmann S, Schott R, Winkler B, Schaper W. Effect of "stunning" on myocardial oxygen consumption (MVO_2) in pigs. Z Kardiol 1989; 78(Suppl 1):135.

57. Fleckenstein A, Janke J, Döring HJ, et al. Myocardial fibre necrosis due to intracellular Ca^{++} overload—a new principle in cardiac pathophysiology. In: Dhalla NS, ed. Myocardial Biology. Baltimore: University Park Press. 1972; pp 563–580.

58. Schaper J, Schaper W. Reperfusion of ischemic myocardium: ultrastructural and biochemical aspects. J Am Coll Cardiol 1983; 1:1037–1046.

59. Williamson JR, Schaffer SW, Ford C, Safer B. Contribution of tissue acidosis to ischemic injury in the perfused rat heart. Circulation 1976; 53(Suppl I):I-3–I-13.

60. Julia P, Young HH, Buckberg GD, Kofsky ER, Bugyi HI. Studies of myocardial protection in the immature heart. IV. Improved tolerance of immature myocardium to hypoxia and ischemia by intravenous metabolic support. J Thorac Cardiovasc Surg 1991; 101:23–32.

61. Lucas SK, Kanter KR, Schaff HV, Elmer EB, Glower DD, Gardner TJ. Reduced oxygen extraction during reperfusion: a consequence of global ischemic arrest. J Surg Res 1980; 28:434–441.

62. Svedjeholm R, Ekroth R, Joachimsson PO, Ronquist G, Svensson S, Tyden H. Myocardial uptake of amino acids and other substrates in relation to myocardial oxygen consumption four hours after cardiac operations. J Thorac Cardiovasc Surg 1991; 101:688–694.

63. McCord JM. Oxygen derived free radicals in postischemic tissue injury. N Engl J Med 1985; 312:159–163.

64. Zweier JL, Flaherty JT, Weisfeldt ML. Direct measurement of free radical generation following reperfusion of ischemic myocardium. Proc Natl Acad Sci USA 1987; 84:1404–1407.

65. Arroyo CM, Kramer JH, Dickens BF, Weglicki WB. Identification of

free radicals in myocardial ischemia/reperfusion by spin trapping with nitrone DMPO. FEBS Lett 1987; 221:101–104.

66. Garlick PB, Davies MJ, Hearse DJ, Slater TF. Direct detection of free radicals in the reperfused rat heart using electron spin resonance spectroscopy. Circ Res 1987; 61:757–760.

67. Braunwald E, Kloner RA. Myocardial reperfusion: a double-edged sword? J Clin Invest 1985; 76:1713–1719.

68. Engler RL, Schmid-Schönbein GW, Pevelec RS. Leukocyte capillary plugging in myocardial ischemia and reperfusion in the dog. Am J Physiol 1986; 84:815–822.

69. Becker LC, Schaper J, Jeremy R, Schaper W. Severity of ischemia determines the occurrence of myocardial reperfusion injury. Circulation 1991; 84(Suppl II):II–254.

70. Sharma GP, Varley KG, Kim SW, Barwinsky J, Cohen M, Dhalla NS. Alterations in energy metabolism and ultrastructure upon reperfusion of the ischemic myocardium after coronary occlusion. Am J Cardiol 1975; 36:234–243.

71. Schaper W, Pasyk S. Influence of collateral flow on the ischemic tolerance of the heart following acute and subacute coronary occlusion. Circulation 1976; 53(Suppl I):I-57–I-62.

72. Golino P, Willerson JT. Is thrombolysis alone the best therapy for acute myocardial infarction? Texas Heart Inst J 1991; 18:50–61.

73. Miller HI, Almagor Y, Keren G, et al. Early intervention in acute myocardial infarction: significance for myocardial salvage of immediate intravenous streptokinase therapy followed by coronary angioplasty. J Am Coll Cardiol 1987; 9:608–614.

74. Allen BS, Buckberg GD, Schwaiger M, et al. Studies of controlled reperfusion after ischemia. XVI. Consistent early recovery of regional wall motion following surgical revascularization after eight hours of acute coronary occlusion. J Thorac Cardiovasc Surg 1986; 91(Suppl): 636–648.

75. Beyersdorf F, Sarai K, Maul FD, Wendt T, Satter P. Immediate functional benefits after controlled reperfusion during surgical revascularization for acute coronary occlusion. J Thorac Cardiovasc Surg (in press).

76. Buckberg GD, Allen B, Okamoto F, Leaf J, Bugyi H, et al. Immediate functional recovery after 6 hours coronary occlusion using regional blood cardioplegic reperfusion and total vented bypass without thoracotomy. A new concept (abstr). Circulation 1984;(Suppl 2):172.

77. Follette D, Fey K, Livesay J, Nelson R, Maloney JV Jr, Buckberg GD. The beneficial effects of citrate reperfusion of ischemic heart on cardiopulmonary bypass. Surg Forum 1976; 26:244–246.

78. Follette DM, Fey K, Buckberg GD, Helly JJ Jr, Steed DL, et al. Reducing post-ischemic damage by temporary modification of reperfusate calcium, potassium, pH and osmolarity. J Thorac Cardiovasc Surg 1981; 82:221–238.

79. Rosenkranz ER, Buckberg GD. Myocardial protection during surgical coronary reperfusion. J Am Coll Cardiol 1983; 1:1235–1246.

80. Vinten-Johansen J, Okamoto F, Rosenkranz E, Buckberg GD, Bugyi H, Leaf J. Superiority of surgical vs non-surgical revascularization after acute coronary occlusion. Circulation 1983; 68(Suppl 2–3):57.

81. Lazar HL, Buckberg GD, Manganaro AJ, Becker H, Maloney JV Jr. Reversal of ischemic damage with amino acid substrate enhancement during reperfusion. Surgery 1980; 80:702–709.

82. Quillen J, Kofsky ER, Buckberg GD, Partington MT, Julia PL, Acar C. Studies of controlled reperfusion after ischemia. XXII. Deleterious effects of simulated thrombolysis preceding simulated coronary artery bypass grafting with controlled blood cardioplegic reperfusion. J Thorac Cardiovasc Surg 1991; 101:455–464.

83. Vinten-Johansen J, Rosenkranz ER, Buckberg GD, Leaf J, Bugyi H. Studies of controlled reperfusion after ischemia. IV. Metabolic and histochemical benefits of regional blood cardioplegic reperfusion without cardiopulmonary bypass. J Thorac Cardiovasc Surg 1986; 92:535–542.

84. Allen BS, Rosenkranz ER, Buckberg GD, Vinten-Johansen J, Okamoto F, Leaf J. Studies of controlled reperfusion after ischemia. VII. High oxygen requirements of dyskinetic cardiac muscle. J Thorac Cardiovasc Surg 1986; 92:543–552.

85. Allen BS, Okamoto F, Buckberg GD, Leaf J, Bugyi H. Studies of controlled reperfusion after ischemia. IX. Reperfusate composition: benefits of marked hypocalcemia and diltiazem on regional recovery. J Thorac Cardiovasc Surg 1986; 92:564–572.

86. Allen BS, Okamoto F, Buckberg GD, Leaf J, Bugyi H. Studies of controlled reperfusion after ischemia. XIII. Reperfusion conditions. Critical importance of total ventricular decompression during regional reperfusion. J Thorac Cardiovasc Surg 1986; 92:605–612.

87. Okamoto F, Allen BS, Buckberg GD, Leaf J, Bugyi H, et al. Studies of controlled reperfusion after ischemia. VIII. Regional blood cardioplegic reperfusion during total vented bypass without thoracotomy. A new concept. J Thorac Cardiovasc Surg 1986; 92:553–563.

88. Okamoto F, Allen BS, Buckberg GD, Young H, Bugyi H, Leaf J. Studies of controlled reperfusion after ischemia. XI. Reperfusate composition. Interaction of marked hyperglycemia and marked hyperosmolarity in allowing immediate contractile recovery after four hours of regional ischemia. J Thorac Cardiovasc Surg 1986; 92:583–593.

89. Okamoto F, Allen BS, Buckberg GD, Bugyi H, Leaf J. Studies of controlled reperfusion after ischemia. XIV. Reperfusion conditions. Importance of ensuring gentle versus sudden reperfusion during relief of coronary occlusion. J Thorac Cardiovasc Surg 1986; 92:613–620.

90. Rosenkranz ER, Vinten-Johansen J, Buckberg GD, Okamoto F, Edwards H, Bugyi H. Benefits of normothermic induction of blood cardioplegia in energy-depleted hearts with maintenance of arrest by multidose cold blood cardioplegic infusions. J Thorac Cardiovasc Surg 1982; 84:667–676.

91. Kofsky ER, Julia PL, Buckberg GD, Quillen JE, Acar C. Studies of controlled reperfusion after ischemia. XXII. Reperfusate composition: effects of leucocyte depletion of blood and blood cardioplegic reper-

fusates after acute coronary occlusion. J Thorac Cardiovasc Surg 1991; 101:350–359.

92. Sawatari K, Kadoba K, Bergner KA, Mayer JE. Influence of initial reperfusion pressure after hypothermic cardioplegic ischemia on endothelial modulation of coronary tone in neonatal lambs. J Thorac Cardiovasc Surg 1991; 101:777–782.

93. Lee JC. Effect of hypothermia on myocardial metabolism. Am J Physiol 1965; 208:1253–1258.

94. Allen BS, Okamoto F, Buckberg GD, Leaf J, Bugyi H. Studies of controlled reperfusion after ischemia. XII. Effects of "duration" of reperfusate administration versus reperfusate "dose" on regional functional, biochemical, and histochemical recovery. J Thorac Cardiovasc Surg 1986; 92:594–604.

95. Rosenkranz ER, Okamoto F, Buckberg GD, Robertson JM, Vinten-Johansen J, Bugyi HI. Safety of prolonged aortic clamping with blood cardioplegia. III. Aspartate enrichment of glutamate-blood cardioplegia in energy-depleted hearts after ischemic and reperfusion injury. J Thorac Cardiovasc Surg 1986; 91:428–435.

96. Okamoto F, Allen BS, Buckberg GD, Leaf J, Bugyi H. Studies of controlled reperfusion after ischemia. X. Reperfusate composition: supplemental role of intravenous and intracoronary coenzyme Q_{10} in avoiding reperfusion damage. J Thorac Cardiovasc Surg 1986; 92:573–582.

97. Weiss J, Hilbrand B. Functional compartmentalization of glycolytic vs oxidative metabolism in isolated rabbit heart. J Clin Invest 1985; 55:436–447.

98. Peng CF, Murphy ML, Colwell K, Straub KD. Controlled vs hyperemic flow during reperfusion of jeopardized ischemic myocardium. Am Heart J 1989; 117:515–522.

99. Swanson DK, Myerowitz PD. Effect of reperfusion temperature and pressure on the functional and metabolic recovery of preserved hearts. J Thorac Cardiovasc Surg 1983; 86:242–251.

100. Nayler WG. The role of calcium in the ischemic myocardium. Am J Pathol 1981; 102:262–270.

101. Shine KI, Douglas AM. Low calcium reperfusion of ischemic myocardium. J Mol Cell Cardiol 1983; 15:251–260.

102. Shine KI, Douglas AM, Ricchiuti NV. Calcium, strontium, and barium movements during ischemia and reperfusion in rabbit ventricle. Circ Res 1978; 43:712–720.

103. Pich S, Klein HH, Lindert S, Nebendahl K, Warneke G, Kreuzer H. Therapie des Reperfusionsschadens mit Calcium Antagonisten und verminderter freier coronarer Calcium Konzentration beim experimentellen Myokardinfarkt. Z Kardiol 1989; 78(Suppl 1):137.

104. Melendez FJ, Gharagozloo F, Sun SC, Benfell K, Austin RE, et al. Effects of diltiazem cardioplegia on global function, segmental contractility, and the area of necrosis after acute coronary artery occlusion and surgical reperfusion. J Thorac Cardiovasc Surg 1988; 95:613–617.

105. Haan C, Lazar H, Yang X, Rivers S, Bernard B, Shemin R. Reduction of infarct size with substrate enhanced coronary venous retroperfusion. Circulation 1991; 84(Suppl II):II–716.
106. Haas GS, DeBoer LWV, O'Keefe DD, Bodenhamer RM, Geffin GA, et al. Reduction of postischemic myocardial dysfunction by substrate repletion during reperfusion. Circulation 1984; 70(Suppl I):I-65–I-74.
107. Engelman RM, Rousou JA, Flack JE III, Iyengar J, Kimura Y, Das DK. Reduction of infarct size by systemic amino acid supplementation during reperfusion. J Thorac Cardiovasc Surg 1991; 101:855–859.
108. Laschinger JC, Grossi EA, Cunningham JN, Krieger KH, Baumann FG, et al. Adjunctive left ventricular unloading during myocardial reperfusion plays a major role in minimizing myocardial infarct size. J Thorac Cardiovasc Surg 1985; 90:80–85.
109. Gharagozloo F, Melendez FJ, Hein RA, Austin RE, Shemin RJ, et al. The effect of oxygen free radical scavengers on the recovery of regional myocardial function after acute coronary occlusion and surgical reperfusion. J Thorac Cardiovasc Surg 1988; 95:631–636.
110. Ohara H, Kanaide H, Yoshimura R, Okada M, Nadamura M. A protective effect of coenzyme Q_{10} on ischemia and reperfusion of the isolated perfused rat heart. Gen Mol Cell Cardiol 1981; 13:65–74.
111. Digerness SB, Kirklin JW, Naftel DC, Blackstone EH, Kirklin JK, Samuelson PN. Coronary and systemic vascular resistance during reperfusion after global myocardial ischemia. Ann Thorac Surg 1988; 46:447–454.
112. Kirklin JK, Neves J, Naftel DC, Digerness SB, Kirklin JW, Blackstone EH. Controlled initial hyperkalemic reperfusion after cardiac transplantation: coronary vascular resistance and blood flow. Ann Thorac Surg 1990; 49:625–631.
113. Kirklin JK. The science of cardiac surgery. Eur J Cardiothorac Surg 1990; 4:63–71.
114. Fujiwara T, Kurtts T, Silvera M, Mayer JE. Physical and pharmacological manipulation of reperfusion conditions in neonatal myocardial preservation. Circulation 1988; 78(Suppl II):II–444.
115. Lazar HL, Wei J, Dirbas FM, Haasler GB, Spotnitz HM. Controlled reperfusion following regional ischemia. Ann Thorac Surg 1987; 44:350–355.
116. Vinten-Johansen J, Faust KB, Mills SA, Cordell AR. Surgical revascularization of acute evolving infarction without blood cardioplegia fails to restore postischemic function in the involved segment. Ann Thorac Surg 1987; 44:66–72.
117. Cheung EH, Arcidi JM, Dorsey LMA, Vinten-Johansen J, Hatcher CR, Guyton RA. Reperfusion of infarcting myocardium: Benefit of surgical reperfusion in a chronic model. Ann Thorac Surg 1989; 48:331–338.
118. Vinten-Johansen J, Edgerton TA, Howe HR, Gayheart PA, Mills SA, et al. Immediate functional recovery and avoidance of reperfusion injury with surgical revascularization and short-term coronary occlusion. Circulation 1985; 72:431–439.
119. Bottner RK, Wallace RB, Visner MS, Stark KS, Recientes E, et al.

Reduction of myocardial infarction after emergency coronary artery bypass grafting for failed coronary angioplasty with use of normothermic reperfusion cardioplegia protocol. J Thorac Cardiovasc Surg 1991; 101:1069–1075.

120. Teoh KH, Christakis GT, Weisel RD, et al. Accelerated myocardial metabolic recovery with terminal warm blood cardioplegia. J Thorac Cardiovasc Surg 1986; 91:888–895.

121. Geltman EM, Ehsani AA, Campbell MK, Schechtman K, Roberts R, Sobel BE. The influence of location and extent of myocardial infarction on long-term ventricular dysrhythmia and mortality. Circulation 1979; 60:805–814.

122. Herlitz J, Hjalmarson A, Waldenstrom J. Relationship between enzymatically estimated infarct size and short- and long-term survival after acute myocardial infarction. Acta Med Scand 1984; 216:261–267.

123. Thanavaro S, Kleiger RE, Province MA, et al. Effect of infarct location on the in-hospital prognosis of patients with first transmural myocardial infarction. Circulation 1982; 66:742–747.

124. Schuster EH, Buckley BH. Early post-infarction angina: ischemia at a distance and ischemia in the infarct zone. N Engl J Med 1981; 305:1102–1105.

125. Wyatt HL, Forrester JS, da Luz PL, Diamond GA, Chagrasulis R, Swan HJC. Functional abnormalities in nonoccluded regions of myocardium after experimental coronary occlusion. Am J Cardiol 1976; 37:366–372.

126. Rosenkranz ER, Buckberg GD, Laks H, Mulder DG. Warm induction of cardioplegia with glutamate-enriched blood in coronary patients with cardiogenic shock who are dependent on inotropic drugs and intra-aortic balloon support: initial experience and operative strategy. J Thorac Cardiovasc Surg 1983; 86:507–518.

127. Stack RS, Califf RM, Hinohara T, et al. Survival and cardiac event rates in the first year after emergency coronary angioplasty for acute myocardial infarction. J Am Coll Cardiol 1988; 11:1141–1149.

128. Rothbaum DA, Linnemeier T, Landin RJ, et al. Emergency percutaneous transluminal coronary angioplasty in acute myocardial infarction: a 3 year experience. J Am Coll Cardiol 1987; 10:264–272.

129. Miller PF, Brodie BR, Weintraub RA, LeBauer J, Katz JD, et al. Emergency coronary angioplasty for acute myocardial infarction. Arch Intern Med 1987; 147:1525–1527.

130. Erbel R, Pop T, Henrichs KJ, v. Olshausen K, Schuster KJ, et al. Percutaneous transluminal coronary angioplasty after thrombolytic therapy: a prospective controlled randomized trial. J Am Coll Cardiol 1986; 8:485–495.

131. Rogers WJ. Update on recent clinical trials of thrombolytic therapy in myocardial infarction. J Invasive Cardiol 1991; 3:11A–19A.

132. Bush LR, Buja LM, Samowitz W, Rude RE, Wathen M, et al. Recovery of left ventricular segmental function after long term reperfusion following temporary coronary occlusion in conscious dogs: comparison of 2- and 4-hour occlusion. Circ Res 1983; 53:248–263.

133. Braunwald E, Kloner RA. The stunned myocardium. Prolonged, postischemic ventricular dysfunction. Circulation 1982; 66:1146–1149.

134. Kennedy JW, Ritchie JL, Davis KB, Fritz JK. Western Washington randomized trial of intracoronary streptokinase in acute myocardial infarction. N Engl J Med 1983; 309:1477–1482.

135. Khaja F, Walton JA, Brymer JF, Lo E, Osterberger L, et al. Intracoronary fibrinolytic therapy in acute myocardial infarction: report of a prospective randomized trial. N Engl J Med 1983; 308:1305–1310.

136. Ritchie JL, Davis KB, Williams KL, Caldwell JH, Kennedy JW. Global and regional left ventricular function and tomographic radionuclide perfusion. The Western Washington intracoronary streptokinase in acute myocardial infarction trial. Circulation 1984; 70:867–875.

137. Leiboff RH, Katz RJ, Wasserman AG, Bren GB, Schwartz H, et al. A randomized angiographically controlled trial of intracoronary streptokinase in acute myocardial infarction. Am J Cardiol 1984; 53:404–407.

138. Stratton JR, Speck SM, Caldwell JH, Stadius ML, Maynard C, et al. Late effects of intracoronary streptokinase on regional wall motion, ventricular aneurysm and left ventricular thrombus in myocardial infarction. Results from the Western Washington randomized trial. J Am Coll Cardiol 1985; 5:1023–1028.

139. Krebber HJ, Schofer J, Mathey D, Montz R, Kalmar P, Rodewald G. Intracoronary thallium 201 scintigraphy as an immediate predictor of salvaged myocardium following intracoronary lysis. J Thorac Cardiovasc Surg 1984; 87:27–34.

140. Sheehan FH. Determinants of improved left ventricular function after thrombolytic therapy in acute myocardial infarction. J Am Coll Cardiol 1987; 9:937–944.

141. Rentrop KP, Feit F, Blanke H, Stecy P, Schneider R, et al. Effects of intracoronary streptokinase and intracoronary nitroglycerin infusion on coronary angiographic patterns and mortality in patients with acute myocardial infarction. N Engl J Med 1984; 311:1457–1463.

142. DeWood MA, Heit J, Spores J, Berg R, Selinger SL, et al. Anterior transmural myocardial infarction. Effects of surgical coronary reperfusion on global and left ventricular function. J Am Coll Cardiol 1983; 1:1223–1234.

143. Berg RJ, Selinger SL, Leonard JJ, Grunwald RP, O'Grady WP. Surgical management of acute myocardial infarction. In: McGoon D, ed. Cardiac Surgery. Philadelphia: F. A. Davis Company. 1982; pp 61–74.

144. Scheidt S, Ascheim R, Killip T. Shock after acute myocardial infarction: a clinical and hemodynamic profile. Am J Cardiol 1970; 26:556–564.

145. Rackley CE, Russell RO, Mantle JA, Reegers WJ. Cardiogenic shock. Cardiovasc Clin 1981; 11:15–24.

146. Goldberg RJ, Gore JM, Alpert JS, Osganian V, DeGroot J, et al. Cardiogenic shock after acute myocardial infarction. N Engl J Med 1991; 325:1117–1122.

147. Hines GL, Mohtashemi M. Delayed operative intervention in cardiogenic shock after myocardial infarction. Ann Thorac Surg 1980; 33: 132–138.
148. Hiller CD, Braunwald E. Myocardial ischemia. N Engl J Med 1977; 296:971–976.
149. Braunwald E. The aggressive treatment of acute myocardial infarction. Circulation 1985; 71:1087–1092.
150. Lee L, Erbel R, Brown TM, Laufer N, Meyer J, O'Neill WW. Multicenter registry of angioplasty therapy of cardiogenic shock: initial and long-term survival. J Am Coll Cardiol 1991; 17:559–603.
151. Dunkman WB, Leinbach RC, Buckley MJ, et al. Clinical and hemodynamic results of intraaortic balloon pumping and surgery for cardiogenic shock. Circulation 1972; 46:465–477.
152. Leinbach RC, Gold HG, Dinsmore RE, et al. The role of angiography in cardiogenic shock. Circulation 1973; 47(Pt 2):III95.
153. Braasch W, Gudbjarnason S, Puri PS, Ravens KG, Bing RJ. Early changes in energy metabolism in the myocardium following acute coronary artery occlusion in anesthetized dogs. Circ Res 1968; 23:429–438.
154. Buckberg GD. Antegrade/retrograde blood cardioplegia to ensure cardioplegic distribution: operative techniques and objectives. J Card Surg 1989; 4:216–238.
155. Drinkwater DC, Laks H, Buckberg GD. A new simplified method of optimizing cardioplegic delivery without right heart isolation. Antegrade/retrograde blood cardioplegia. J Thorac Cardiovasc Surg 1990; 100:56–64.
156. Partington MT, Acar C, Buckberg GD, Julia PL. Studies of retrograde cardioplegia. II. Advantages of antegrade/retrograde cardioplegia to optimize distribution in jeopardized myocardium. J Thorac Cardiovasc Surg 1989; 97:613–622.
157. Masuda M, Yonenaga K, Shiki K, et al. Myocardial protection in coronary occlusion by retrograde cardioplegic perfusion via the coronary sinus in dogs. J Thorac Cardiovasc Surg 1986; 92:255–263.
158. Flameng W, Sergeant P, Vanhaecke J, Suy R. Emergency coronary bypass grafting for evolving myocardial infarction: effects on infarct size and left ventricular function. J Thorac Cardiovasc Surg 1987; 94:124–131.
159. Buckberg GD, Brazier JR, Nelson RL, Goldstein SM, McConnell DH, Cooper N. Studies of the effect of hypothermia on regional myocardial blood flow and metabolism during cardiopulmonary bypass. I. The adequate perfused beating, fibrillating and arrested heart. J Thorac Cardiovasc Surg 1977; 73:87–94.
160. Allen BS, Rosenkranz E, Buckberg GD, Davtyan H, Laks H, et al. Studies on prolonged acute regional ischemia. VI. Myocardial infarction with left ventricular power failure: a medical/surgical emergency requiring urgent revascularization with maximal protection of remote muscle. J Thorac Cardiovasc Surg 1989; 98:691–703.
161. Schuster EH, Buckley BH. Ischemia at a distance after acute myocar-

dial infarction: a cause of early postinfarction angina. Circulation 1980; 62:509–515.

162. Killip T III, Kimball JT. Treatment of myocardial infarction in a coronary care unit: a two-year experience with 250 patients. Am J Cardiol 1967; 20:457–464.

163. Binder MJ, Ryan JA, Marcus S, Mugler T, Strange D, Agress CM. Evaluation of therapy in shock following acute myocardial infarction. Am J Med 1955; 18:622–632.

Chapter 6

Emergency Coronary Artery Bypass Graft Surgery After Failed Percutaneous Transluminal Coronary Angioplasty

Harold L. Lazar

Introduction

Percutaneous transluminal coronary angioplasty (PTCA) has emerged as an alternative method of revascularization to coronary artery bypass grafting (CABG) in the treatment of ischemic myocardial syndromes.[1] Despite improvements in catheter design and angioplasty techniques, it is estimated that 5% of patients undergoing PTCA will develop an occlusion, dissection, or perforation of a coronary vessel resulting in myocardial ischemia unresponsive to medical management.[2,3] Emergent CABG has been demonstrated to be the accepted therapy for patients with acute ischemia after a failed PTCA.[2,4–6] As the number of patients undergoing PTCA

Lazar HL (editor): *Current Therapy for Acute Coronary Ischemia,* © Futura Publishing Co., Inc., Mount Kisco, NY, 1993.

continues to increase, more emergency CABG procedures will be performed when acute ischemia develops after an unsuccessful PTCA.

Emergent CABG surgery for a failed PTCA has resulted in a unique population of patients posing both technical and logistical problems for cardiac surgeons. Unlike patients undergoing CABG for unstable angina, it is estimated that 40% of these patients will develop a perioperative myocardial infarct despite prompt and expeditious surgical revascularization.[2] In addition, the surgeon must contend with mechanical trauma to the vessel being grafted, including dissection and perforation. This chapter reviews the Boston University Medical Center's experience with emergent CABG after an unsuccessful PTCA as well as the experience of other centers. In addition to documenting the profiles and clinical outcomes of these patients, those factors responsible for perioperative myocardial necrosis and the effects of changing risk factors also are reviewed.

Management of Failed PTCA Patients at the Boston University Medical Center

From March 1980 through December 1988, 2900 PTCAs were performed at the Boston University Medical Center. In 53 (1.8%) of these patients, an emergent CABG was required because of acute myocardial ischemia during or immediately after the PTCA. During this period, standard protocols were established for surgical support of all PTCA procedures. All patients were prepared for surgery the night before their PTCA and were seen in consultation by a member of the surgical team. From 1980 to 1986, a specific operating room was made available during all PTCA procedures for possible surgical intervention. This was supplemented by teams of nurses, surgeons, perfusionists, and anesthesiologists on call for PTCA backup. In 1987, this policy was changed such that all CABG procedures performed following an unsuccessful PTCA followed in the next available operating room. Since all operating rooms were capable of supporting cardiopulmonary bypass equipment, all rooms in the operating suite could be used even when the designated "heart rooms" were being used.

Acute myocardial ischemia during or after PTCA was evaluated immediately by coronary angiography. Patients with ischemia were treated by a variety of methods including sublingual, intravenous, and intracoronary administration of nitroglycerin, sublingual administration of nifedipine, repeat angioplasty, and intracoronary infusion of thrombolytic agents. Patients with hemodynamic instability and ongoing ischemia despite maximal medical management received an intra-aortic balloon pump (IABP). In 1987, reperfusion catheters became available at the Boston University Medical Center to establish temporary reperfusion to areas of the myocardium distal to the occlusion.[7] These were inserted whenever technically possible in the presence of a total occlusion and were removed during CABG. Percutaneous bypass techniques were instituted in 1989 and were not used in any of the patients in this series. A coronary occlusion during PTCA was defined as a vessel that became occluded during the PTCA and that remained occluded at the end of cardiac catheterization. If the PTCA was unsuccessful but the patient remained pain free, or if the lesion could not be crossed without any change in clinical symptoms, CABG was performed on an elective date. These patients were not included in this study. Myocardial ischemia that was refractory to medical management with an inadequate angioplasty outcome resulted in emergent CABG.

Patients were rapidly transported to the operating room, cannulated, and placed on cardiopulmonary bypass. The decision to use an internal mammary artery (IMA) graft was based on the coronary anatomy, segmental wall motion of the region being grafted, and the hemodynamic stability of the patient. A variety of cold blood and crystalloid cardioplegic solutions were employed as well as antegrade and retrograde delivery systems supplemented with topical and systemic hypothermia. All vessels with at least a 50% lesion were bypassed. All distal anastomoses were performed during one period of ischemic arrest with the anastomosis to the vessel involved during the PTCA performed first. Cardioplegic solution was given down each vein graft after the completion of each distal anastomosis. The time to revascularization was defined as that period from the start of coronary occlusion in the cath lab to the restoration of blood through all the completed bypass grafts in the operating room. A perioperative myocardial infarction was diagnosed either by the appearance of new electrocardiogram (ECG) changes using the Minnesota Code or by the elevation of the myocardial fractions of creatine kinase (CK-MB) to >50 IU in the immediate 24-hour period after surgery.

Statistical analysis was performed using chi-square testing, nonpaired Student's t tests, and Wilcoxon Nonparametric tests. All data presented represents the mean ± standard error and was considered significant when p values were < 0.05.

Emergent CABG After Unsuccessful PTCA

Patient Profiles

The results of patients undergoing emergent CABG at the Boston University Medical Center from 1980 through 1988 are summarized in Tables 1 through 9. The profiles of these patients are displayed in Table 1. The mean age of the 53 patients in this series was 60 ± 2 years, although 34% were 65 years and older. There were twice as many men as women and 60% had unstable angina at the time of their PTCA. The mean ejection fraction before PTCA was 56 ± 3% and none of the patients were in congestive heart failure.

Table 1

Emergent CABG After Unsuccessful PTCA: 1980–1988 Patient Profiles

Variable	
Number	53 (1.8%)
Mean age*	60 ± 2
Age > 65	18 (34%)
Men/women	35/18
Unstable angina	32 (60%)
Hypertension	19 (36%)
Congestive heart failure	0 (0%)
Diabetes	7 (13%)
EF*·†	56 ± 3%

*Data represented as mean ± the standard error.
†Ejection fraction was based on preoperative ventriculograms.
CABG = coronary artery bypass graft; PTCA = percutaneous transluminal coronary angioplasty; EF = ejection fraction.

PTCA and Catheterization Profiles

In this series (Table 2), the mean number of vessels that had at least a 50% stenosis was 2.0 ± 0.1. A multivessel PTCA was attempted in eight patients (15%). The most common type of PTCA complication was a coronary occlusion, which occurred in 22 patients (42%). Dissections occurred in 15 patients (28%) and 16 patients (30%) had a combination of occlusions and dissections. A successful insertion of a reperfusion catheter was possible in seven patients (13%). An IABP was inserted in 43 patients (81%) and 10 patients (19%) also required some form of inotropic support in the catheterization laboratory after their PTCA. ECG changes were noted in 27 patients (51%) after their unsuccessful PTCA, of which 22 patients ultimately went on to have a perioperative myocardial infarction by either enzyme or ECG criteria.

Operative Data

Nineteen patients (36%) in this series had a single-vessel CABG, whereas 34 patients (64%) had a multivessel CABG (see Table 3). The mean number of vessels bypassed was 2.0 ± 0.1 and 15 patients (28%) received an IMA graft. The crossclamp time was 36.0 ± 2.2 minutes and the mean total time to revascularization was 160 ± 6 minutes.

Table 2

Emergent CABG After Unsuccessful PTCA: 1980–1988 PTCA and Catheterization Profiles

Variable		
Vessels with ≥50% stenosis*	2.0 ± 0.1	
Multivessel PTCA	8	(15%)
Coronary occlusion	22	(42%)
Coronary dissection	15	(28%)
Coronary occlusion and dissection	16	(30%)
Insertion of reperfusion catheter	7	(13%)
Preoperative IABP	43	(81%)
Inotropic support after PTCA	10	(19%)
ECG changes after PTCA	27	(51%)

*Data represented as mean ± the standard error.
PTCA = percutaneous transluminal coronary angioplasty; CABG = coronary artery bypass grafting; IABP = intra-aortic balloon pump; ECG = electrocardiogram.

Table 3

Emergent CABG After Unsuccessful PTCA: 1980–1988 Operative Data

Variable	
Mean number of vessels bypassed*	2.0 ± 0.1
Single-vessel CABG	19 (36%)
Multivessel CABG	34 (64%)
Crossclamp time (min)*	36 ± 2
Time to revascularization (min)*	160 ± 6
IMA	15 (28%)

*Data represented as mean ± the standard error.
CABG = coronary artery bypass graft; PTCA = percutaneous transluminal coronary angioplasty; IMA = internal mammary artery.

Surgical Results

The 30-day operative mortality in this series was 11% (see Table 4). Of the six deaths, two were noncardiac related. One patient was a Child's Class "C" cirrhotic who developed hepatic failure postoperatively and died of sepsis and multiorgan failure. Another patient sustained a massive cerebrovascular accident (CVA) and never regained consciousness. All four cardiac-related deaths had cardiac arrests in the catheterization laboratory and were brought to the operating room on large doses of inotropes, an IABP, and in cardiogenic shock. There was evidence for a perioperative myocardial infarction in 29 patients (55%). Of these 29 patients, 20 had evidence of both enzyme elevations and ECG changes. Major complications occurred in nine patients (17%), which included hemorrhage requiring reoperation (four), respiratory insufficiency requiring prolonged intubation (one), sternal infections (three), and a CVA (one).

Changing Profiles of Failed PTCA Patients: Impact on Surgical Results

In 1979, the National Heart, Lung, and Blood Institute established a registry for PTCA patients to evaluate the safety and efficacy of this technique.[3] In 1985, the registry was reopened to

Table 4

Emergent CABG After Unsuccessful PTCA: 1980–1988 Surgical Results

Variable		
30-day mortality	6	(11%)
Cardiac-related mortality	4	
Major complications	9	(17%)
Hemorrhage	4	
Respiratory insufficiency	1	
Sternal infection	3	
CVA	1	
Myocardial infarction	29	(55%)
Enzyme elevation	9	(17%)
Enzyme elevations and ECG changes	20	(38%)

CABG = coronary artery bypass graft; PTCA = percutaneous transluminal coronary angioplasty; CVA = cerebrovascular accident; ECG = electrocardiogram.

document changes in angioplasty strategies and outcomes.[8] This study compared patients undergoing PTCAs in the period 1985–1986 with the earlier registry patients from 1977 to 1981. Patients undergoing PTCA in 1985–1986 were older and had a higher incidence of unstable angina, a significantly higher proportion of multivessel disease, poorer left ventricular (LV) function, and a higher incidence of previous myocardial infarctions. These patients also had more complex coronary lesions and more multilesion angioplasties. As more of these high-risk patients undergo PTCA, the changing profiles of angioplasty patients who might require emergent CABG surgery after a failed PTCA may alter operative morbidity and mortality. To study this issue further, the patients in this series were divided into two groups based on the year of their PTCA. Group I comprised 18 patients who required emergent CABG after a failed PTCA in the years 1980 to 1985. Group II consisted of 35 patients requiring an emergent CABG in the years 1986 to 1988. The results are summarized in Tables 5 through 8.

Table 5 reviews the patient profiles of the two groups. The incidence of emergent CABG after a failed PTCA was similar for both groups (2.1% Group I vs. 1.9% Group II; NS). Although there was no significant difference in mean age between the groups, Group II had a significantly higher percentage of patients >65 years (46%

Table 5

Patient Profiles

Variable	Group I: 1980–1985	Group II: 1986–1988	p Value
Number	18 (2.1%)	35 (1.9%)	—
Mean age*	58 ± 2	61 ± 2	NS
Age ≥65	2 (11%)	16 (46%)	<0.03
Men/women	12/6	23/12	NS
Unstable angina	6 (33%)	26 (74%)	<0.004
Hypertension	5 (28%)	14 (40%)	NS
Congestive heart failure	0 (0%)	0 (0%)	NS
Diabetes	2 (11%)	5 (14%)	NS
EF (%)*,†	63 ± 5	53 ± 2	<0.05

*Data represented as mean ± the standard error.
†Ejection fraction was based on preoperative ventriculograms.
NS = not significant; EF = ejection fraction.

vs. 11%; $p<0.03$). Group II patients also tended to have more symptomatic coronary disease as seen by a significantly higher percentage of patients with unstable angina (75% vs. 33%; $p<0.004$). The incidence of risk factors such as hypertension, congestive heart failure, and diabetes was similar in both groups. Group II patients, however, did have significantly lower ejection fractions on their preoperative ventriculogram (53 ± 2% vs. 63 ± 5%; $p<0.05$).

The PTCA and catheterization profiles are listed in Table 6. Group II patients had a significantly greater number of vessels with ≥50% stenosis (2.1 ± 0.2 vs. 1.6 ± 0.2; $p<0.05$); however, the incidence of attempted multivessel PTCAs was similar in both groups. PTCA failures were more likely to result from coronary occlusion in Group II patients (54% vs. 22%; $p<0.05$), whereas Group I patients were more likely to have a combination of occlusion and dissections (55% vs. 17%; $p<0.05$). None of the patients in Group I had the insertion of a reperfusion catheter, whereas this device was used in seven patients in Group II (20%; $p<0.05$ from Group I). The incidence of insertion of a preoperative IABP, the need for inotropic support in the catheterization laboratory, and the presence of ECG changes after the unsuccessful PTCA were not significantly different between the two groups.

Table 6

PTCA and Catheterization Profiles

Variable	Group I: 1980–1985		Group II: 1986–1988		p Value
Number	18		35		—
Vessels with ≥50% stenosis*	1.6 ± 0.2		2.1 ± 0.2		<0.05
Multivessel PTCA	3	(17%)	5	(14%)	NS
Coronary occlusion	4	(22%)	18	(54%)	<0.05
Coronary dissection	4	(22%)	11	(31%)	NS
Coronary occlusion and dissection	10	(55%)	6	(17%)	<0.05
Insertion of reperfusion catheter	0	(0%)	7	(20%)	<0.05
Preoperative IABP	16	(80%)	27	(70%)	NS
Inotropic support after PTCA	2	(11%)	8	(23%)	NS
ECG changes after PTCA	10	(56%)	17	(49%)	NS

*Data represented as mean ± the standard error.
NS = not significant; PTCA = percutaneous transluminal coronary angioplasty; IABP = intra-aortic balloon pump; ECG = electrocardiogram.

Table 7 reviews the results of the intraoperative data. The mean number of vessels bypassed, the incidence of multivessel CABG, and the crossclamp times were not significantly different between Group I and Group II patients. The time to revascularization was, however, more prolonged for patients in Group II (144 ± 5 min vs. 168 ± 8 min; $p<0.02$). The IMA was used more frequently for grafting in Group II patients (40% vs. 6%; $p<0.008$).

The surgical outcomes are listed in Table 8. Thirty-day operative mortality was identical in both groups (11% vs. 11%; NS) and the incidence of major complications was not statistically different (22% Group I vs. 14% Group II; NS). The patterns and incidence of myocardial infarctions also was not statistically different between the two groups.

Table 7

Operative Data

Variable	Group I: 1980–1985	Group II: 1986–1988	p Value
Number	18	35	—
Mean number of vessels bypassed*	1.7 ± 0.5	2.1 ± 0.1	NS
Single-vessel CABG	9 (50%)	10 (28%)	NS
Multivessel CABG	9 (50%)	25 (72%)	NS
Crossclamp time (min)*	33.8 ± 3.7	36.4 ± 3.2	NS
Time to revascularization (min)*	144 ± 0.5	168 ± 8	<0.02
IMA	1 (6%)	14 (40%)	<0.008

*Data represented as mean ± the standard error.
CABG = coronary artery bypass graft; IMA = internal mammary artery.

Table 8

Surgical Results

Variable	Group I: 1980–1985		Group II: 1986–1988		p Value
Number	18		35		—
30-day mortality	2	(11%)	4	(11%)	NS
Cardiac related	1		3		NS
Major complications	4	(22%)	5	(14%)	NS
Hemorrhage	2		2		NS
Respiratory insufficiency	1		0		NS
Sternal infection	1		2		NS
CVA	0		1		NS
Myocardial infarction	12	(67%)	17	(49%)	NS
Enzyme elevation	5	(28%)	4	(11%)	NS
Enzyme elevation and ECG changes	7	(39%)	13	(37%)	NS

NS = not significant; CVA = cerebrovascular accident; ECG = electrocardiogram.

Risk Factors Associated with Myocardial Necrosis After Emergent CABG for a Failed PTCA

In addition to reviewing the effects of changing patient profiles in surgical outcomes after a failed PTCA, a univariate analysis also was performed to identify those risk factors associated with a perioperative myocardial infarction. These are summarized in Table 9. There was no significant difference in mean age between the two groups; however, there was a significantly higher incidence of women in the myocardial infarction group. Although there was no significant difference in the incidence of unstable angina or preoperative ejection fractions between the groups, patients who developed myocardial infarction had significantly more coronary vessels that had lesions with greater than 50% stenosis (2.0 ± 0.1; $p<0.05$). The particular vessel dilated and type of injury (occlusion vs. dissection) did not determine the incidence of perioperative infarctions. However, patients in whom a multivessel PTCA was attempted had a significantly higher incidence of myocardial infarction (28% vs. 9%; $p<0.01$). The presence of ECG changes after a failed PTCA and the need for inotropic support were significantly higher in those patients who developed a perioperative myocardial infarction. In this series, neither the insertion of an IABP nor a reperfusion catheter decreased the incidence of preoperative myocardial necrosis. In addition, the time to revascularization was not statistically significant between the two groups.

Discussion

Although the incidence of emergency CABG after a failed PTCA is relatively low, averaging between 3% and 5% in most series, these patients provide unique technical, logistical, and management problems for the cardiac surgeon.[2] Recent and evolving changes in the practice of cardiology, emphasizing PTCA for multivessel disease and extending periods of medical therapy, have resulted in significant changes in the profiles of patients now presenting for medical and surgical revascularization.[8,9] The changing profiles of our most recent failed PTCA patients (Group II: 1986–1988) were similar to those seen in the recent national PTCA registry study.[8] A higher percentage of these patients were older than 65 years and had

Table 9

Risk Factors Associated with Myocardial Necrosis After Emergent CABG for Failed PTCA

Variable	MI Group		No MI Group		p Value
Number	29		24		—
Mean age*	61 ± 2		59 ± 2		NS
Men/women	16/13		19/5		<0.05
Unstable angina	15	(52%)	11	(46%)	NS
Vessels with ≥50% stenosis*	2.0 ± 0.1		1.2 ± 0.1		<0.05
Preoperative EF*,†	54 ± 2		59 ± 4		NS
Multivessel PTCA	8	(28%)	0	(0%)	<0.01
LAD dilatation	17	(58%)	11	(46%)	NS
RCA dilatation	6	(21%)	7	(29%)	NS
CX dilatation	6	(21%)	6	(25%)	NS
Coronary occlusion	10	(34%)	12	(50%)	NS
Coronary dissection	8	(28%)	7	(29%)	NS
Coronary occlusion and dissection	11	(38%)	5	(21%)	NS
ECG changes after PTCA	22	(76%)	5	(21%)	<0.02
Preoperative IABP	26	(90%)	17	(71%)	NS
Preoperative inotropic support	9	(31%)	1	(4%)	<0.01
Insertion of reperfusion catheter	3	(10%)	4	(17%)	NS
Time to revascularization (min)	148 ± 8		164 ± 8		NS
IMA	6	(21%)	9	(38%)	NS

*Data represented as mean ± the standard error.
†Ejection fraction was based on preoperative ventriculogram.
NS = not significant; PTCA = percutaneous transluminal coronary angioplasty; MI = myocardial infarction; EF = ejection fraction; LAD = left anterior descending artery; RCA = right coronary artery; CX = circumflex artery; IABP = intra-aortic balloon pump; ECG = electrocardiogram; IMA = internal mammary artery.

a significantly higher incidence of unstable angina, their preoperative ejection fractions were lower, and they had more extensive coronary disease. Despite the more complex and extensive coronary lesions, the incidence of unsuccessful PTCAs was only 1.9%, which reflects improvements in catheter designs, angioplasty techniques, and the skills of the interventional cardiologists.

The most common indication for proceeding to CABG emergently after a PTCA was the presence of refractory ischemia associated with a coronary occlusion or dissection. Other indications include perforated arteries associated with tamponade, broken guidewires trapped in the distal vessel, and persistent ventricular arrhythmias.[2,6] It is important to note that the Boston University series includes only patients who went directly to the operating room from the catheterization laboratory because of either pain or ECG changes associated with an anatomical problem as a result of the PTCA. This is opposed to other series where the indications included patients in whom the lesion could not be crossed or the desired decrease in the diameter of the lesion was not obtained.[2,6] Many of these patients had no evidence of ischemic changes and this may explain the higher incidence of ECG changes and IABP insertions in the Boston University series. Certain lesions are more likely to result in failed anoplasties. In a recent multicenter review, Cowley and his associates found that eccentric lesions, nondiscrete lesions, and lesions with ≥90 stenosis were more likely to result in a failed PTCA leading to an emergent CABG.[6] In addition, they found that the incidence of emergent CABG declined with the increasing experience of the individual performing the PTCA.

Once coronary blood flow is interrupted after a failed PTCA, time becomes a critical factor in determining how much myocardium can be salvaged. Experimental studies in a canine model and clinical experience with intracoronary thrombolysis in patients with an acute myocardial infarction demonstrated salvage of ischemic myocardium when coronary reperfusion was achieved in less than 4 hours after the onset of ischemia.[10,11] The average time to revascularization in the Boston University series was 160 minutes. Revascularization time has ranged from 142 to 180 minutes in other series.[2,4,5] Although the time to revascularization was significantly longer in Group II patients in our series, the incidence of myocardial infarction was not significantly different. This is consistent with our findings that time to revascularization was not a univariate risk factor for the presence of perioperative myocardial necrosis and is in agreement with the findings of Murphy et al. and Pelletier et al.[4,5] The longer time to revascularization in the Group II patients may be reflective of our change in operating room standby policy adapted in 1987 where emergent CABGs after a failed PTCA were triaged to the next available operating room. The fact that the mean difference between the two groups was only 24 minutes and that this "delay" resulted in no further increase in mortality or infarct rate tends to support the "next available room" backup system provided that there is close communication between the catheterization laboratory and the operating room.[12]

The emergent CABG after a failed PTCA poses certain unique technical problems for the surgeon. In recent years, the incidence of multivessel disease has increased in patients with failed PTCA requiring emergent CABG. Hence, a multivessel CABG usually is required. At the Boston University Medical Center, we have made every attempt to utilize the IMA and, like Ferguson and his co-workers, have not found it to be a risk factor for perioperative myocardial necrosis.[13] Saphenous veins alone have been used only for distal obtuse marginal, posterolateral and posterior descending vessels, and in the presence of cardiogenic shock. We have left the reperfusion catheter in the angioplasty vessel during cardiopulmonary bypass. Some surgeons have found it useful to deliver cardioplegia through the catheter so that the area of risk is perfused and to define the proper vessel lumen in the presence of a dissection.[14] The important principles of myocardial protection in these patients include grafting the vessel at risk first and ensuring that the graft is perfused with cardioplegic solution as soon as possible. We have used blood cardioplegia, which is administered through the completed vein graft or through a retrograde cardioplegia catheter when an IMA graft is used. Occasionally, the dissection will extend throughout the course of the vessel to be grafted. Helpful technical maneuvers to ensure that the proper lumen is grafted include retroperfusion with cardioplegia and perfusion through the reperfusion catheter if it is available. In general, we keep these patients on lidocaine and intravenous nitroglycerin for the first 12 postoperative hours to decrease the incidence of malignant arrhythmias.

The 30-day operative mortality in this series was 11% and remained constant despite the increased incidence of risk factors in the Group II patients. Of the six deaths in this series, four occurred in patients who were in cardiogenic shock after their failed PTCA. In a recent review, Cameron et al. noted that the average operative mortality in the literature for these patients was 6.4%, with a range of 0% to 12%.[12] In our series, we have not included those patients in whom a PTCA was not attempted for technical reasons or in whom a guidewire could not be inserted across the lesion. These patients remained stable without ischemia and underwent CABG on an elective basis. In addition, we also have included patients who underwent PTCA on an emergent basis for postinfarction angina. The occlusion and inclusion of these patient groups may have accounted for our higher mortality rate. Major complications excluding myocardial infarction occurred in 17% of our patients compared to a range of 10% to 50% reported by other authors.[2,4,15-17]

The most common complication in these patients was the development of a perioperative infarction. In our series, 55% of the patients had some evidence of myocardial necrosis but only 38% had ECG changes and enzyme elevations to document an infarct. Perioperative infarct rates have ranged from 18% to 63% with an average of 40% in the literature.[2,4-6,13,15-18] In our series, women tended to have a higher infarct rate than men, which may reflect the smaller caliber of coronary vessels in women and the more diffuse nature of their disease. As in other series, we found that patients who developed a perioperative myocardial infarction had a higher incidence of multivessel disease and attempted multivessel PTCA.[2,15] One possible explanation for this finding is that the presence of partial stenosis in other vessels may limit the amount of collateral flow to the ischemic myocardium. As in other series, the particular vessel dilated, and the nature of the injury (occlusion vs. dissection) did not predict the development of a perioperative myocardial infarction.[2] A significant predictor of the development of myocardial infarction was the presence of ECG changes after the failed PTCA.[4] Although the IABP had been noted to decrease the incidence of Q-wave infarcts in some series, we could not demonstrate a decrease in the incidence of myocardial necrosis with the IABP in our patients.[4,18] Similarly, we found that in the seven patients in whom reperfusion catheters were inserted in this study, three went on to develop myocardial infarction as evidenced by ECG and enzyme changes. These findings are similar to those of Douglas and his colleagues, who failed to show any difference in the frequency of Q-wave infarcts and peak CPK-MB levels in patients with reperfusion catheters.[19] Nevertheless, Ferguson and associates found that these catheters helped to reverse the ECG changes seen after a failed PTCA and reduced the incidence of myocardial necrosis.[14] Despite our findings, we continue to advocate the use of the IABP and reperfusion catheters in the face of ongoing ischemia after a failed PTCA. Our current methods of determining myocardial necrosis may not accurately reflect the true size of the infarct. There is evidence that the higher levels of CK-MB seen in CABG patients after a failed PTCA actually may reflect better washout of previously underperfused areas of the myocardium, thus leading to an overestimation of the actual infarct size.[20]

Conclusion

Although improvements in catheter design and angioplasty techniques have reduced the incidence of PTCA complications, it is estimated that 5% of all patients undergoing PTCA will require emergency CABG for acute myocardial ischemia. Urgent surgical revascularization is the accepted therapy for the patient with acute ischemia after a failed PTCA. Despite prompt surgical revascularization, these patients continue to have mortality and infarct rates that are significantly higher than for elective revascularization. Variables that predispose to a perioperative myocardial infarction in these patients include female gender, multivessel PTCA, the presence of multiple vessels with at least 50% stenoses, and the presence of new ECG changes immediately after the failed PTCA. The development of cardiac shock in the catheterization laboratory increases operative mortality. Despite the changing profiles of patients undergoing PTCA, which reveal older patients with more extensive coronary artery disease and lower ejection fractions, operative results remain unchanged. The next chapter examines the therapeutic interventions and strategies being developed to attempt to decrease the morbidity and mortality in these patients requiring emergent surgical revascularization after acute coronary ischemia.

References

1. Gruentzig A, Senning A, Siegenthaler W. Non-operative dilatation of coronary artery stenosis: percutaneous transluminal coronary angioplasty (PTCA). N Engl J Med 1979; 301:61–68.
2. Greene MA, Gray LA, Slater AD, Ganzel BL, Mavroudis C. Emergency aortocoronary bypass after failed angioplasty. Ann Thorac Surg 1991; 51:194–199.
3. Detre KM, Myler RK, Kelsey SF, Van Raden M, To T, Mitchell H. Baseline characteristics of patients in the National Heart, Lung, and Blood Institute Percutaneous Transluminal Coronary Angioplasty Registry. Am J Cardiol 1984; 53:7–11.
4. Murphy DA, Craver JM, Jones EL, et al. Surgical management of acute myocardial ischemia following percutaneous transluminal coronary angioplasty: role of the intra-aortic balloon pump. J Thorac Cardiovasc Surg 1984; 87:332–339.
5. Pelletier LC, Pardini A, Renkin J, et al. Myocardial revascularization

after failure of percutaneous transluminal coronary angioplasty. J Thorac Cardiovasc Surg 1985; 90:265–271.

6. Cowley MJ, Dorros G, Kelsey SF, Raden MV, Detre KM. Emergency coronary bypass surgery after coronary angioplasty: the National Heart, Lung, and Blood Institute's percutaneous transluminal coronary angioplasty registry experience. Am J Cardiol 1984; 53:22C–26C.

7. Hinohara, T, Simpson JB, Phillips HR, et al. Transluminal catheter reperfusion: a new technique to re-establish blood flow after coronary occlusion during percutaneous transluminal coronary angioplasty. Am J Cardiol 1986; 57:684–686.

8. Detre K, Holubkov R, Kelsey S, et al. Percutaneous transluminal coronary angioplasty in 1985–1986 and 1977–1981. N Engl J Med 1988; 318:265–270.

9. Jones EL, Weintraub WS, Craver JM, Guyton A, Cohen CL. Coronary bypass surgery: is the operation different today? J Thorac Cardiovasc Surg 1991; 101:108–115.

10. Reimer KA, Lowe JE, Rasmussen MM, Jennings RB. The wave-front phenomenon of ischemic cell death: I. Myocardial infarct size vs duration of coronary occlusion in dogs. Circulation 1977; 56:786–791.

11. Anderson JL, Marshall HW, Bray BE, et al. A randomized trial of intracoronary streptokinase in the treatment of acute myocardial infarction. N Engl J Med 1983; 308:1312–1317.

12. Cameron DE, Stinson DC, Greene PS, Gardner TJ. Surgical standby for percutaneous transluminal coronary angioplasty: a survey of patterns of practice. Ann Thorac Surg 1990; 50:35–39.

13. Ferguson TB, Muhlbaier LH, Salai DL, Wechsler AS. Coronary bypass grafting after failed elective and failed emergent percutaneous angioplasty. J Thorac Cardiovasc Surg 1988; 95:761–772.

14. Ferguson TB, Hinohara T, Simpson J, Stack RS, Wechsler AS. Catheter reperfusion to allow optimal coronary bypass grafting following failed transluminal coronary angioplasty. Ann Thorac Surg 1986; 42:399–405.

15. Golding LA, Loop FD, Hollman JL, et al. Early results of emergency surgery after coronary angioplasty. Circulation 1986; 74(Suppl 3):26–29.

16. Brahos GJ, Baker NH, Ewy GG, et al. Aortocoronary bypass following unsuccessful PTCA: experience in 100 consecutive patients. Ann Thorac Surg 1985; 40:7–10.

17. Parsonnet V, Fisch D, Gielchinsky I, et al. Emergency operation after failed angioplasty. J Thorac Cardiovasc Surg 1988; 96:198–203.

18. Alcan KE, Stertzer SH, Wallsh E, DePasquale NP, Bruno MS. The role of intra-aortic balloon counterpulsation in patients undergoing percutaneous transluminal coronary angioplasty. Am Heart J 1983; 105:527–530.

19. Douglas JS, King SB, Roubin GS, et al. Efficacy of coronary artery perfusion catheters in patients with failed angioplasty and acute myocardial ischemia. J Am Coll Cardiol 1987; 9:105A.

20. Jarmakani JM, Limbard L, Graham TC, Marks RA. Effect of reperfusion on myocardial infarct and the accuracy of estimating infarct size from serum creatinine phosphokinase in the dog. Cardiovasc Res 1976; 10:245–252.

Chapter 7

Methods of Reducing Myocardial Necrosis After Failed Percutaneous Transluminal Coronary Angioplasty in Patients Undergoing Emergent Coronary Artery Bypass Surgery

Harold L. Lazar

Introduction

As noted in the previous chapter, despite prompt and expedient surgical revascularization, acute coronary ischemia after a failed percutaneous transluminal coronary angioplasty (PTCA) results in significant myocardial ischemia and necrosis. In most series reviewed, 50% of all patients will have some evidence of myocardial

Lazar HL (editor): *Current Therapy for Acute Coronary Ischemia,* © Futura Publishing Co., Inc., Mount Kisco, NY, 1993.

necrosis by either electrocardiographic (ECG) or enzyme criteria.[1–3] The presence of new ECG changes and the need for inotropic support immediately after coronary occlusion in the catheterization laboratory have emerged as factors that predispose to a perioperative infarction.[1–3] This suggests that strategies aimed at reducing myocardial necrosis after a failed PTCA must begin immediately after coronary occlusion in the catheterization laboratory. If the surgeon or cardiologist waits to reverse this ischemic damage by interventions during the periods of cardioplegic arrest and reperfusion, much of this damage may be irreversible. This chapter reviews the interventions that can be performed by both cardiologists and surgeons in the catheterization laboratory immediately after a failed PTCA to help decrease myocardial necrosis.

When the clinician is confronted with acute coronary ischemia after a failed PTCA, there are several treatment strategies that can be employed (Table 1). Systemic medications may be given to more favorably alter the myocardial supply-demand balance. Coronary blood flow may be increased by antegrade coronary arterial or retrograde coronary venous techniques. Myocardial energy demands may be reduced by devices that either partially or totally support the circulation. Finally, combinations of techniques that work on various aspects of the supply-demand equation may be used to decrease myocardial necrosis. Each of these interventions has its own advantages and disadvantages and its use may be limited by anatomical factors. The clinician must rapidly assess the etiology of the ischemia, the anatomical severity of the underlying lesions, and its effect on the overall ventricular function before deciding which technique will work best for the patient.

Systemic Medical Management

The least invasive method of reducing ischemic damage is systemic medical management. This involves the intravenous and intracoronary administration of nitroglycerin, inderal, and calcium channel blockers. While some patients may respond rapidly to these pharmacological agents, the results after a failed PTCA are not as predictable as for patients with unstable angina in a coronary care unit (CCU) setting.[4] Nevertheless, the ease by which these agents

Table 1

Methods of Reducing Myocardial Necrosis After a Failed PTCA in Preparation for Emergent CABG

Systemic Medical Management
Intravenous or intracoronary
    Nitroglycerin
    Inderal
    Calcium channel blockers
L-glutamate
Methods to Increase Coronary Blood Flow
Antegrade coronary perfusion
    "Bailout" catheters
    Autoperfusion dilatation catheters
    Stents
Retrograde coronary sinus perfusion
    SRP
    PICSO
Reduction of Myocardial Demands and Circulatory Support
    IABP
    PB
    Nimbus hemopump
    Percutaneous left heart bypass
Combination of Techniques to Increase Supply and Decrease Demands
    IABP + PB
    IABP + PICSO
    PICSO + PB

PTCA = percutaneous transluminal coronary angioplasty; CABG = coronary artery bypass grafting; SRP = synchronized retroperfusion; PICSO = pressure-controlled intermittent coronary sinus occlusion; IABP = intra-aortic balloon pump; PB = percutaneous bypass.

can be administered make them the initial intervention of choice. Recent experimental evidence also has shown that the intravenous administration of the amino acid L-glutamate during a period of left anterior descending artery (LAD) occlusion also may decrease infarct size.[5] Substrate enhancement with L-glutamate is thought to replenish Krebs' cycle intermediates lost during ischemia, thus increasing high energy phosphate levels. These reactions take time and while ultimately decreasing the extent of myocardial necrosis, L-glutamate does not acutely reverse the ischemic process and has no immediate effect on ventricular performance.

Methods to Increase Coronary Blood Flow

Current methods available to increase coronary blood flow after a failed PTCA may be done antegrade through the coronary artery or retrograde through the coronary sinus.

Antegrade Coronary Perfusion

Antegrade coronary perfusion techniques employ catheters that restore arterial blood flow to the distal ischemic myocardium. The "bailout catheter" consists of a 4.3F coronary infusion catheter with multiple proximal and distal side holes. It can provide up to 80 ml/min of passive blood flow across the coronary stenosis. In experimental studies involving LAD occlusions in dogs, these "bailout" catheters have restored nearly 70% of coronary flow to the ischemic myocardium with minimal necrosis.[6] The "bailout" catheter was designed to provide some distal perfusion during the time necessary to perform emergency bypass surgery.[7] The use of this catheter in clinical practice has had mixed results. In a nonrandomized study involving 31 patients with abrupt closure after a PTCA, Sundram and his co-workers were able to place a "bailout" catheter in 61% of the patients attempted.[8] This resulted in a significant decrease in Q-wave infarcts from 75% to 9%. In the Boston University series, we could not demonstrate a decrease in the incidence of myocardial necrosis using "bailout" catheters.[1] Similar results were obtained by Murphy and his colleagues.[9] A newer technique of antegrade perfusion employs the "perfusion balloon dilatation catheter." This 4.5F catheter consists of a 20-mm balloon and 10 proximal and 4 distal side holes. The catheter is advanced across the stenosis and the central guidewire is withdrawn to a position just proximal to the side holes. When the balloon is inflated, blood enters the proximal side holes, flows through the central lumen, and leaves the catheter beyond the coronary stenosis. Unlike the bailout catheter, this catheter not only provides antegrade coronary perfusion but also allows for additional dilation of the lesion. There is some experimental evidence to suggest that this catheter results in better perfusion than the standard "bailout catheter"[10] and that balloon inflations using this technique result in fewer ECG changes, angina, or enzymatic evidence of necrosis during PTCA.[11] Despite these theoretical advantages, there are several limitations to using these catheters in clinical practice. It is not possible to cross all types of lesions safely using the guidewire. The stiffness of the catheter may make it hard to negotiate lesions at bend points or in tortuous, smaller diffusely diseased vessels. It may be ineffective in preventing ischemia in the distribution of side branches at the lesion or in vessels straddled by the balloon catheter. An adequate perfusion pressure (>80 mm Hg) is required since passive flow in the face of hypotension is insufficient to prevent ischemic damage. Finally, these catheters may be ineffective in restoring flow in arteries with long areas of distal dissections. Nevertheless, when these catheters can be inserted successfully, they do allow for more controlled conditions, during which time the patient can be transferred to the operating room. Although we and others have not seen a decrease in the incidence of ischemic necrosis using these catheters, it may well be that newer diagnostic techniques will show that the actual size of the infarct is significantly decreased.

As noted above, one of the disadvantages of antegrade perfusion catheters is that there is compromised flow to side branches that straddle the lesion. Recently, a 4F stainless steel retrievable mesh stent has been developed that can maintain vessel patency without compromising side branch perfusion.[12] Preliminary clinical trials using these stents have shown no evidence of myocardial ischemia for up to 90 minutes. Further clinical investigation will be necessary before the role of transient stenting is defined.

Adjuvants to Antegrade Coronary Perfusion

Another disadvantage to antegrade coronary perfusion techniques is the limited flow rates achieved if systemic hypotension is present. The concept of hemoperfusion attempts to overcome this by pumping blood obtained from the venous or arterial sheath directly through the central lumen of the angioplasty catheter. This can be done either by hand injection[13] or by roller pump or angiographic power injector.[14] Several clinical studies employing hemoperfusion during balloon inflation have shown less chest pain, fewer ECG changes, and better preservation of wall motion.[15–17] However, similar to the autoperfusion catheter, blood flow to coronary side branches that are occluded by the inflated balloon remains compromised.

To increase further tissue oxygenation to the ischemic myocardium, fluosol, a biologically inert perfluorocarbon emulsion with an oxygen-carrying capacity of 7 ml O_2/dl at 600 mm Hg, recently has been introduced as a distal coronary perfusate during coronary angioplasty. Its low viscosity and absence of hemolysis at high flow rates make it especially desirable for perfusion of ischemic myocardium. Experimental and clinical studies have shown that fluosol limits infarct size and improves regional wall motion during periods of coronary occlusion associated with PTCA.[18–20] However, other studies comparing blood reperfusion versus fluosol infusions suggest that blood is a better perfusate.[21] Furthermore, the 30 to 60 minutes needed to prepare and oxygenate the fluosol limit its effectiveness during abrupt coronary occlusions.

Retrograde Coronary Sinus Perfusion

Because of the limitations of antegrade perfusion after an acute coronary occlusion, there has been a renewed interest in protecting jeopardized myocardium with coronary sinus retroperfusion. Synchronized retrograde perfusion (SRP) and pressure-controlled intermittent coronary sinus occlusion (PICSO) have emerged as techniques by which blood can be redirected through the coronary sinus to nourish ischemic myocardium beyond a coronary occlusion.

The SRP technique consists of pumping blood obtained from a peripheral artery into the coronary sinus via a catheter during diastole. An 8.5F retroperfusion catheter is introduced into the coronary sinus through the internal jugular vein and advanced into the great cardiac vein. This catheter has side holes near the tip surrounded by a 10-mm autoinflatable balloon and an end hole where arterial blood is ejected in a retrograde fashion. The side holes allow inflation of the balloon in diastole and deflation in systole. The catheter is advanced into the coronary sinus and its position can be verified by coronary sinus saturations, fluoroscopy, or hand injection of contrast medium. Arterial blood is obtained from a catheter in the femoral artery and is delivered to a pump that pumps the blood into the coronary sinus catheter. A monitoring console in the pump permits ECG synchronization of blood flow. Flow rates of up to 250 ml/min have been obtained with this technique.[22] Experimental studies involving LAD occlusions in dogs have shown that SRP significantly decreases infarct size and significantly increases blood flow to the myocardium at risk.[23] In addition, these studies showed an increased uptake of F-18 deoxyglucose, suggesting that SRP not only provides increased delivery of oxygenated blood to the ischemic myocardium but that the flow is also nutritive and results in increased myocardial metabolism. These findings were reflected in clinical studies with SRP in patients with unstable angina undergoing LAD angioplasty.[24-26] SRP resulted in a lower incidence of angina pain, less depression of global ejection fraction and stroke work, and better preservation of regional wall motion.

Whereas SRP directly shunts oxygenated blood retrograde to areas of ischemic myocardium, PICSO redistributes coronary venous blood by changes in pressure gradients throughout the coronary venous system. A balloon-tipped catheter is positioned in the orifice of the coronary sinus and connected to a pneumatic pump. The pump automatically inflates and deflates the balloon according to a preset cycle of 10 seconds of inflation and 4 seconds of deflation. During the period of coronary sinus occlusion, blood is redistributed retrograde to ischemic areas of the myocardium. Balloon deflation results in drainage of the coronary sinus. The intermittent nature of the inflation-deflation cycle avoids the complications of hemorrhage, edema, thrombosis, and arrhythmias seen when the coronary sinus is occluded for prolonged periods. Unlike SRP, PICSO does not require catheterization of the femoral artery and is ideal for patients with peripheral vascular disease. Our previous experimental studies and those of others have shown that PICSO results in improved wall motion, less tissue acidosis, and decreased infarct size after LAD occlusion.[27-29] Furthermore, using PICSO during cardioplegic arrest allowed for better distribution of antegrade cardioplegia beyond a coronary occlusion.[30] We now employ a retrograde cardioplegia catheter for the PICSO technique so that in addition to PICSO, retrograde cardioplegic techniques can be employed. To determine PICSO's role in reversing ischemic damage, we recently developed an experimental model to simulate the events after the surgical revascularization of an unsuccessful PTCA.[31] In adult pigs, the second and third diagonal vessels just beyond the takeoff of the LAD were occluded with snares for 90 minutes to simulate the period of ischemia after a failed PTCA. The animals were then placed on cardiopulmonary bypass, arrested for 30 minutes with antegrade, crystalloid cardioplegia, and then reperfused for 180 minutes with the coronary artery snares released. During the period of coronary occlusion before cardioplegic arrest, 10 pigs received PICSO and 10 others had no intervention. PICSO-treated hearts had significantly less tissue acidosis, better wall motion scores, and the least necrosis ($73 \pm 4\%$ vs. $27 \pm 4\%$; $p < 0.5$).

Despite these improvements in reversing ischemic damage using SRP and PICSO, considerable ventricular dysfunction still remains. This suggests that SRP and PICSO alone will not completely protect jeopardized myocardium during acute coronary occlusion. In addition to increasing blood flow, pharmacological manipulations also may be necessary to allow for maximal protection of ischemic myocardium. Recent experimental studies in totally occluded LAD vessels have shown that the retroinfusion of various pharmacological agents such as streptokinase,[32] procainamide,[33] oxygen free radical scavengers,[34] metoprolol,[35] and deferoxamine[36] resulted in higher drug concentrations in the ischemic myocardium that could be achieved with systemic intravenous administration. This has resulted in decreased infarct size and improved ventricular function. In a recent experimental study using the same model previously described, we also found that combining coronary venous substrate enhancement using L-glutamate with PICSO resulted in the most optimal recovery of acutely ischemic myocardium.[37]

In summary, retrograde coronary sinus perfusion techniques offer several advantages over antegrade perfusion after acute coronary artery occlusion. Perfusion to the ischemic myocardium is still possible even when the occluded lesion cannot be opened or a guidewire cannot be passed. Circulation to side branches is maintained, which otherwise might be compromised by angioplasty or "bailout" catheters. There are, however, several disadvantages. Retroperfusion to areas supplied by the circumflex and right coronary arteries may not be as adequate as the LAD. As noted above, ischemic damage is not totally reversed and may be incomplete. In addition, in 10% to 15% of patients, it may not be possible to cannulate the coronary sinus.[26] While retrograde perfusion techniques may increase blood flow, they do not support the circulation when hemodynamic deterioration is present. Nevertheless, these techniques should be considered when restoration of coronary arterial flow is not possible.

Reduction of Myocardial Demands and Circulatory Support

Despite all attempts to restore blood flow to the acutely ischemic myocardium, hemodynamic deterioration may occur. Prompt institution of devices that aid in circulatory support may be essential in decreasing myocardial demands, limiting the size of the infarct, and supporting systemic functions so that the patient can be transported safely to the operating room.

Intra-Aortic Balloon Pump

Since its introduction to clinical practice by Kantrowitz et al. in 1968,[38] the intra-aortic balloon pump (IABP) has been shown to benefit ischemic myocardium by decreasing afterload and augmenting diastolic pressure.[39-43] Microsphere studies in animals with acute coronary artery occlusions have demonstrated that this augmented diastolic perfusion pressure results in increased blood flow to all layers of the ischemic myocardium.[40,44,45] When IABP support was begun immediately after LAD occlusion in the dog, collateral coronary blood flow increased significantly in areas of ischemic myocardium.[45] This increased collateral flow was not evident when IABP support was delayed 20 minutes after LAD ligation. This favorable alteration of the supply-demand balance by the IABP has been shown in several experimental studies to reduce the area of infarction in animals undergoing acute coronary occlusion.[46-49] Similar results were seen by Alcan and his co-workers.[50] These findings would indicate that early insertion of the IABP in patients after a failed PTCA results in a more favorable supply-demand balance, which leads to decreased ischemic damage. The IABP, however, has several limitations in treating coronary ischemia after a failed PTCA. It has minimal effect on preload and cannot independently support the systemic circulation should cardiopulmonary arrest occur. It is ineffective in the presence of severe arrhythmias and cannot be inserted in the presence of severe peripheral vascular disease. It also can be associated with arterial trauma at the insertion site, resulting in leg ischemia. Nevertheless, in those patients with evidence of ischemia unresponsive to medical management or in patients with deteriorating hemodynamics requiring inotropic support, it remains a very effective method of stabilizing patients in preparation for surgery. By decreasing afterload and increasing diastolic pressure, thus increasing coronary blood flow, the IABP is unique in that it favorably alters both myocardial supply and demand. In the Boston University series, 81% of patients requiring an emergent CABG after a failed PTCA received an IABP in the catheterization laboratory.[1]

Percutaneous Bypass

Percutaneous bypass has emerged recently as an alternative means of mechanical support during periods of hemodynamic instability after a failed PTCA. This technique reduces both preload and afterload, is not rhythm dependent, and can completely support the systemic circulation should a cardiopulmonary arrest occur.[51] In this technique, a 1-cm skin incision is made over the femoral artery and vein. A guidewire is used to puncture the vessels followed by sequential dilators. A 17F arterial cannula is then inserted, followed by a 21F venous catheter that is positioned in the right atrium. The patient is anticoagulated with intravenous heparin so that the activated clotting time is greater than 400 seconds. A perfusionist monitors the membrane oxygenator pump, which consists of a Vortex pump, heat exchange unit, and membrane oxygenator. Flow rates of 3.5 to 5.0 liters/min can be achieved with this system. Arterial blood gases and mixed venous oxygen saturations are monitored carefully to ensure the physiological adequacy of flow. Mean aortic pressures can range from between 50 and 75 mm Hg. Percutaneous bypass currently has been used for elective high-risk PTCA support or as a resuscitative tool for patients in cardiogenic shock or cardiac arrest. Although the elective use of percutaneous bypass has resulted in acceptable morbidity and mortality,[51] the emergency application of percutaneous bypass has had poor results, with survival ranging from 4% to 21%.[52–54] Furthermore, patients brought to the emergency room in cardiac arrest or who experienced a cardiac arrest outside the catheterization laboratory had an extremely poor prognosis. In contrast, survival is significantly better if the arrest occurs in the catheterization laboratory and percutaneous bypass is instituted within 20 minutes of the event.[55,56] In the initial report of the National Registry of Supported Angioplasty Participants, 34% of patients were long-term survivors if percutaneous bypass was established within 20 minutes of cardiac arrest.[57] In contrast, only 12% of patients survived if percutaneous bypass was instituted after 20 minutes of resuscitation. In the entire series, only 29% of patients who underwent a cardiothoracic surgical procedure survived. In addition to a short period of cardiac arrest (<20 min), increased survival also has been noted in patients who have anatomically correctable lesions.[55,56] Hence, patients with poor distal vessels or cardiomyopathies with low ejection fractions are not acceptable candidates for surgery after institution of percutaneous bypass. In published series, operative survival after percutaneous bypass for cardiogenic shock has ranged from 0% to 64%.[55,56,58] Like the IABP, percutaneous bypass is limited by the presence of peripheral vascular disease and has the potential for arterial, venous, and nerve injuries at the cannulation site. In the initial report of the National Registry of Elective Cardiopulmonary Bypass Supported Coronary Angioplasty, 50% of patients had some type of complication related to percutaneous bypass and 50% of those involved arterial, venous, or nerve injury at the cannulation site.[51] Since it requires an oxygenator, percutaneous bypass is more expensive than the IABP, requires a perfusionist, and necessitates additional surgery to repair the cannulated vessels.

While percutaneous bypass has been shown to stabilize patients with circulatory collapse after a failed PTCA, its role in reversing regional ischemia has not been defined.[51,52,56,57] Although percutaneous bypass effectively reduces myocardial demands and prevents ventricular distention, there is no direct augmentation of coronary perfusion as might occur during IABP support. Preliminary studies obtained during supported angioplasty have shown that 20% of patients will have chest pain, ECG changes, or echocardiographic evidence of segmental myocardial dysfunction during balloon inflation.[51] To define better the role of percutaneous bypass after a failed PTCA, we undertook an experimental study to determine its effectiveness compared to the IABP.[59] In 30 adult pigs, the second and third diagonal vessels were occluded with snares for 90 minutes followed by 30 minutes of cardioplegic arrest and 180 minutes of reperfusion, during which time the snares were released. During the period of coronary occlusion prior to the institution of cardiopulmonary bypass, 10 pigs were placed on percutaneous bypass (PB), 10 pigs received an IABP, and 10 others received no intervention (unmodified). Ischemic damage in the area at risk was assessed by echo wall motion scores ($4 =$ normal to $-1 =$ dyskinesia), changes in myocardial tissue pH (ΔpH) from preischemia, and the area of necrosis/area of risk (AN/AR). Hearts treated with the IABP had the highest wall motion scores (1.27 ± 0.33 unmodified vs. 1.40 ± 0.30 PB vs. 2.04 ± 0.30 IABP), the least change in pH values from preischemia (ΔpH $= 0.41 \pm 0.13$ unmodified vs. 0.60 ± 0.10 PB vs. $0.25 \pm 0.09^{+}$ IABP; $^{+}p < 0.05$ from PB), and the least amount of myocardial necrosis in the area of risk ($73 \pm 4\%$ unmodified vs. $43 \pm 2^{*}$ PB vs. $27 \pm 4^{*+}$ IABP; $^{*}p < 0.05$ from unmodified; $^{+}p < 0.05$ from PB). Although percutaneous bypass resulted in less myocardial necrosis than the unmodified group, the most optimal recovery occurred in the IABP group. The fact that percutaneous bypass reduces demands but does not effectively increase myocardial oxygen supply explains why it is not as effective as the IABP during periods of myocardial ischemia in the absence of circulatory collapse. The findings of this experimental study have helped us to formulate a plan for the use of percutaneous bypass in the management of patients who require emergent CABG after a failed PTCA at the Boston University Medical Center. Patients who are hemodynamically stable without any ECG evidence of myocardial ischemia have been managed without any mechanical support. In those patients with ECG evidence of ischemia or hemodynamic deterioration requiring inotropic support, an IABP is inserted. We reserve the insertion of percutaneous bypass for those instances of hemodynamic instability unresponsive to the IABP.

Nimbus Hemopump

The Nimbus hemopump is a catheter-mounted left ventricular assist device that withdraws blood directly from the left ventricle and propels it into the descending aorta. In this technique, a 21F flexible inflow cannula is inserted through a cutdown in the femoral artery and passed retrograde across the aortic valve into the left ventricle. A miniature Archimedes spiral vane screw pump at the base of the cannula rotates at 27,000 rpm, producing nonpulsatile flow rates up to 3.5 liters/minute, which is independent of underlying venticular function or cardiac rhythm. Experimental studies in dogs with LAD occlusions have shown that the hemopump provided superior hemodynamic support and resulted in less regional wall motion abnormalities as compared to the IABP.[60] Initial clinical studies in patients with refractory cardiogenic shock after a myocardial infarction or during cardiac surgical procedures showed that the insertion of the hemopump significantly improved ventricular function and patient survival.[61] Despite the encouraging results of these initial clinical studies, there are several disadvantages to this technique. As in all devices that must be inserted through the femoral artery, the presence of significant peripheral vascular disease limits its use and may increase the risk of leg ischemia. The unit is extremely expensive and the cardiac output is limited to 3.5 liters/minute. In addition, its position in the left ventricle raises the possibility of dislodging mural thrombi and inducing arrhythmias. These limitations have kept this technique from gaining widespread use as a left ventricular assist device.

Percutaneous Left Heart Bypass

In the percutaneous left heart bypass technique, a 14F to 20F catheter is introduced through the femoral vein, punctures the atrial septum, and is positioned in the left atrium. Oxygenated blood is then returned to the circulation via a femoral arterial cannula. The advantage of this technique over conventional percutaneous bypass is that an oxygenator is not required. This technique has been used recently for circulatory support during high-risk angioplasties.[62] The experience with this device is limited and its insertion is technically more complex than standard percutaneous bypass techniques. Furthermore, the long-term hemodynamic effects of the atrial septal defect created with this catheter are unknown.

Combinations of Techniques to Increase Supply and Decrease Demands

Acute coronary occlusion after a failed PTCA results in an acute decrease in myocardial oxygen supply, forcing other regions of the myocardium to increase their demands. If additional coronary lesions are present in those areas or if these regions are already hypokinetic, a severe supply-demand imbalance will occur. Interventions that may increase blood to the ischemic myocardium have no effect on preload or afterload and cannot independently support the circulation should severe mechanical failure occur. In contrast, devices that may adequately decrease demands by supporting the systemic circulation and unloading the ventricle are ineffective in increasing blood flow to areas of ischemic myocardium. This implies that prompt intervention by techniques that more favorably alter both supply and demand after an acute coronary occlusion would result in a significant reduction in myocardial ischemic damage. To test this hypotheses, we undertook a series of experiments in the pig using the model of 90 minutes of coronary occlusion, 30 minutes of cardioplegic arrest, and 180 minutes of reperfusion to simulate a failed PTCA undergoing surgical revascularization. During the 90-minute period of coronary occlusion, hearts were treated with several combinations of interventions that effected supply and demand. These included

1. intra-aortic balloon pump + percutaneous bypass (IABP + PB)
2. intra-aortic balloon pump + pressure-controlled intermittent coronary sinus occlusion (IABP + PICSO)
3. pressure-controlled intermittent coronary sinus occlusion + percutaneous bypass (PICSO + PB).

The results of the percent AN/AR at the end of 180 minutes of reperfusion are summarized in Table 2. The addition of the IABP to both percutaneous bypass and pressure-controlled intermittent coronary artery occlusion significantly decreased the infarct size. Similarly, the addition of PICSO to percutaneous bypass also significantly reduced the AN. These experimental studies lend further support to the premise that combinations of techniques that act at both spectrums of the supply/demand equation result in the most optimal salvage of ischemic myocardium after an unsuccessful PTCA.

Table 2

Reduction of Myocardial Necrosis After Coronary Occlusion and Reperfusion

Intervention	Area of Necrosis/Area at Risk (%)
Unmodified	73 ± 4
PB	$43 \pm 2^*$
IABP	$27 \pm 4^{*+}$
IABP + PB	$25 \pm 4^{*+}$
IABP + PICSO	$15 \pm 1^{*+\#}$
PB + PICSO	$14 \pm 2^{*+\#}$

All results are mean $\pm$ standard error.
*$p < 0.05$ from unmodified.
+$p < 0.05$ from PB.
#$p < 0.05$ from IABP, IABP + PB.
PB = percutaneous bypass; IABP = intra-aortic balloon pump; PICSO = pressure-controlled intermittent coronary sinus occlusion.

Conclusions

This chapter has summarized the various methods available to both cardiologists and surgeons in reducing ischemic damage after an unsuccessful PTCA in preparation for an emergent CABG. Once the decision has been made to proceed with a CABG, all attempts should be made to cross the lesion with a "bailout" or perfusion catheter. In the absence of chest pain or ECG changes, systemic coronary vasodilatation (i.e., nitroglycerin) may be all that is necessary. If, however, chest pain or ECG changes persist, an IABP should be inserted if technically feasible. Retrograde coronary sinus perfusion is another option if the lesion cannot be crossed using antegrade techniques. Percutaneous bypass should be considered when hemodynamics deteriorate despite IABP and inotropic support. In the Boston University series, the condition of the patient upon leaving the catheterization laboratory strongly influenced the operative outcome.[1] This suggests that strategies aimed at reducing myocardial necrosis must begin immediately after coronary occlusion in the catheterization laboratory in order to achieve the greatest salvage of ischemic myocardium.

References

1. Lazar HL, Faxon DP, Paone G, Khorasani AR, Jacobs AK, et al. Changing profiles of failed coronary angioplasty patients: impact on surgical results. Ann Thorac Surg 1992; 53:269–273.
2. Lazar HL, Haan CK. Determinants of myocardial infarction following emergency coronary artery bypass for failed percutaneous coronary angioplasty. Ann Thorac Surg 1987; 44:646–650.
3. Green MA, Gray LA, Slater AD, Ganzel BL, Mavroudis C. Emergency aortocoronary bypass after failed angioplasty. Ann Thorac Surg 1991; 51:194–199.
4. Zalowski A, Savage M, Goldberg S. Protection of the ischemic myocardium during percutaneous transluminal coronary angioplasty. Am J Cardiol 1988; 61:54–60.
5. Engelman RM, Rousou JA, Flack JE, Iyengar J, Kimura Y, Das DK. Reduction of infarct size by systemic amino acid supplementation during reperfusion. J Thorac Cardiovasc Surg 1991; 101:855–859.
6. Christensen CW, Lasser TA, Daley LC, Reider MA, Schmidt DH. Regional myocardial blood flow with a reperfusion catheter and an autoperfusion balloon catheter during total coronary occlusion. Am Heart J 1990; 119:242–248.

7. Hinohara T, Simpson JB, Phillips HR, et al. Transluminal catheter reperfusion: a new technique to reestablish blood flow after coronary occlusion during percutaneous transluminal coronary angioplasty. Am J Cardiol 1986; 57:684–686.

8. Sundram P, Harvey JR, Johnson RG, Schwartz MJ, Baim DS. Benefit of the perfusion catheter for emergency coronary artery grafting after failed percutaneous transluminal coronary angioplasty. Am J Cardiol 1989; 63:282–285.

9. Murphy DA, Craver JM, Jones EL. Surgical management of acute myocardial ischemia following percutaneous transluminal coronary angioplasty: role of the intra-aortic balloon pump. J Thorac Cardiovasc Surg 1984; 87:332–338.

10. Turi ZG, Campbell CA, Gottimukkala MV, Kloner RA. Preservation of distal coronary perfusion during prolonged balloon inflation with an autoperfusion angioplasty catheter. Circulation 1987; 75:1273–1280.

11. Quigley PG, Kereiakes DJ, Abbottsmith CW, et al. Prolonged autoperfusion angioplasty: immediate clinical outcome and angiographic follow-up. J Am Coll Cardiol 1989; 13:155A.

12. Gaspard PE, Didier BP, Delsanti GL. The temporary stent catheter: a non-operative treatment for acute occlusion during coronary angioplasty. J Am Coll Cardiol 1990; 15:118A.

13. Banka VS, Trivedi A, Patel R, Ghusson M, Voci G. Prevention of myocardial ischemia during coronary angioplasty: a simple new method for distal antegrade arterial blood perfusion. Am Heart J 1989; 118:830–836.

14. Heibig J, Angelini P, Leachman R, Beall MM, Beall AC. Use of mechanical devises for distal hemoperfusion during balloon catheter coronary angioplasty. Cathet Cardiovasc Diagn 1988; 15:143–149.

15. Lehmann KG, Atwood JE, Synder EL, Ellison RL. Autologous blood perfusion for myocardial protection during coronary angioplasty: a feasibility study. Circulation 1987; 76:312–323.

16. Tokioka H, Miyazaki A, Fung P, et al. Effects of intracoronary infusion of arterial blood or Fluosol-DA 20% on regional myocardial metabolism and function during brief coronary artery occlusion. Circulation 1987; 75:473–481.

17. Maniet AR, Lehmann D, Banka VS. Prevention of regional wall motion abnormalities during coronary angioplasty. J Am Coll Cardiol 1988; 11:195A.

18. Bajaj AK, Cobb AM, Virman R, Gay JC, Light RJ, Forman MB. Limitation of myocardial reperfusion injury by intravenous perfluorochemicals: role of neutrophil activation. Circulation 1989; 79:645–656.

19. Cleman M, Jaffee CC, Wohlgelernten D. Prevention of ischemia during percutaneous transluminal coronary angioplasty by transcatheter infusion of oxygenated fluosol DA 20%. Circulation 1986; 74:555–562.

20. Anderson HV, Leimgruber PP, Roubin GS, Nelson DL, Gruentzig AR. Distal coronary artery perfusion during percutaneous transluminal coronary angioplasty. Am Heart J 1985; 110:720–726.

21. Christensen CV, Reeves WC, Lassar TA, Schmidt DH. Inadequate

subendocardial oxygen delivery during perfluorocarbon perfusion in a canine model of ischemia. Am Heart J 1988; 115:30–37.

22. Hajduczki I, Kar S, Areeda J, et al. Reversal of chronic regional myocardial dysfunction (hibernating myocardium) by synchronized diastolic coronary angioplasty. J Am Coll Cardiol 1990; 15:238–242.

23. O'Byrne GT, Nienaber CA, Miyasaki A, Araugo L, Fishbein MC, et al. Positron emisson tomography demonstrates that coronary sinus retroperfusion can restore regional myocardial perfusion and preserve metabolism. J Am Coll Cardiol 1991; 18:257–270.

24. Kar S, Drury JK, Hajduczki I, Eigler N, Wakida Y, et al. Synchronized coronary venous retroperfusion for support and salvage of ischemic myocardium during elective and failed angioplasty. J Am Coll Cardiol 1991; 18:271–282.

25. Costantino C, Sampaolegi A, Serra CM, Pacheco G, Neuburger J, et al. Coronary venous retroperfusion support during high risk angioplasty in patients with unstable angina: preliminary experience. J Am Coll Cardiol 1991; 18:283–292.

26. Corday E, Kar S, Drury JK, et al. Coronary venous retroperfusion for support of ischemic myocardium. Cardiovasc Rev Rep 1988; 9:50–53.

27. Mohl W, Punzengruber C, Moser M. Effects of pressure-controlled intermittent coronary sinus occlusion on regional ischemic myocardial function. J Am Coll Cardiol 1985; 5:939–945.

28. Mohl W, Glogar DH, Mayr H. Reduction of infarct size induced by pressure-controlled intermittent coronary sinus occlusion. Am J Cardiol 1984; 53:923.

29. Lazar HL, Rajaii A, Roberts AJ. Reversal of reperfusion injury following ischemic arrest with pressure-controlled intermittent coronary sinus occlusion. J Thorac Cardiovasc Surg 1988; 95:637–642.

30. Lazar HL, Khoury T, Rivers S. Improved distribution of cardioplegia with pressure-controlled intermittent coronary sinus occlusion (PICSO). Ann Thorac Surg 1988; 46:202–207.

31. Lazar HL, Haan C, Bernard S, Rivers S, Shemin RJ. Reduction of infarct size following revascularization of an acute coronary occlusion with pressure-controlled intermittent coronary sinus occlusion (PISCO). J Moll Cell Cardiol 1990; 22:515.

32. Meerbaum S, Lang TW, Pouzhitkov M. Retrograde lysis of coronary artery thrombus by coronary venous streptokinase administration. J Am Coll Cardiol 1983; 1:1262–1267.

33. Karagueuzian HS, Ohta M, Drury JK. Coronary venous retroinfusion of procainamide: a new approach for the management of spontaneous and inducible sustained ventricular tachycardia during myocardial infarction. J Am Coll Cardiol 1986; 7:551–563.

34. Hatori N, Miyazaki A, Tadokoro H. Beneficial effects of coronary venous retroinfusion of superoxide dismutase and catalase on reperfusion arrhythmias, myocardial function and infarct size in dogs. J Cardiovasc Pharmacol 1989; 14:396–404.

35. Ryden L, Tadokoro H, Sjoquist PO, Regardh C, Kobayashi S, et al. Pharmacokinetic analysis of coronary venous retroinfusion: a compari-

son with antegrade coronary artery drug administration using metoprolol as a tracer. J Am Coll Cardiol 1991; 18:603–612.
36. Kobayashi S, Tadokoro H, Wakida Y, Kar S, Nordlander R, et al. Coronary venous retroinfusion of deferoxamine reduces infarct size in pigs. J Am Coll Cardiol 1991; 18:621–627.
37. Haan C, Lazar H, Yang X, Rivers S, Bernard S, Shemin R. Reduction of infarct size with substrate enhanced coronary venous retroperfusion. Circulation 1991; 84II:717.
38. Kantrowitz A, Tjonneland S, Freed PS, Phillips SJ, Butner AN, Sherman JL. Initial clinical experience with intra-aortic balloon pumping in cardiogenic shock. JAMA 1968; 203:135–140.
39. Buckley MJ, Leinbach R, Kaster J, Laird J, Kantrowitz AR, et al. Hemodynamic evaluation of intra-aortic balloon pumping in man. Circulation 1970; 46:130–136.
40. Weber KT, Janick JS. Intra-aortic balloon counterpulsation: a review of physiological principles, clinical results, and device safety. Ann Thorac Surg 1974; 17:602–636.
41. Bolooki H, Williams W, Thurer RJ, Vargas A, Kaiser GA, et al. Clinical and hemodynamic criteria for use of intra-aortic balloon pump in patients requiring cardiac surgery. J Thorac Cardiovasc Surg; 62:678–756.
42. Hood WB, Joison J, Kumar R, Norman JC, Tyberg JF, Vachel CW. Experimental myocardial infarction: VII. Effects of intra-aortic balloon pump counterpulsation on cardiac performance in intact conscious dogs with left ventricular failure due to coronary insufficiency. Cardiovasc Res 1971; 5:103–112.
43. Powell WJ, Daggett WM, Magro AE, Gianco JA, Buckley MJ, et al. Effects of intra-aortic balloon counterpulsation on cardiac performance, oxygen consumption, and coronary blood flow in dogs. Circ Res 1970; 26:753–764.
44. Gill C, Wechsler A, Newman G, Oldhan H. Augmentation and redistribution of myocardial blood flow during acute ischemia by intra-aortic balloon pumping. Ann Thorac Surg 1975; 16:445–453.
45. Watson JT, Willerson JT, Fixler DE, Sugg NL. Temporal changes in collateral coronary blood flow in ischemic myocardium during intra-aortic balloon pumping. Circulation 1974; 50:249–254.
46. Roberts AJ, Alonso DR, Combes JR, Jacobstein J, Post M, et al. Role of delayed intra-aortic balloon pumping in the treatment of experimental myocardial infarction. Am J Cardiol 1978; 41:1202–1208.
47. Feola M, Haiderer O, Kennedy JH. Intra-aortic balloon pumping at different levels of experimental acute left ventricular failure. Chest 1971; 59:68–76.
48. Nachlas MN, Siedband MP. The influence of diastolic augmentation on infarct size following coronary artery ligation. J Thorac Cardiovasc Surg 1967; 53:698–703.
49. Sugg WL, Webb WR, Ecker RR. Reduction of extent of myocardial infarction by counterpulsation. Ann Thorac Surg 1969; 7:310–316.
50. Alcan KE, Stertzer SH, Wallsh E, DePasquale NP, Bruno MS. The role of intra-aortic balloon counterpulsation in patients undergoing per-

cutaneous transluminal coronary angioplasty. Am Heart J 1983; 105:527–530.

51. Vogel RA, Shawl F, Tommaso C, et al. Initial report of the National Registry of Elective Cardiopulmonary Bypass Supported Coronary Angioplasty. J Am Coll Cardiol 1990; 15:23–29.

52. Phillips SJ, Zeff RH, Kongtahworn C, et al. Percutaneous cardiopulmonary bypass: application and indication for use. Ann Thorac Surg 1989; 47:121–123.

53. Hartz R, LoCicero J, Sanders JH, Frederiksen JW, Joob AW, Michaelis LL. Clinical experience with portable cardiopulmonary bypass in cardiac arrest patients. Ann Thorac Surg 1990; 51:437–441.

54. Overlie RA, Reichman RT, Smith SC, et al. Emergency use of portable cardiopulmonary bypass in patients with cardiac arrest. J Am Coll Cardiol 1989; 13:160A.

55. Mooney MR, Arom KV, Joyce LD, et al. Emergency cardiopulmonary bypass support in patients with cardiac arrest. J Thorac Cardiovasc Surg 1991; 101:450–454.

56. Shawl FA, Comansi MJ, Wish MH, Davis M, Punga A, Hernandez TJ. Emergency cardiopulmonary bypass support in patients with cardiac arrest in the catheterization laboratory. Cathet Cardiovasc Diagn 1990; 19:8–12.

57. Overlie PA, Vogel RA, O'Neill WW, Smith S, Mooney MR, et al. Emergency cardiopulmonary bypass: initial report of the National Registry of Supported Angioplasty Participants. Circulation 1991; 84:II 132.

58. Sugimato JT, Baird E, Bruner C. Percutaneous cardiopulmonary support in cardiac arrest. ASAIO Transactions 1991; 37:282–283.

59. Lazar HL, Yang XM, Rivers S, Treanor P, Shemin J. Role of percutaneous bypass in reducing infarct size following revascularization for acute coronary insufficiency. Circulation 1991; 84:III:416–421.

60. Smalling RW, Cassidy DB, Merhige M, et al. Improved hemodynamic and left ventricular unloading during acute ischemia using the hemopump left ventricular assist device compared to intra-aortic balloon counterpulsation. J Am Coll Cardiol 1989; 13:160A.

61. Frazier OH, Nalcatan T, Duncan JM, Parnis SM, Fugua JM. Clinical experience with the hemopump. ASAIO Transactions 1989; 35:604–606.

62. Babic UU, Grujicic S, Djurisic Z, Vucinic M. Percutaneous left atrial-aortic bypass with a roller pump. Circulation 1989; 80 II:272.

Chapter 8

Surgical Revascularization for Refractory Unstable Angina

Gabriel S. Aldea and Richard J. Shemin

Introduction

Unstable angina (UA) represents an important link in the spectrum of acute coronary syndromes and is critical in our understanding of the progression of coronary artery disease from chronic stable angina to acute myocardial infarction (AMI). It is a common and quite serious condition. As many as 30% to 60% of patients with AMI present initially with a prodrome of UA.[1] Despite improvement in medical therapy, patients with UA remain at high risk for subsequent fatal and nonfatal ischemic events (10% incidence of AMI, 12% mortality within 1 year), and only a minority of patients recover without any further sequelae.[2–4] UA is responsible for more than 750,000 hospital admissions annually in the U.S.,[5] with a mean duration of hospitalization of 10 days.[6] Most patients undergo coronary angiography, 86% of responders and 96% of patients

Lazar HL (editor): *Current Therapy for Acute Coronary Ischemia,* © Futura Publishing Co., Inc., Mount Kisco, NY, 1993.

refractory to medical therapy undergo either elective or urgent PTCA or surgical revascularization,[7] representing a significant social and economic burden.[8] Surgical revascularization for unstable angina represents 7% to 33%[9-11] of all isolated coronary artery bypass grafting (CABG) procedures performed. In our own institution, this incidence has increased progressively and currently exceeds 50% of all CABG procedures, an increase of 27% since the late 1980s. In part this reflects changes in referral patterns to a tertiary care institution and the emerging aggressive role of percutaneous transluminal coronary angioplasty (PTCA) in the management of angina.

Varied pathophysiological processes and clinical syndromes continue to be lumped under this heading, confounding the selection of appropriate treatment modalities for these patients. Despite attempts to develop a standardized classification of UA,[12] medical and surgical series continue to differ in their individual inclusion and exclusion criteria, and in patient profiles, resulting in radically varied risks and reported outcomes.

Definition

Under current classifications, UA includes a spectrum of clinical conditions ranging from new-onset angina, crescendo angina, to rest angina. Patients are treated aggressively with oral antianginal therapy (nitrates, beta blockers, and calcium antagonists), often in the setting of an intensive care unit, while the diagnosis of an AMI is excluded by cardiac isoenzymes and electrocardiogram (ECG) criteria. Patients who become asymptomatic with such treatment can undergo revascularization with an operative mortality virtually identical to that of patients undergoing elective CABG.[13,14] On the other hand, the patients who are refractory to such measures and in whom an AMI has been excluded require intravenous nitroglycerin or heparin, or both, and represent the higher risk subset, which is the subject of this chapter. Included in this high-risk subset are patients with postinfarction angina (within 30 days of a subendocardial or transmural AMI). In contrast to the first group, patients with refractory UA undergo medical or surgical interventions (including catheterization, PTCA, or CABG) at the same hospitalization, underlining the urgency of the condition. Excluded from this discussion are the highest risk patients with acute ongoing infarction, cardiogenic shock, or structural cardiac abnormalities resulting from AMI. Also excluded are patients undergoing emergency surgical revascularization for acutely failed PTCA, whose management is discussed in the following chapters.

Pathophysiology and Rationale for Medical Therapy

Background

When compared to patients with stable angina (SA), those with UA tend to be older, with a higher ratio of female and diabetic patients, lower ejection fraction, and greater incidence of previous infarction with a more complex morphology of angiographic lesions.[9–11] Although some studies demonstrate a similar distribution of single- and multivessel disease among patients with SA and UA (with a predominance of multivessel disease in both), series with more stringent inclusion criteria and higher risk patients document a higher incidence of angiographically significant ($>$50%) left main (LM) disease (15–33%) and three-vessel disease (53–70%) in patients with UA.[9–11,14]

Patients with UA represent a high-risk subgroup with severe multivessel coronary disease, compromised collaterals, and partially occlusive thrombi. In the absence of adequate medical therapy, 5% to 50% of patients with UA progress to an AMI.[2–4] Pathological,[15,16] coronary angiographic,[17,18] and coronary angioscopic[19,20] studies have extended the role of progression of atherosclerotic disease to include dynamic components to explain this unstable condition. These dynamic components include rapid progression of atherosclerotic coronary disease, plaque fissuring or rupture, active vasomotion and spasm, and formation of thrombus and platelet aggregates.[21,22] Although described as independent factors, there are undoubtedly important interactions whereby activation of one mechanism triggers activation of another.

In its early presentation, UA is difficult to distinguish from acute evolving myocardial infarction, and individual contributing pathophysiological components cannot be discerned by current clinical and laboratory evaluation. Medical therapy therefore tends to be broad, nonspecific, and all-encompassing in an attempt to treat multiple pathophysiological mechanisms.[23–25]

Medical Therapy

Experimental and clinical evidence demonstrate that intravenous nitroglycerin can alter hemodynamic and coronary flow characteristics to limit infarct size.[26–28] Beta blockers and calcium antagonists are equally effective in preventing progressive ischemia and cardiac events in UA by decreasing myocardial oxygen demand.[29–31] Beta blockers are especially effective when tachycardia is present and calcium antagonists are preferred when the underlying mechanism is suspected to be spasm. Low-dose aspirin inhibits platelet aggregation with the subsequent production of thromboxane A_2 without inhibition of the potent endothelial synthesized vasodilator prostacyclin, and has been shown to decrease significantly the rate of AMI in patients with UA by 51% (from 7% to 3.4%, $p<0.05$) as well as decrease death after an AMI by 50% (from 10% to 5%, $p<0.05$).[32–34] Intravenous heparin has been shown to be effective in preventing the evolution of transmural AMI in patients with UA, perhaps by preventing the propagation of thrombus proximal to a critical coronary lesion.[35] Lytic agents have been demonstrated to decrease myocardial injury and preserve left ventricular function in patients with AMI. Although these agents have resulted in angiographic modification of thrombi present in patients with UA, clinical outcome (incidence of AMI, ratio of patients refractory to medical therapy, rate of emergency revascularization procedures, and mortality) was not influenced by thrombolytic therapy.[6] However, since UA and AMI are clinically indistinguishable in their early presentation, patients often are subjected to lytic therapy. This combination of antihemostatic agents [aspirin, heparin, streptokinase-tissue plasminogen activator (SK/t-PA), and calcium antagonists] have resulted in a two- to fourfold increase in perioperative bleeding, transfusion requirement, and surgical re-exploration in patients undergoing surgical revascularization for UA.[36,37]

Outcome

A recent study demonstrates that less than 33% of patients admitted to the coronary care unit (CCU) with UA receive optimal "maximal" medical therapy.[38] Even when optimal triple drug antianginal therapy (intravenous nitroglycerin, beta blockers, and calcium antagonists) as well as antihemostatic therapy (aspirin and heparin) is tolerated at "maximal" doses, as many as 20% to 44% of patients with UA continue to have recurrent, stuttering episodes of angina.[7,14,25] Clinical tolerance of "maximal" triple drug anti-anginal therapy (intravenous nitroglycerin, beta blockers, and calcium antagonists) often is limited by the patient's hemodynamic status, further limiting their use and desired effects. In this setting, when possible, intra-aortic balloon pump (IABP) counterpulsation is used to stabilize the patient's condition (congestive failure or persistent angina) before urgent revascularization.[39]

Patients who fail to respond to medical therapy have a fourfold incidence of AMI compared to responders (13% vs. 3%, $p<0.01$).[2–4,7,14,24] Refractory patients with UA are subjected to urgent coronary angiography. Nearly 90% of the patients go on to urgent revascularization and are nearly equally divided between PTCA and CABG; the remaining 10% receive intensified medical therapy.[7] The overall in-hospital mortality of all patients presenting with UA is 4% to 8%, most of which occur in patients refractory to medical therapy.[7,24] Patients treated medically for UA, particularly those with diminished left ventricular function, have a high incidence of rehospitalization (>60% in 3 yr), and often cross over to surgical revascularization (38% in 3 yr, 43% at 5 yr).[40,41] More than 50% of patients who cross over to surgical revascularization do so within 3 months of being assigned to medical therapy. Patients refractory to medical therapy who cross over to revascularization therapy have a significantly higher mortality (10.3% vs. 4.1%, $p<0.05$) than those assigned primarily to revascularization.[40] This baseline information is particularly important when results of different therapeutic interventions are compared.

PTCA in Patients with UA

Background

With advances in catheter design, operator experience, improved success rate, and diminishing rate of acute complications,[42–48] PTCA has emerged as an attractive alternative in *selected* patients with isolated, discrete, concentric, proximal stenoses in single coronary arteries. Prompted by the development and widespread use of the Stack perfusion balloon catheter, which significantly decreased the need for emergency surgical revascularization (from 23% to 5%),[45] this enthusiasm has translated to more frequent use of PTCA in all patients, including those with multivessel disease and those requiring acute revascularization for UA.

Patient Selection

Patients with UA who are unresponsive to maximal medical therapy requiring revascularization are roughly equally divided between PTCA and CABG.[7] Currently nearly 60% of all patients undergoing PTCA have UA,[45,48] and nearly 87% of all lesions subjected to PTCA in the setting of UA are either complex, long (>10 mm), irregular, eccentric, or associated with intraluminal filling defects.[42] Frequent use of PTCA for UA is especially perplexing given the predominance of multivessel coronary disease, advanced age with its associated multiple comorbid factors, and ventricular impairment after previous myocardial infarction in this patient subset. Although no clinical factor is strong enough as a predictive parameter to be considered alone, these are well recognized to increase the risk and compromise the long-term outcome of an acute PTCA intervention in the setting of UA.[42–48] This approach is explained primarily by the frequently applied strategy of "culprit lesion" angioplasty over that of multiple dilations. Favorable long-term outcome has been previously related to complete revascularization in both surgical and medical literature[43,45,49] and has guided the strategy for elective PTCA. This strategy is readily abandoned in favor of "culprit lesion" angioplasty when PTCA is performed urgently or emergently for UA.[43] Despite a distinct selection bias in referral patterns, complete revascularization is more likely in patients undergoing surgical revascularization compared to those undergoing PTCA (88% vs. 66%).[7] The practice of "culprit lesion" angioplasty for UA supplants previous recommendations and guidelines of the American College of Cardiology/American Heart Association[50] to evaluate coronary lesions in the context of the global severity of the patients condition, making *any* individual lesion eligible for consideration. Long-term outcome of this new approach is largely unknown.

Outcome

Complete *or* partial angiographic success *per lesion* can be expected in 84% to 90% of patients with UA[42–48] (and vary with the angiographic definition of "success"). Success diminishes and serious complications increase dramatically with advanced patient age, urgency of revascularization, multivessel disease, impaired ventricular function, and number of occluded vessels.[42-48] In patients undergoing angioplasty for UA in the recent NHLBI PTCA registry (1985–1986), severity of coronary artery disease was as follows: 46.6% single (SVD), 31.6% double (DVD), and 21.7% triple (TVD) vessel disease.[46] In the same series, in only 14.9% of patients was the ejection fraction less than 0.50, and none had LM disease. Other series of PTCA in patients with UA have an even higher incidence of SVD (72–86%) and a lower incidence of TVD (7–10.5%).[43,48] Because of the therapeutic approach in the NHLBI registry of "culprit lesion" angioplasty, only 26.2% of all double and only 8.2% of all triple-vessel disease had attempted PTCA of all diseased vessels. Despite this selective approach, complete success *in the vessels attempted* was influenced by severity of coronary artery disease: 83.1% for SVD, 76.4% for DVD, and 75.8% for TVD. Furthermore, severity of coronary artery disease also influenced the rate of complicated failure: 7.4% for SVD, 11.3% for DVD, and 12.1% in TVD.[46] Despite careful patient selection and lower risk profile in the NHLBI PTCA registry, patients with UA undergoing PTCA had a 38% higher complication rate when compared with patients with SA (9.7% vs. 6.0%, $p<0.01$). The incidence of AMI (5% vs. 2%), need for emergency CABG (4.4% vs. 2.2%), and death (1.3% vs. 0.5%) were nearly doubled in the SA group.[43] This disparity between the UA and SA groups is demonstrated even more dramatically in other series with less selective inclusion criteria, with as much as a fourfold increase in the rate of complications, with an incidence of myocardial infarction ranging between 7% and 10%, and a mortality between 1.3% and 16%.[47,48] Patients requiring emergency CABG for failed angioplasty carry a significantly higher mortality than those undergoing urgent revascularization for UA, and have a higher incidence of perioperative AMI.[51] Finally, when compared to patients with SA, those with UA had a significantly longer duration of angioplasty-related hospital stay (4.4 vs 2.9 days, $p<0.01$).[8]

In a large PTCA series with a high-risk population (more comparable to CABG population), a significant increased incidence of vessel occlusion (36.4% vs. 19.2%), previous myocardial infarction (32.8% vs. 22%), three-vessel disease (24.9% vs. 9.5%), impaired ventricular function (6.8% vs. 3.2%), and age greater than 70 (22.7% vs. 10.7%) were noted in patients with UA compared to those with

SA (all $p<0.001$).[47] When compared to patients with SA undergoing PTCA, patients with UA had a higher rate of complications from AMI (6.8% vs. 2.6%, $p<0.01$) and mortality (3.2% vs. 0.8%, $p<0.01$).[47] The lowest failure rate and mortality were noted in young patients (age <60) undergoing elective PTCA for single-vessel disease (93% and 0%, respectively). Success rate decreased (80%) and mortality increased (11%) significantly ($p<0.001$) in patients with UA and three-vessel disease undergoing urgent PTCA.[47] Mortality was highest in patients with UA undergoing PTCA with three-vessel disease with depressed ventricular function (16%) and cardiogenic shock (33%).[47]

Although the incidence of abrupt closure is somewhat higher in patients with UA,[42] the rate of restenosis is similar to that of PTCA in SA, and ranges between 30% and 40%.[45,52] Despite an excellent initial outcome in selected patients, long-term cardiovascular free survival in patients subjected to PTCA for UA is more modest. After an initial successful PTCA, as many as 40% of patients suffer a cardiovascular complication: late death (4%), AMI (6%), and require a CABG (16%) or repeat PTCA (20%) within 5 years.[48,52] Only 50% of patients are symptom free with no evidence of myocardial ischemia on stress test.[48,52]

Surgical Revascularization in Patients with UA

Background

Published results of outcome of surgical revascularization in patients with UA often do not reflect the evolution of myocardial protection and revascularization techniques, the growing surgical and anesthetic experience with revascularization of unstable patients, or improved patency and long-term prognosis with increased usage of arterial conduits and antiplatelet agents. On the other side of the spectrum, nor do these series reflect the relentless, progressive increase of perioperative comorbid risks in patients undergoing CABG. Previously published results therefore should be interpreted with caution.

When compared with patients with SA, those presenting for

surgical revascularization with UA are older, have a lower ejection fraction (EF), and have a higher incidence of recent AMI.[9–11,14,49,51,53] In addition, as many as 36% of these patients are women, 63% are hypertensive, 15% are diabetic, 13% have significant peripheral vascular disease, 12% have significant chronic obstructive pulmonary disease (COPD), and 14% have a history of a cerebrovascular accident (CVA).[10] These comorbid factors have been shown to result in an increased risk for postoperative complications including death, stroke, wound infection, reoperations for bleeding, need for inotropic support, prolonged ventilation, and postoperative hospital stays.[54]

Patient Selection and Preoperative Therapy

Indications for CABG for patients with UA are similar to those in SA. Patients who are refractory to medical therapy and who are poor PTCA candidates frequently are referred for CABG. Patients with UA are treated initially with triple drug antianginal therapy. After an initial satisfactory response, these patients may be evaluated for surgical revascularization on a relatively elective basis. Patients refractory to oral medical therapy are treated with intensified medical therapy (intravenous nitroglycerin and heparin) and frequently are supported with an intra-aortic balloon pump (IABP),[39] while urgent surgical revascularization is planned after careful evaluation of angiographic pathology. Many studies demonstrated enhanced morbidity and mortality with urgent surgical interventions,[4,7,9–11,49,51,53–56] especially in the setting of postinfarction UA. This leads to a practice of deferring surgery, whenever clinically possible, until after "medical stabilization" for a period of unclear duration. However, in series in which surgery urgency was carefully evaluated as an independent predictor of outcome using multivariate analysis (step-wise linear regression), a clear relationship was not found.[10,14] After a brief effort at medical stabilization, extended attempts at medical control and avoidance of surgery in such high-risk patients may be associated with exceedingly poor results.[14] The main role of preoperative therapy, therefore, is to stabilize and reverse any adverse preexisting problems (renal, respiratory, infectious, etc.), allow complete assessment of the patient's condition, and prevent myocardial damage before cardioplegic arrest.

Intraoperative Management

Intraoperative advances include improved anesthetic management and monitoring of patients with UA. In addition to the more traditional monitoring with continuous arterial pressure transducers and pulmonary artery catheters, we now routinely use transesophageal echocardiography (TEE) to monitor these critical patients. TEE has been demonstrated to detect myocardial ischemia before electrocardiographic (ECG) or global cardiac output measurements.[57] Significant laboratory advances have been made to enhance myocardial protection and have been applied with increasing success clinically to the acutely ischemic myocardium.[58] These techniques include use of retrograde blood cardioplegia as an adjuvant to antegrade delivery, substrate-enhanced cardioplegia, "hot" shot, as well as the addition of superoxide radical scavengers and leukocyte depletion, among many advances.[59–61] Clinical series have demonstrated the superiority of blood over crystalloid cardioplegia in patients with UA with significant reductions in operative death (0% vs. 5%, $p<0.05$), low cardiac output (10% vs. 19%, $p<0.05$), and perioperative mortality rates (4% vs. 13.5%, $p<0.05$).[62]

The use of the IMA conduit has been demonstrated convincingly to improve graft patency, decrease subsequent cardiac events, and improve long-term survival even in the high-risk patient subset.[63,64] This has resulted in a marked change in the use of arterial conduit for urgent CABG in these patients from 0%[14] to its nearly universal use,[10] despite the urgency and complexity of the surgical revascularization or advanced patient age. The effects of routine use of aspirin to enhance vein graft patency has been documented in elective CABG for SA. These advances are not reflected in any of the earlier series of surgical revascularization for UA, making accurate interpretation of current outcomes more difficult, and are expected to result in improved long-term outcomes.

Immediate Outcome

Perioperative mortality for surgical revascularization of patients with UA varies from 2.8% to 8.5%,[9–11,13,14,49,51,53,55] depending on patient acuity, and ratio of urgent and postinfarction patients included in individual series. Increased mortality is strongly associated with advanced age, urgency of surgery, coronary reoperation, depressed EF, recently of AMI (especially transmural), female gender, LM disease, and crossclamp and total bypass times. Contribution of individual factors assessed as independent predictors in multivariate analyses are less dramatic.[10,14] Only age is a clear *independent* predictor of operative mortality.[10,54] More than 37% of deaths were due to noncardiac causes[10] reflecting the multiplicity of comorbid factors in this aged, high-risk patient subset.

Low cardiac output syndrome, defined as need for significant inotropic or IABP support for more than 24 hours postoperatively, is especially pronounced in patients requiring urgent surgical revascularization in the setting of postinfarction angina, and varies between 11% and 17%.[10] Low cardiac output is statistically more frequent in patients with a depressed preoperative EF and in those requiring preoperative IABP.[10]

The incidence of perioperative myocardial infarction varies from 7% to 12.5%,[9,10,14,49,51,53,62] and does not differ from the incidence of myocardial infarction in patients with UA unresponsive to medical therapy.[10,49,65,66] Perioperative myocardial infarction is highest among patients with depressed EFs and insulin-dependent diabetes.[10,11]

Additional complications are common in this high-risk patient subset. More than 24% of patients have one or more major complications.[49] These include stroke (3%), renal failure (1%), postoperative bleeding (4%), sternal problems (4%), ventricular arrhythmias (20%), and respiratory complications (16%).[10]

Long-Term Outcome

Long-term outcome in patients undergoing surgical revascularization with UA have been uniformly excellent. Five-year survival is most influenced by the individual patient's comorbid factors, especially left ventricular function, and is approximately 95%, with more than 95% of survivors relieved of their chest pain or congestive heart failure and are NYHA and CSCC class I or II.[10,14,53,55] The significance of depressed EF on long-term outcome has been further challenged, suggesting that an acutely depressed EF in patients with UA may represent myocardial stunning, and may not impact significantly on long-term outcome.[14,67]

Comparison of Surgical Revascularization with Medical Therapy

Initial comparisons of medical and surgical therapy of patients with UA demonstrated no differences in 2-year survival (91% vs. 92%) or incidence of AMI (11.7% vs. 12%).[41,65,66] These studies have excluded high-risk patients (such as patients with LM disease, postinfarction angina, women, or patients over 70 years old or with EF <0.25). Less than 20% of patients studied had truly refractory (type II) UA.[65] However, even in this lower risk patient population, patients with depressed left ventricular function (EF <0.50) demonstrated a 71.7% reduction in 8-year cumulative mortality with surgical revascularization when compared to medical therapy (13% vs. 46%, $p<0.04$).[65] Noteworthy is a 2-year cumulative crossover rate from medical to surgical therapy in patients with UA of 34% at 3 years, which increased to 43% by 5 years.[41] The crossover rate from medical to surgical therapy within 30 days of therapy was more than threefold in the refractory type II UA group (19.8% vs. 5.1%, $p<0.05$). Patients who crossed over to surgical therapy had a 2.5-fold increase in operative morality in these patients (10.3% vs. 4.1%) compared to patients treated initially with surgical revascularization.[45,65]

CABG does not seem to reduce the incidence of myocardial infarction in patients with UA, compared to their medically treated refractory cohorts,[45] although older series may not reflect advances in myocardial protection techniques. Laboratory studies have documented that although the incidence of AMI (documented by ECG and enzyme criteria) may not be reduced by urgent surgical revascularization, the size of the resulting infarct (area at risk vs. area of necrosis) is clearly diminished.[58] The presence or absence of a perioperative AMI therefore is a crude assessment of the potential benefits of coronary revascularization for UA and more sensitive clinical tests and follow-up are needed.

Patients with moderately depressed left ventricular function and UA followed for 3 years had a 65% reduction in mortality (6.1% vs. 17.6%, $p<0.04$), and nearly half the rate of hospitalization (31% vs. 60.5%, $p<0.02$) when compared to patients treated with medical therapy.[66] Surgical patients, when compared to their medically treated cohorts, also are less likely to require medications and more likely to have an improved treadmill performance.[41] Finally, work status, which is best predicted by activity level before hospitalization, was similar in the medically and surgically treated groups.[41]

Comparison of Surgical Revascularization with PTCA

There are no large series randomizing patients with UA to either PTCA or CABG. Existing series reflect patient referral bias for each procedure, and are modest in size and limited in follow-up.[49] Accurate comparison of revascularization procedures therefore is not possible. However, when compared to patients with UA referred for angioplasty, patients referred for CABG have more extensive disease (with a preponderance of LM and three-vessel disease) and lower left ventricular function. Despite these selection biases, patients undergoing surgical revascularization have an improved disease-free survival.[49,52]

Conclusion

The wide use of lytic therapy may affect the incidence and progression of AMI resulting in a rapidly increasing incidence of patients with persistent or residual UA. Despite advances in medical therapy, because of the complex, multivessel nature of these patients' coronary artery disease, many patients will fail medical therapy, thereby requiring urgent revascularization. PTCA has emerged as a successful alternative therapy in *selected* patients with UA, with preserved myocardial function and single-vessel coronary disease. No controlled randomized series comparing PTCA and surgical revascularization exist. Given the complexity, urgency, and multitude of comorbid factors, it is unlikely that therapy can be truly randomized in this high-risk patient subset. However, from the existing data we can conclude that an aggressive surgical approach and meticulous operative management of patients with UA result in acceptable morbidity and mortality, with a gratifying long-term prognosis. Surgical advances in myocardial protection and the use of arterial conduits are expected to enhance this outcome further.

References

1. Harper RW, Kennedy G, DeSanctis RW, et al. The incidence and pattern of angina prior to acute myocardial infarction: a study of 577 cases. Am Heart J 1979; 97:178–183.
2. Julian DG. The natural history of unstable angina. In: Hugenholtz PG, Goldman BS, eds. Unstable Angina: Currents Concepts and Management. Stuttgart: Schattauer. 1985; pp 65–70.

3. Gazes PC, Mobley EM, Faris HM, et al. Preinfarction (unstable) angina—a prospective study—ten year follow-up. Circulation 1973; 48:331–337.
4. Rahimtoola SH. Coronary bypass surgery for unstable angina. Circulation 1984; 69:842–848.
5. National Center for Health Statistics. Vital and health statistics: detailed diagnosis and procedures for patients discharged from short stay hospitals. Series 13, no. 90. Hyattsville, MD: US Department of Health and Human Services, Public Health Service, 1987.
6. Brunelli C, Spallarossa P, Ghigliotti G, et al. Thrombolysis in refractory unstable angina. Am J Cardiol 1991; 68:110B–118B.
7. Leeman DE, McCabe CH, Faxon DP, et al. Use of percutaneous coronary angioplasty and bypass surgery despite improved medical therapy for unstable angina pectoris. Am J Cardiol 1988; 61:38G–44G.
8. Wittels EH, Hay JW, Cotto AM Jr. Medical cost of coronary artery disease in the United States. Am J Cardiol 1990; 65:432–440.
9. Fremes SE, Goldman BS, Christakis GT, et al. Current risk of coronary bypass surgery for unstable angina. Eur J Cardiothorac Surg 1991; 5:235–243.
10. Naunheim KS, Fiore AC, Arango DC, et al. Coronary artery bypass grafting for unstable angina: risk analysis. Ann Thorac Surg 1989; 47:569–574.
11. Huttunen K, Rehnberg S, Huttunen H, et al. Clinical characteristics and coronary anatomy in refractory unstable angina pectoris leading to coronary artery bypass grafting. Scand J Thorac Surg 1989; 23:19–23.
12. Braunwald E. Unstable angina. A classification. Circulation 1989; 80:410–414.
13. Teoh KH, Christakis GT, Weisel RD, et al. Increased risk of urgent revascularization. J Thorac Cardiovasc Surg 1987; 93:291–299.
14. Rankin JS, Newton JR Jr, Califf RM, et al. Clinical characteristics and current management of medically refractory unstable angina. Ann Surg 1986; 200:457–465.
15. Davies MJ, Thomas AC. Plaque fissuring—the cause of acute myocardial infarction, sudden ischaemic death, and crescendo angina. Br Heart J 1985; 53:363–373.
16. Falk E. Unstable angina with fatal outcome: dynamic coronary thrombosis leading to infarction and/or sudden death. Circulation 1985; 71:699–708.
17. Ambrose JA, Winters SL, Arora RR, et al. Angiographic evolution of coronary artery morphology in unstable angina. J Am Coll Cardiol 1986; 7:472–478.
18. Gotoh K, Minamino T, Katoh O, et al. The role of intracoronary thrombus in unstable angina: angiographic assessment and thrombolytic therapy during ongoing anginal attacks. Circulation 1988; 77:526–534.
19. Sherman CT, Litvack F, Grundfest W, et al. Coronary angioscopy in patients with unstable angina pectoris. N Engl J Med 1986; 315:913–919.
20. Chaux A, Lee ME, Blanche C, et al. Intraoperative coronary angioscopy.

Technique and results in 58 patients. J Thorac Cardiovasc Surg 1986; 92:972–976.

21. Fitzgerald DJ, Roy L, Catella F, et al. Platelet activation in unstable coronary disease. N Engl J Med 1986; 315:983–989.

22. Fuster V, Badimon L, Cohen M, et al. Insight into the pathogenesis of acute ischemic syndromes. Circulation 1988; 76:1213–1220.

23. Epstein SE, Palmeri ST. Mechanisms contributing to precipitation of unstable angina and acute myocardial infarction: implication regarding therapy. Am J Cardiol 1984; 54:1245–1252.

24. Theroux P. A pathophysiologic basis for the clinical classification and management of unstable angina. Circulation 1987; 75(Suppl V):V103–V109.

25. Becker CR, Gore JM, Lapert JS. Postinfarction unstable angina. Pathophysiologic basis for current treatment modalities. Cardiology 1989; 76:144–157.

26. Epstein SE, Borer JS, Kent KM, et al. Protection of the ischemic myocardium by nitroglycerin: experimental and clinical results. Circulation 1976; 53(Suppl I):I-191–I-197.

27. Nordlander R. Use of nitrates in the treatment of unstable and variant angina. Drugs 1987; 33(Suppl 4):131–139.

28. Bussmar WD, Passek D, Seidel W, et al. Reduction of CK and CK-MB indexes of infarct size by intravenous nitroglycerin. Circulation 1981; 63:615–622.

29. The International Collaborative Study Group. Reduction of infarct size with early use of timolol in acute myocardial infarction. N Engl J Med 1984; 310:9–15.

30. Gottlieb SO, Weisfeldt ML, Arynag P, et al. Effect of the addition of propranolol to therapy with nifedipine for unstable angina pectoris: a randomized, double blind, placebo controlled trial. Circulation 1986; 73:331–337.

31. Blaustein AS, Heller GV, Kolman BS. Adjunctive nifedipine therapy in high-risk, medically refractory, unstable angina pectoris. Am J Cardiol 1983; 52:950–956.

32. Lewis HD, Davis JW, Archibald DJ, et al. Protective effect of aspirin against acute myocardial infarction and death in men with unstable angina. N Engl J Med 1983; 309:396–403.

33. Cairns JA, Gent M, Singer J, et al. Aspirin, sulfipyrazone, or both for unstable angina: results of the Canadian Multicenter Trial. N Engl J Med 1985; 313:1369–1375.

34. Lewis HD. Unstable angina: status of aspirin and other forms of therapy. Circulation 1985; 72(Suppl V):V155–V160.

35. Theroux P, Quimet H, McCans J, et al. Aspirin, heparin or both to treat acute unstable angina. N Engl J Med 1988; 313:1105–1111.

36. Becker RC, Alpert JS. The impact of medical therapy on hemorrhagic complications following coronary artery bypass grafting. Arch Intern Med 1990; 150:2016–2021.

37. Barner HB, Jea JW, Naunheim KS, et al. Emergency coronary bypass not associated with preoperative cardiogenic shock in failed an-

gioplasty, after thrombolysis, and for acute myocardial infarction. Circulation 1989; 79(Suppl I):I152–I159.

38. Conti RR, Hill JA, Mayfield WR. Unstable angina pectoris: pathogenesis and treatment. Curr Probl Cardiol 1989; 14:609–613.

39. Creswell LL, Rosenbloom M, Cox JL, et al. Intraaortic balloon counterpulsation: patterns of usage and outcome in cardiac surgery patients. Ann Thorac Surg 1992; 54:11–20.

40. Scott SM, Luchi RJ, Deupree RH, et al. Veterans Administration Cooperative Study for the treatment of patients with unstable angina. Results in patients with abnormal left ventricular function. Circulation 1988; 78(Suppl I):I-113–I-121.

41. Booth DC, Deupree RH, Hultgren HN, et al. Quality of life after bypass surgery for unstable angina. Five-year follow-up results of the Veterans Affairs Cooperative Study. Circulation 1991; 83:87–95.

42. Myler RK, Shaw RE, Stertzer SH, et al. Unstable angina and coronary angioplasty. Circulation 1990; 82(Suppl II):II-88–II-95.

43. DeFeyter PJ, Suryapranata H, Serruys PW, et al. Coronary angioplasty for unstable angina: immediate and late results in 200 consecutive patients with identification of risk factors for unfavorable early and late outcomes. J Am Coll Cardiol 1988; 12:324–333.

44. DeFeyter PJ, Serruys PW, Van Den Brand M, et al. Emergency coronary angioplasty in refractory unstable angina. N Engl J Med 1985; 313:342–346.

45. Faxon DP. Percutaneous coronary angioplasty in stable and unstable angina. Cardiol Clin 1991; 9(1):99–113.

46. Bentivoglio LG, Holubok R, Kelsey SF, et al. Short and long term outcome of percutaneous transluminal coronary angioplasty in unstable angina versus stable angina: a report of the 1985–1986 NHLBI PTCA Registry. Cathet and Cardiovasc Diagn 1991; 23:227–238.

47. Colle JP, Delarche N. Clinical factors affecting the immediate outcome of PTCA patients with unstable angina and poor candidates for surgery. Cathet and Cardiovasc Diagn 1991; 23:155–163.

48. Talley JD, Hurst JW, King SB 3rd, et al. Clinical outcome 5 years after attempted transluminal angioplasty in 427 patients. Circulation 1988; 77(4):820–829.

49. Hammermeister KE, Morrison DA. Coronary artery bypass surgery for stable and unstable angina. Cardiol Clin 1991; 9(1):135–155.

50. Ryan TJ, Faxon DP, Gunnar RM, et al. Guidelines for percutaneous transluminal coronary angioplasty: a report of the American College of Cardiology/American Heart Association Task Force on the assessment of diagnostic and therapeutic cardiovascular procedures (subcommittee of percutaneous transluminal angioplasty). Circulation 1988; 78:486–502.

51. Lazar HL, Faxon DP, Paone G, et al. Changing profile of failed coronary angioplasty: impact on surgical results. Ann Thorac Surg 1992; 53:269–273.

52. Steffenino G, Meier B, Finchi L, et al. Follow up results of the treatment

of unstable angina by coronary angioplasty. Br Heart J 1987; 57(5): 416–419.

53. Connoly MW, Gelbfish JS, Rose DM, et al. Early coronary artery bypass grafting for complicated acute myocardial infarction. J Cardiovasc Surg 1988; 29(4):375–382.

54. Horneffer PJ, Gardner TJ, Manolio TA, et al. The effect of age on outcome after coronary bypass surgery. Circulation 1987; 76(Suppl V):V6–V12.

55. Stuart RS, Baumgartner WA, Soule S, et al. Predictors of perioperative mortality in patients with unstable postinfarction angina. Circulation 1988; 78(Suppl I):I-163–I-165.

56. Curtis JJ, Walls JT, Salam NH, et al. Impact of unstable angina on operative mortality with coronary revascularization at varying time intervals after myocardial infarction. J Thorac Cardiovasc Surg 1991; 102(6):867–873.

57. Smith JS, Cahalan MK, Benefiel DJ, et al. Intra-operative detection of myocardial ischemia in high-risk patients; electrocardiography versus two dimensional echocardiography. Circulation 1985; 72(5):1015–1021.

58. Buckberg GD. Strategies and logic of cardioplegia delivery to prevent, avoid and reverse ischemic and reperfusion damage. J Thorac Cardiovasc Surg 1987; 93:127–139.

59. Julia PL, Buckberg GD, Acar C, et al. Studies of controlled reperfusion after ischemia. XXI. Reperfusate composition: superiority of blood cardioplegia over crystalloid cardioplegia limiting reperfusion damage-importance of endogenous oxygen free radical scavengers in red blood cells. J Thorac Cardiovasc Surg 1991; 101(2):303–313.

60. Kofsky ER, Julia PL, Buckberg GD, et al. Studies of controlled reperfusion after ischemia. XXII. Reperfusate composition: effects of leukocyte depletion of blood and blood cardioplegic reperfusate after acute coronary occlusion. J Thorac Cardiovasc Surg 1991; 101(2):350–359.

61. Rosenkrantz ER, Okamoto F, Buckberg GD, et al. Safety of prolonged aortic clamping with blood cardioplegia. III. Aspartate enrichment of glutamate-blood cardioplegia in energy depleted hearts after ischemic and reperfusion injury. J Thorac Cardiovasc Surg 1986; 91(3):428–435.

62. Christakis GT, Fremes SE, Weisel RD, et al. Reducing the risk of urgent revascularization for unstable angina: a randomized clinical trial. J Vasc Surg 1986; 3(5):764–772.

63. Loop FD, Lytle BW, Cosgrove DM, et al. Influence of the internal mammary-artery on 10-year survival and other cardiac events. N Engl J Med 1986; 314:1–6.

64. Azariasdes M, Fessler CL, Floten HS, et al. Five year results of coronary artery bypass grafting for patients older than 70 years: role of the internal mammary artery. Ann Thorac Surg 1990; 50(6):940–945.

65. Luchi RJ, Scott RM, Deupree RH, et al. Comparison of medical and surgical therapy for unstable angina pectoris. Results of the Veteran Administration Cooperative Study. N Engl J Med 1987; 316:977–984.

66. Scott SM, Luchi RJ, Deupree RH, et al. Veterans Administration Cooperative Study for the treatment of patients with unstable angina. Results in patients with abnormal left ventricular function. Circulation 1988; 78(Suppl I):I-113–I-121.

67. Cobanoglu A, Freimanis I, Grunkemeir G, et al. Enhanced late survival following coronary artery bypass graft operation for unstable versus chronic angina. Ann Thorac Surg 1984; 37(1):53–58.

Chapter 9

The Surgeon's Role in the Management of Acute Myocardial Infarction

Robert J. Rizzo and Lawrence H. Cohn

Introduction

Experimental and clinical results suggest that acute reperfusion of ischemic or infarcted myocardium limits the extent of damage and minimizes the early and late complications of acute myocardial infarction (AMI).[1-5] Based on the advances in medical and surgical reperfusion techniques, an aggressive, integrated, multimodality approach has been developed for the treatment of myocardial infarction, the most common cause of death in the United States.[6] Medical methods of reperfusion now include thrombolysis, percutaneous transluminal coronary angioplasty (PTCA), laser angioplasty, and coronary atherectomy. Surgical reperfusion now includes coronary bypass with saphenous vein or with multiple arterial conduits, along with improved methods of myocardial

Lazar HL (editor): *Current Therapy for Acute Coronary Ischemia,* © Futura Publishing Co., Inc., Mount Kisco, NY, 1993.

protection. Surgical management of patients with irreversible cardiogenic shock after AMI also includes use of ventricular assist devices as bridges to cardiac transplantation. In this chapter we review the role of the surgeon in the management of AMI.

History of Surgery for AMI

It was not long after Favalaro first introduced coronary artery bypass grafting in 1967 for coronary artery disease that this technique was applied to patients with acute coronary ischemia.[7–9] Clinical experience in the early 1970s suggested that patients developing thrombosis of a coronary artery during cardiac catheterization and thus with known coronary anatomy could be surgically revascularized with low morbidity and mortality. In a small series of eight patients who had emergency coronary bypass grafting for acute coronary occlusion noted at the time of catheterization at the Peter Bent Brigham Hospital, there were no perioperative deaths, infarctions were prevented in more than 50% of cases, and those who sustained an AMI had uncomplicated courses if reperfused surgically within 12 hours.[10] The NIH unstable angina study demonstrated in the mid-1970s that most patients with unstable angina could be stabilized and then operated on semielectively.[11] Those patients demonstrating persistent hemodynamic or electrical instability despite maximal medical therapy could be operated on urgently with reasonable success. Transmural myocardial infarction usually was not considered a surgical indication in the 1970s, unless patients were in cardiogenic shock requiring intra-aortic balloon counterpulsation.[9] Most clinicians felt patients who had an uncomplicated transmural myocardial infarction should not have coronary bypass surgery for at least 6 weeks unless a complicating mechanical defect became evident.[12]

In an effort to limit infarct size, several clinicians beginning in the late 1970s performed emergent surgical reperfusion for patients with evolving AMI.[13,14] Phillips et al., from Des Moines, Iowa, reported a series in which coronary bypass grafting was performed within 6.5 hours of the onset of chest pain.[13] The hospital mortality was 1.3% and the late mortality was 2.8%. All of the mortalities occurred in hemodynamically unstable patients, and this group had a combined early and late mortality risk of 18%. DeWood and Berg from Spokane, Washington, reported 187 patients who had emergency coronary bypass surgery for AMI and a hospital mortality of 5.8% compared with a control group treated medically that had an 11.5% mortality.[14] In 1981, Berg et al. reported a hospital mortality of 2% for patients having emergency coronary bypass surgery less than 6 hours after the onset of acute anterior myocardial infarction and a late mortality at 43 months of only 5%.[15] This compared favorably with medical treatment in that same hospital where the hospital mortality was 15.7% and the late mortality was 28%. In a follow-up study of this Spokane emergency coronary bypass surgery experience, DeWood et al. in 1983 noted that the hospital mortality rate for a patient with acute infarction was related to the severity of coronary disease.[16] The hospital mortality for patients with myocardial infarction and single-vessel disease was 2.3%, for double-vessel disease it was 4.4%, and for those with triple-vessel disease it was 9%. Patients with anterior infarction and triple-vessel disease had a 12% hospital mortality, and if they had Canadian Heart Classification (CHC) IV angina as well, the hospital mortality rate was 28% within the first 24 hours.[17] Thus, the hospital mortality rate appeared related to the severity of coronary artery disease and the degree of preoperative myocardial dysfunction.

In both the Spokane and Des Moines experiences rapid revascularization was associated with improved results. Phillips et al. in 1986 noted that recovery of left ventricular wall motion was improved with rapid surgical reperfusion, subtotal occlusion of the infarct-related artery, and the presence of collateral vessels.[18] Rogers et al. in 1984 had already noted that regional wall motion improved after either angioplasty or coronary bypass only in patients with subtotally occluded arteries or in patients with angiographic evidence of collateral blood flow to the infarct region.[19] The benefits of early reperfusion were particularly noticeable for anterior myocardial infarction. The enthusiasm for emergent surgical reperfusion for AMI was tempered by several reports suggesting surgical reperfusion of infarctions in evolution resulted in hemorrhagic myocardial infarctions.[20,21] Hemorrhagic infarction after reperfusion appeared most related to situations where reperfusion occurred late. All of these studies strongly supported the need for rapid reperfusion to optimize salvage of myocardium and decrease long-term mortality, which is known to be related to ventricular function.

Laboratory investigations of reperfusion published during a similar time period suggested a time limit of about 6 hours beyond which there appeared to be minimal reduction in the ultimate size of the myocardial infarction after acute reperfusion.[22] Riemer et al. noted that myocardial infarct size was directly related to the duration of coronary occlusion in dogs.[23] Although early reperfusion appeared to salvage ischemic myocardium, some concern was raised that late reperfusion may increase the amount of myocardial damage through a mechanism referred to as reperfusion injury. Myocardial reperfusion was thus thought possibly to represent a "double-edged sword."[24] Reperfusion of ischemic myocardium does result in cellular swelling, which may disturb microvascular blood flow and create more ischemic damage.[25] The mechanism underlying ischemic reperfusion injury is thought to involve release of oxygen-derived free radicals and other inflammatory mediators including stimulated leukocytes.[26] Experimental reperfusion of ischemic myocardium, like in the clinical studies, appeared beneficial when instituted early but not late.

Since speed of reperfusion of ischemic myocardium appeared critical in efforts to limit the extent of damage from myocardial infarction, the stimulus was provided for development of more rapid means of reperfusion than was possible by surgery. Nonsurgical means of coronary reperfusion were thus intensively developed and applied in the late 1970s. Although the feasibility of thrombolysis for AMI was first demonstrated in 1958 by Fletcher et al.,[27] the current era of nonsurgical reperfusion was initiated by Chazov et al. in 1976 using intracoronary administration of fibrinolysin,[28] and by Rentrop et al. in 1978, who relieved thrombotic obstruction via guidewire recanalization.[29] The large European trial of streptokinase (SK) in 1979 reported reduced mortality at 6 months if SK was given within 12 hours of AMI.[30] The success of intravenous SK reported in a large GISSI trial with reduced mortality for AMI if given within 6 hours of the onset of symptoms established the routine use of thrombolytic therapy for AMI.[31] The finding by DeWood et al. in 1980 that acute coronary angiography in patients with acute transmural myocardial infarction revealed infarct-related total coronary occlusion in 87% of cases, of which many were found to contain coronary thrombosis, provided much optimism for the use of thrombolytic therapy to establish acute and rapid reperfusion for AMI.[32] Treatment with recombinant tissue-type plasminogen activator (rt-PA) achieved patency of the infarct-related artery in 75% to 85% of patients and provided improvement in left ventricular function as well as survival.[33]

Gruntzig et al. introduced PTCA in 1978 for the treatment of coronary arterial stenosis, and shortly thereafter wire-guided balloon angioplasty was applied to achieve prompt reperfusion of infarct-related arteries during AMI.[34] Although PTCA is less easily available than thrombolytic therapy, PTCA has been used both in lieu of thrombolytic therapy or after failed thrombolysis, or when a severe stenosis remains after successful thrombolysis. The hospital mortality rate for emergency PTCA for AMI has been reported to be 1% for patients with single-vessel disease and 12% for patients with multivessel disease.[35,36] Although primary PTCA may result in less subsequent ischemia than thrombolysis alone, it has not been shown to be superior to an initial attempt at reperfusion with thrombolytic therapy.[37] Early emergency PTCA after thrombolysis has not been shown to be better than delayed PTCA, which was used only if ischemia was documented later in the postinfarction course.[38] Rescue angioplasty has been used for patients in whom thrombolytic therapy has failed to achieve reperfusion and has been successful in more than 75% of cases.[39] PTCA also has been applied in patients with severe hemodynamic compromise and appears to have provided substantial benefit, although at relatively high risk.[40]

The evolution of thrombolysis and PTCA has relegated surgery to a secondary yet vital role in the management of AMI. This includes cases in which thrombolysis or PTCA failed or were not applicable, and cases complicated by mechanical defects necessitating ventricular repair, assistance, or replacement.

Postinfarction Angina

In the late 1970s and early 1980s, experience accumulated regarding the course and optimal management of postinfarction angina, or angina that occurs hours to days after AMI. Postinfarction angina often heralds extension of an uncomplicated AMI into a complicated one, which may lead to further loss of myocardium, hemodynamic collapse, or death. Extension of an AMI occurs in 8% to 30% of cases and may occur in a stuttering fashion over several days, and be associated with intermittent release of myocardial enzymes, loss of myocardium, and eventually cardiogenic shock.[41,42] Patients who presented in acute cardiogenic shock after extension of AMI in the 1970s and were revascularized emergently suffered a high mortality.[43] The poor late prognosis of patients after non–Q wave myocardial infarction due to subtotal occlusion of the infarct-related artery may be accounted for by infarct extension occurring due to the presence of significant residual myocardium at risk in the ischemic zone distal to the subtotal occlusion of the infarct-related artery.[44] Postinfarction angina may be caused by ischemic myocardium adjacent to the site of the recent infarct or in areas distant to the recent infarct, where inadequate perfusion exists because of additional coronary artery disease.[45]

In the early 1980s it became obvious that patients with postinfarction angina treated medically had a nearly 50% mortality[45]; thus, aggressive surgical revascularization was employed and resulted in low morbidity and mortality, and appeared to decrease the number of patients presenting in cardiogenic shock after extension of AMI.[46–48] In some cases of postinfarction angina, aggressive medical therapy may alleviate the symptoms and ECG changes, and revascularization may be recommended after semi-elective cardiac catheterization and a period of evaluation. However, aggressive medical therapy often fails to stabilize postinfarction angina, necessitating aggressive medical or surgical reperfusion therapy.[38,47] Patients with single-vessel disease and those with minimal multivessel disease and a dominant "culprit" lesion are candidates for PTCA. In those who are not candidates for PTCA, particularly those with triple-vessel disease, and in those who failed PTCA, urgent CABG may be considered at any time after AMI for continued postinfarction angina.[48] Several early experiences with CABG for postinfarction angina reported operative mortalities of 2% to 3% and 5-year survivals of between 85% and 90%, similar to those of elective coronary bypass surgery.[46–48]

The results of CABG for postinfarction angina have been analyzed in several large series for predictors associated with increased mortality. Gardner et al. reported a retrospective multivariate analysis of 300 patients who had a 5% hospital mortality. This study identified the presence of an anterior transmural myocardial infarction and preoperative need for intra-aortic balloon pump (IABP) as significant independent predictors of mortality.[49] Kennedy et al. reviewed 793 patients operated on within 30 days of AMI and reported a 5.7% operative mortality.[50] They found increased age, the degree of surgical urgency, prior coronary bypass surgery, congestive heart failure, and a Q-wave myocardial infarction were associated with increased mortality. Kouchoukos et al. reported a 3.3% 30-day mortality for 240 patients operated on within 30 days of

AMI: left main coronary disease, female sex, and left ventricular (LV) dysfunction were independent predictors of death.[51] Naunheim et al. reviewed 336 patients having isolated CABG after AMI and found advanced age, decreased LV function, and worse clinical group to be independent predictors of mortality after multivariate analysis.[52] The mortality for patients with mild stable angina was 2%, with rest angina 6%, with angina requiring IABP for pain control 10%, and for patients with postinfarction ischemia or infarct extension complicated by cardiogenic shock 48%. Overall, these studies indicate the results of CABG for postinfarction angina are good compared with medical therapy, but increased operative risk can be expected in patients with advanced age or worse LV function, particularly those in cardiogenic shock.

CABG is not necessary after AMI for all patients, but should be considered for patients with viable myocardium at risk even when classic postinfarction angina is not evident.[53] Theroux et al. described the prognostic value of exercise testing soon after AMI, and was able to identify patients at high risk for sudden death after AMI.[54] For patients who display greater than 1 mm ST depression during or immediately after submaximal ETT within 2 weeks of AMI, the 1-year mortality was 27% (13-fold higher) compared with the 2% mortality risk for patients with a normal ETT after AMI. In addition to exercise stress testing, positron emission tomography (PET) has proved useful for recognizing viable ischemic myocardium after AMI.[55] Early dipyridamole-thallium imaging also may help predict further postinfarct ischemia.[56] Patients with evidence of easily inducible postinfarct ischemia may be an important subgroup that may benefit from coronary bypass surgery, particularly considering the proven benefits for surgery in patients with depressed LV function.[57]

PTCA Failures

Emergency CABG after failure or complication of PTCA initially was required in up to 14% of cases, but as interventional cardiologists have gained experience, the need for emergency CABG after PTCA has dropped to below 5%.[58,59] Ferguson et al. reported no difference in operative mortality after emergency CABG for failed elective or emergency PTCA.[60] A coronary reperfusion catheter, also known as a Stack catheter, was used in more than half of the emergency PTCA failures to help alleviate myocardial ischemia during preparation for surgery.[61] Talley et al. reviewed the Emory University experience with emergency CABG after failed PTCA, which was most commonly due to coronary artery dissection.[58] Their mortality rate for emergency CABG was 2.5%, and analysis of their surgical technique revealed frequent use of IABP support, less use of internal mammary artery (IMA) grafts, and the focus was on expeditious institution of cardiopulmonary bypass with systemic cooling and rapid revascularization. A summary of published reports of emergency CABG for failed PTCA revealed an average mortality of 6% and an average incidence of Q-wave myocardial infarction of 29%.[58]

Evolving AMI

The goal for therapy of patients with evolving AMI is now rapid reperfusion, usually accomplished via thrombolysis but complemented by PTCA and CABG. Acute reperfusion is now considered for almost every patient with evolving AMI, particularly involving the anterior wall, provided there are no serious medical or surgical contraindications. Reperfusion should be achieved within 4 to 6 hours of the onset of ischemia to salvage sufficient myocardium to improve long-term survival.[2,3] Emergent CABG plays a significant role in the present treatment of AMI, particularly in patients with complicated multivessel disease, in whom acute reperfusion has not been established by thrombolysis or PTCA.[4,5,62]

Recent experiences have shown that reperfusion of AMI via thrombolysis has been quite effective, and the need for emergency CABG has been limited by the application of thrombolysis and PTCA.[5,62] Emergency CABG is indicated in the setting of evolving AMI for patients with single- or multivessel disease not amenable to or having failed reperfusion via thrombolysis or PTCA, and in whom myocardial ischemia persists and enough time remains for surgical reperfusion to occur before myocardial necrosis in the infarct zone is completed. Immediate CABG after failed thrombolysis can be performed successfully, but there is increased bleeding and blood transfusion requirement. CABG performed 12 hours and later after thrombolysis has been associated with minimal bleeding problems and excellent results, similar to those for elective CABG.[63,64]

Although some have advocated routine early prophylactic

CABG after successful thrombolysis to prevent reinfarction due to delayed thrombotic occlusion,[65] others have applied a more selective approach to emergency CABG after successful thrombolysis.[62–64] Data from The Thrombolysis and Angioplasty in Myocardial Infarction Trial (TAMI) revealed that only 6% of patients required emergency CABG in this trial, with indications including left main disease, unsuitable anatomy for PTCA, and unsuccessful PTCA.[62] There were no operative deaths and three (12.5%) hospital deaths, all in patients in cardiogenic shock preoperatively. Global and regional LV function was found to be preserved by emergency CABG. Late in-hospital CABG was performed on 15% of the patients in the TAMI trial, and there were no operative deaths and two (3.4%) in-hospital deaths, again in patients with preoperative cardiogenic shock. Although patients in the surgical group, which comprised 21% of the TAMI trial, were older, had more extensive CAD, and had a higher incidence of anterior myocardial infarction, the hospital mortality (6%), 1-year mortality (2.5%), event-free survival, and anginal and general health status were similar to patients who did not require surgery. CABG is indicated during evolving AMI after thrombolysis when important residual stenoses remain that are less suitable to PTCA than CABG, such as left main or extensive triple-vessel coronary disease, or when CABG would be recommended even outside the setting of AMI.

Emergency surgical revascularization has been applied successfully to patients during AMI even without prior use of thrombolysis. Phillips et al., DeWood et al., and Berg et al. were the first to attempt this logistically difficult plan, but both groups were able to report good results when reperfusion occurred within 6 hours, particularly in patients who were not in cardiogenic shock.[13–15] These and other groups have since reported low mortality and improved ventricular function and survival in patients undergoing CABG for AMI.[62,66,67] In a review of the literature by Barner et al. in 1989, the overall 1-month mortality for emergency CABG for AMI without cardiogenic shock was estimated at 5%.[63] Late follow-up of emergency CABG has revealed improved LV function, particularly after anterior AMI, and improved functional class and survival.[2,3]

Emergency CABG for cardiogenic shock due to AMI is associated with increased mortality relative to patients with stable hemodynamics, but may be lifesaving often enough to make this aggressive approach worthwhile. Bolooki reviewed the literature regarding CABG for cardiogenic shock in 1989 and found the overall survival to be 66%, and 80% of survivors were New York Heart Association (NYHA) functional class I or II.[68] Survival appears better in patients who respond favorably to insertion of an IABP, and emergency coronary artery bypass surgery in this group appears to improve early and late survival. If the patient in cardiogenic shock after AMI is not a candidate for CABG due to irreversible end-stage ventricular dysfunction, yet relatively young and otherwise healthy, then cardiac transplantation should be considered.[69] If the patient's condition deteriorates despite IABP support while awaiting a donor heart, then a mechanical ventricular assist device may be employed as a bridge to cardiac transplantation.

Acute Mechanical Complications of AMI

After AMI, necrosis of myocardium may lead to myocardial rupture, which may involve the LV free wall, the interventricular septum, or the papillary muscle of the mitral valve. Rupture of the LV free wall causes pericardial tamponade, rupture of the interventricular septum causes acute congestive heart failure, and rupture of the papillary muscle causes acute mitral regurgitation and pulmonary edema. All of these myocardial ruptures represent acute mechanical complications of AMI that usually cause cardiogenic shock, which may be correctable.[12]

LV Free Wall Rupture (Cardiorrhexis)

Rupture of the LV free wall has been reported to be the cause of death in 5% to 10% of patients dying in-hospital of AMI, and this usually occurs within 2 weeks after the AMI.[70] The diagnosis of LV free wall rupture often is made at autopsy and is actually three to four times more common than postinfarction ventricular septal defects (VSD). Rupture of the LV free wall usually results in sudden hemopericardium with development of acute cardiac tamponade. The clinical presentation may be marked by acute onset of chest pain and profound cardiogenic shock with marked venous distention, pulsus paradoxus, and eventual electromechanical dissociation.[71] Diagnosis before death requires a high degree of clinical suspicion and emergency pericardiocentesis may be lifesaving. Some patients may leak blood slowly into the pericardium before frank rupture, and in these patients echocardiography and angiography may assist in the diagnosis. Salvage of patients with LV free wall rupture after AMI requires emergency sternotomy, relief of cardiac tamponade, institution of cardiopulmonary bypass, repair of the rupture, and sometimes coronary bypass grafting. The actual site of rupture usually is at the junction of the infarcted and normal myocardium. Repair of the rupture may require resection of the necrotic myocardium or infarctectomy followed by closure of the LV free wall defect with a patch similar to that for a LV aneurysm repair.[72,73] However, some sites of rupture have been expeditiously and successfully repaired without infarctectomy by closing the rupture site with heavy suture supported by Teflon strips parallel to the linear tear. In patients in whom coronary angiography was unable to be obtained preoperatively, some consideration should be given to blind coronary bypass if atherosclerotic lesions are palpable in any of the major coronary arteries. In a review by Bolooki of cases of surgical treatment for LV free wall rupture after AMI, the overall survival was 65%.[68]

Incomplete rupture of the LV free wall may occur when a slow leak is contained by organizing thrombus and hematoma which, combined with adhesions to pericardium, may seal the rupture and prevent the development of hemopericardium and tamponade. Over time, the area of partial rupture may become a small LV diverticulum or a large pseudoaneurysm.[74] There is a propensity for LV pseudoaneurysm eventually to rupture, which may occur weeks or months after the initial infarction.[75] Once the diagnosis of LV pseudoaneurysm is made, surgical repair is indicated to prevent acute rupture. Surgical repair involves resection of the pseudoaneurysm with care being taken to avoid systemic embolization of thrombus within the false aneurysm sac.[76] Once debrided, the edges of the LV free wall defect may be repaired either primarily or via patch with the purpose being maintenance of LV geometry.

LV Aneurysm

AMI is complicated by the development of left ventricular aneurysm (LVA) in approximately 10% to 15% of cases, but varies depending on the criteria used for diagnosis.[77] LVAs occur after total occlusion of the infarct-related artery in areas that have sustained transmural AMI. Anterior LVAs are the most common. In patients who develop an LVA after AMI, the infarct region loses its ability to contract and becomes healed with a scar. Then, due to the wall stresses imposed by forceful contraction of the remaining viable myocardium, the scarred area of infarction becomes dyskinetic, thins out, and eventually bulges enough paradoxically during systole to be considered an aneurysm. The development of an LVA after AMI is associated with a poor prognosis regarding both morbidity and mortality. In a necropsy series by Schlichter et al., 88% of these patients died after the diagnosis of LVA was made less than 5 years previously.[78] Morbid complications of LVA in decreasing order of frequency include congestive heart failure, angina, ventricular arrhythmias, and arterial embolization, and all may be considered indications for repair.[79]

Likoff and Bailey first performed a surgical excision of postinfarction LVA in 1955,[80] and the first LVA resected using cardiopulmonary bypass was performed by Cooley et al. in 1958.[81] The use of a Dacron patch for repair of a postinfarct VSD by Daggett et al.[82] in 1977 was then applied by Jatene to the repair of LVA.[83] Preservation of LV geometry has been emphasized by Jatene, who has also introduced circular reduction followed by linear or patch closure. Surgical results depend on the severity of associated coronary artery disease, completeness of revascularization, function of the residual LV myocardium, and the ability to reconstruct the LV geometry properly.

Acute early repair of LVA after AMI with or without postinfarction angina is required infrequently, but excellent results have been reported when done within 8 weeks after an AMI. In 1980, Walker et al. reported 20 patients who required acute aneurysmectomy for severe congestive heart failure or serious tachyarrhythmia with only one operative death.[84] The principles of surgical treatment for acute and chronic LVA are the same. The patient is placed on cardiopulmonary bypass and cooled systemically. The left ventricle is vented to define the edges of the aneurysm and then the aneurysm sac is opened and all of the thrombus is removed, with care taken to avoid spillage into the LV cavity, which could result in systemic embolization. A central portion of the aneurysm sac is excised and an attempt is then made to recreate preinfarction ventricular geometry during closure of the defect. Small defects can be closed in a linear fashion, but larger aneurysms may require narrowing of the defect size via circumferential purse string suture around the base of the

LVA, as described by Jatene,[83] followed by a Dacron patch closure of the defect. Operative mortality for LVA repair has ranged between 4% and 50%.[79–86] Long-term survival after surgical repair of LVA has been between 50% and 70%,[79,86] and is much improved over medical management of LVA.

LVA sometimes is associated with recurrent ventricular arrhythmias, which also need to be addressed at the time of surgical repair of the aneurysm. Results of LV aneurysmectomy with or without CABG have not been consistently satisfactory.[87] With the development of intraoperative endocardial and epicardial mapping techniques, the area of irritability could be excised more reliably. Harken et al. reported in 1980 that blind LV aneurysmectomy for ventricular tachycardia had an associated operative mortality of 42%, with all but one postoperative death due to uncontrolled ventricular arrhythmias.[88] In contrast, directed endocardial resection after endocardial mapping and LVA repair was associated with an operative mortality of 7%, and 27 of the 30 patients had ablation of their ventricular tachycardia. Guiraudon et al. reported the use of encircling endocardial ventriculotomy for relief of inducible ventricular tachycardia for patients in whom the site of the tachycardia could not be elucidated by mapping techniques.[89] The development of the automatic implantable cardioverter defibrillator now provides one of the most effective therapies for treatment of recurrent sustained ventricular arrhythmias and has improved survival markedly.[90]

Rupture of the Interventricular Septum

Postinfarction VSD is responsible for 1% to 2% of deaths after AMI.[91] Rupture of the interventricular septum usually occurs within the first week, an average of 2.6 days after AMI.[92] An autopsy study found 66% of infarct VSDs located in the low anterior septum, 17% in the posterior septum, 13% in the mid-portion, and 4% in the upper septum.[93] Without operative intervention, postinfarct VSD results in death in 65% of patients within 2 weeks and in 90% at 1 year.[94] Diagnosis should be suspected in patients after transmural AMI who suddenly develop congestive heart failure and have been found to have a holosystolic murmur at the lower mid-left sternal border. Bedside right heart catheterization can easily demonstrate an oxygen step-up in the right ventricle associated with right ventricular (RV) and PA hypertension.[92] Inotropic medication, afterload reduction, and intra-aortic balloon counterpulsation often are needed to help stabilize the patient before surgery.

In the past, surgical therapy for a ruptured ventricular septum was delayed in hopes that scarring of the defect would occur over time, which would allow earlier suturing and repair of the defect. Unfortunately, most patients cannot survive much delay even with IABP support. If clinical stability allows, coronary angiography should be performed before repair of the defect. Urgent surgical repair of postinfarct VSD is now considered optimal treatment, since further delay merely prolongs the period of cardiogenic shock in these patients.[82] Rupture of the interventricular septum usually occurs after the first AMI, and is poorly tolerated because the defect often is associated with a relatively large AMI, acute LV aneurysm, and markedly elevated PA pressures in patients with previously normal pulmonary vascular resistance.

The first successful surgical repair of postinfarct VSD was reported by Cooley et al. in 1957 and was performed via a right ventriculotomy, which was a technique used for repair of congenital VSD.[95] It was found that repair of postinfarct VSD via the RV resulted in further compromise of an often already dysfunctional RV, it left the LV infarct unmanaged, and it often was associated with a high incidence of a residual VSD.[96,97] The postinfarct VSD was more difficult to identify clearly via the right ventriculotomy because of the natural trabeculations within the RV, and also the infarction was more extensive on the LV side of the septum than on the right. Kitamura et al. and Javid et al. first demonstrated the efficacy of the left-sided approach for infarcted VSD.[98,99] Kitamura et al. reported that a residual recurrent shunt occurred in 11% of the patients with a left-sided approach versus 42% of the patients with an RV approach.[98]

Surgical repair of postinfarction VSD now includes the use of bicaval cannulation with snarring of both venae cavae and establishment of total cardiopulmonary bypass. An incision is made through the area of LV infarction and the VSD is inspected. Apical VSDs may be repaired by amputation of the apex including the area of the VSD, and then reapproximation of the RV and LV to the intact residual ventricular septum at the edge of the apical amputation. The less distal VSDs, either anterior or posterior, may require debridement of the necrotic septum with repair of the ventricular septal defect with a Dacron patch. The area of the ventricular free wall infarct may be resected and patched with Dacron, as suggested by Daggett et al.[97] Coronary bypass grafting has been required in one-third of the patients undergoing repair of acute postinfarction VSD.[68] From a summary of several reports of surgery for acute postinfarction VSD, the overall operative survival has been reported at 45% with 84% of survivors being NYHA functional class I or II.[68] A more recent report by Daggett et al. revealed an overall hospital mortality of 25% in patients treated since 1975, and mortality was 34% for posterior defects and 15% for anterior defects.[100]

Ruptured Papillary Muscle

Ischemic mitral regurgitation may occur after AMI due to papillary muscle dysfunction, papillary muscle infarction with rupture, or posterior LV dilatation and mitral valve annular dilatation.[12] Rupture of the papillary muscle after AMI has been reported to account for 1% of deaths after AMI, and it is more commonly related to rupture of the posterior medial papillary muscle.[101] Ruptured papillary muscle usually occurs within the first week after AMI and results in acute pulmonary edema with an associated early mortality of 70% within 24 hours if not corrected. Diagnosis of ruptured papillary muscle should be expected in patients who develop acute pulmonary edema and a loud apical systolic murmur within the first week after posterior or inferior AMI. Although the murmur associated with a postinfarct VSD is louder at the left sternal border and not at the apex, clinical differentiation between ruptured papillary muscle and ruptured interventricular septum may be difficult. Right-heart catheterization will reveal no oxygen step-up within the RV and a profound V wave on the pulmonary capillary wedge tracing. Echocardiography may identify a flail segment of the mital valve including prolapsing of the tip of the papillary muscle. Medical therapy should include stabilization with inotropes, systemic vasodilators, and intra-aortic balloon counterpulsation. Stabilization in this manner may allow coronary angiography and more specifically directed coronary bypass, but continued hemodynamic instability may require surgery without coronary angiography.

Surgical treatment for ruptured papillary muscle after AMI includes bicaval cannulation with establishment of cardiopulmonary bypass with systemic hypothermia; the distal coronary graft anastomoses are performed first, then the left atrium is opened, and the prolapsing papillary muscle tip is resected while preserving the posterior leaflet. Mitral valve replacement usually is performed since reconstruction often is frought with difficulty in the patient with acute mitral regurgitation, due to the small left atrium and quite friable subvalvar tissues.

Surgical repair of ruptured papillary muscle after AMI has been associated with an operative survival of 54% in a summary of multiple series.[68] The first successful reported repair of ruptured papillary muscle was by Austen et al. in 1965.[102] The overall 5-year survival rate is nearly 40% and is related to the functional status of the LV.[103]

Summary

The surgeon's role in the management of AMI has evolved along with the development of new techniques for diagnosis and treatment of this condition.[104] At the present time, surgical treatment of AMI is indicated for:

1. sudden coronary artery occlusion during cardiac catheterization or after PTCA that cannot be reperfused by thrombolysis or PTCA,

2. evolving AMI in patients in whom reperfusion via thrombolysis or PTCA was either not applicable, had failed, or was associated with signs of continuing ischemia, and surgical reperfusion could be performed before completion of the infarction,

3. postinfarction angina not responding to maximal medical therapy and/or PTCA,

4. acute mechanical defects such as LV free wall rupture or aneurysm, rupture of the interventricular septum, or rupture of the papillary muscle, unless there is terminal organ damage,

5. irreversible cardiogenic shock in patients who are candidates for cardiac transplantation and may require LV assist as a mechanical bridge to transplantation.

References

1. Kloner RA, Ellis SG, Lange R, Braunwald E. Studies of experimental coronary artery reperfusion: effects on infarct size, myocardial function, biochemistry, ultrastructure and microvascular damage. Circulation 1983; 68(Suppl I):I-8–15.

2. DeWood MA, Notske RN, Berg R Jr, et al. Medical and surgical management of early Q wave myocardial infarction. I. Effects of surgical reperfusion on survival, recurrent myocardial infarction, sudden death and functional class at 10 or more years of followup. J Am Coll Cardiol 1989; 14:65–77.

3. DeWood MA, Leonard J, Grunwald RP, et al. Medical and surgical management of early Q wave myocardial infarction. II. Effects on mortality and global and regional left ventricular function at 10 or more years of followup. J Am Coll Cardiol 1989; 14:78–90.

4. Phillips SJ, Kongtahworn C, Skinner JR, Zeff RH. Emergency coronary artery reperfusion: a choice therapy for evolving myocardial infarction. J Thorac Cardiovasc Surg 1983; 86:679–688.

5. Califf RM, Topol EJ, George BS, et al. One-year outcome after therapy with tissue plasminogen activator: report from the thrombolysis and angioplasty in myocardial infarction trial. Am Heart J 1990; 119:777–785.

6. Braunwald E. The aggressive treatment of acute myocardial infarction. Circulation 1985; 71:1087–1092.

7. Favaloro RG. Saphenous vein autograft replacement of severe segmental coronary artery occlusion. Operative technique. Ann Thorac Surg 1968; 5:334–339.

8. Favaloro RG, Effler DB, Cheanvechai CH, Quint RA, Sones FM Jr. Acute coronary insufficiency (impending myocardial infarction and myocardial infarction). Surgical treatment by the saphenous vein graft technique. Am J Cardiol 1971; 28:598–607.

9. Mundth ED, Yurchak PN, Buckley MJ, Leinbach RC, Kantrowitz A, Austen WG. Circulatory assistance and emergency direct coronary artery surgery for shock complicating acute myocardial infarction. N Engl J Med 1970; 283:1382–1384.

10. Cohn LH, Gorlin R, Herman MV, Collins JJ Jr. Aorto-coronary bypass for acute coronary occlusion. J Thorac Cardiovasc Surg 1972; 64:503–513.

11. Unstable Angina Pectoris Study Group. Unstable angina pectoris: national cooperative study group to compare surgical and medical therapy. II. In-hospital experience and initial followup results in patients with one, two and three vessel disease. Am J Cardiol 1978; 42:839–848.

12. Cohn LH. Surgical management of acute and chronic cardiac mechanical complications due to myocardial infarction. Am Heart J 1981; 102:1049–1060.

13. Phillips SJ, Kongtahworn C, Zeff RH, et al. Emergency coronary artery revascularization: a possible therapy for acute myocardial infarction. Circulation 1979; 60:241–246.

14. DeWood MA, Speres J, Notske RH, et al. Medical and surgical management of acute myocardial infarction. Am J Cardiol 1979; 44:1356–1364.

15. Berg R Jr, Selinger SL, Leonard JJ, Grunwald RP, O'Grady WP. Immediate coronary artery bypass for acute evolving myocardial infarction. J Thorac Cardiovasc Surg 1981; 81:493–497.

16. DeWood MA, Speres J, Berg R Jr, et al. Acute myocardial infarction: a decade of experience with surgical perfusion. Circulation 1983; 68(Suppl II):II-8–16.
17. DeWood MA, Heit J, Spores J, et al. Anterior transmural myocardial infarction: effects of surgical coronary reperfusion on global and regional left ventricular function. J Am Coll Cardiol 1983; 1:1223–1234.
18. Phillips SJ, Zeff RH, Skinner JR, Toon RS, Grignon A, Kongtahworn C. Reperfusion protocol and results in 738 patients with evolving myocardial infarction. Ann Thorac Surg 1986; 41:119–125.
19. Rogers WJ, Hood WP Jr, Mantle JA, et al. Return of left ventricular function after reperfusion in patients with myocardial infarction: importance of subtotal stenosis or intact collaterals. Circulation 1984; 69:338–349.
20. Montoya A, Mulet J, Pifarre R, et al. Hemorrhagic infarct following myocardial revascularization. J Thorac Cardiovasc Surg 1978; 75:206–212.
21. Lie JT, Lawrie GM, Morris GC Jr, Winters WL. Hemorrhagic myocardial infarction associated with aortocoronary bypass revascularization. Am Heart J 1978; 96:295–302.
22. Maroko PR, Libby P, Ginks WR, et al. Coronary artery reperfusion. I. Early effects on local myocardial function and the extent of myocardial necrosis. J Clin Invest 1972; 51:2710–2716.
23. Reimer KA, Lowe JE, Rasmussen MM, Jennings RB. The wave front phenomenon of ischemic cell death. I. Myocardial infarct size and duration of coronary occlusion in dogs. Circulation 1977; 56:786–794.
24. Braunwald E, Kloner RA. Myocardial reperfusion: a double-edged sword? J Clin Invest 1985; 76:1713–1719.
25. Kloner RA, Ganote CE, Jennings RB. The "no-reflow" phenomenon after temporary coronary occlusion in the dog. J Clin Invest 1974; 54:1496–1508.
26. Forman MB, Virmani R, Puett DW. Mechanism and therapy of myocardial reperfusion injury. Circulation 1990; 81(Suppl IV):IV-69–78.
27. Fletcher AP, Alkjaersig N, Smyriotis FE, Sherry S. The treatment of patients suffering from early myocardial infarction with massive and prolonged streptokinase therapy. Trans Assoc Am Phys 1958; 71:287–296.
28. Chazov EI, Mateeva LS, Mazaev AV, et al. Intracoronary administration of fibrinolysin in acute myocardial infarction. Ter Arkh 1976; 48:8–19.
29. Rentrop P, VeVivie ER, Karsch KR, Keruzer H. Acute coronary occlusion with impending infarction as an angiographic complication relieved by guide-wire recanalization. Clin Cardiol 1978; 1:101–106.
30. European Cooperative Study Group for Streptokinase Treatment in Acute Myocardial Infarction. Streptokinase in acute myocardial infarction. N Engl J Med 1979; 301:797–802.
31. Gruppo Italiano Per Lo Studio Della Streptochinasi Nell'Infarto Mio-

cardico (GISSI). Effectiveness of intravenous thrombolytic treatment in acute myocardial infarction. Lancet 1986; 1:397–402.

32. DeWood MA, Spores J, Notske R, et al. Prevalence of total coronary occlusion during the early hours of transmural myocardial infarction. N Engl J Med 1980; 303:897–902.

33. Collen D. Coronary thrombolysis: streptokinase or recombinant tissue-type plasminogen activator? Ann Intern Med 1990; 112:529–538.

34. Gruntzig AR, Senning A, Siegenthaler WE. Nonoperative dilatation of coronary artery stenosis: percutaneous transluminal coronary angioplasty. N Engl J Med 1979; 301:61–68.

35. Stone GW, Rutherford BD, McConahay DR, et al. Direct coronary angioplasty in acute myocardial infarction: outcome in patients with single vessel disease. J Am Coll Cardiol 1990; 15:534–543.

36. Kahn JK, Rutherford BD, McConahay DR, et al. Results of primary angioplasty for acute myocardial infarction in patients with multivessel coronary artery disease. J Am Coll Cardiol 1990; 16:1089–1096.

37. Brundage BH. Because we can, should we? J Am Coll Cardiol 1990; 15:544–545.

38. Guerci AD, Ross RS. TIMI II and the role of angioplasty in acute myocardial infarction. N Engl J Med 1989; 320:663–665.

39. Stack RS, Califf RM, Hinohara T, et al. Survival and cardiac event rates in the first year after emergency coronary angioplasty for acute myocardial infarction. J Am Coll Cardiol 1988; 11:1141–1149.

40. Ellis SG, O'Neill WW, Bates ER, et al. Implications for patient triage from survival and left ventricular functional recovery analyses in 500 patients treated with coronary angioplasty for acute myocardial infarction. J Am Coll Cardiol 1989; 13:1251–1259.

41. Baker JT, Bramlet DA, Lester RM, et al. Myocardial infarction extension: incidence and relationship to survival. Circulation 1982; 65:918–923.

42. Kagen L, Scheidt S, Butt A. Serum myoglobin in myocardial infarction: the "staccato phenomenon": is acute myocardial infarction in man an intermittent event? Am J Med 1977; 62:86–92.

43. Leinbach RC, Gold HK, Dinsmore RE, et al. The role of angiography in cardiogenic shock. Circulation 1973; 48(Suppl III):III-95–98.

44. Hutter AM Jr, DeSanctis RW, Flynn T, Yeatman LA. Nontransmural myocardial infarction: a comparison of hospital and late clinical course of patients with that of matched patients with transmural anterior and transmural inferior myocardial infarction. Am J Cardiol 1981; 48:595–602.

45. Schuster EH, Bulkley BH. Early postinfarction angina. Ischemia at a distance and ischemia in the infarct zone. N Engl J Med 1981; 305:1101–1105.

46. Nunley DL, Grunkemeier GL, Teply JF, et al. Coronary bypass operation following acute complicated myocardial infarction. J Thorac Cardiovasc Surg 1983; 85:485–491.

47. Singh AK, Rivera R, Cooper GN Jr, Karlson KE. Early myocardial revascularization for postinfarction angina: results and long-term followup. J Am Coll Cardiol 1985; 6:1121–1125.

48. Floten HS, Ahmad A, Swanson JS, et al. Long-term survival after postinfarction bypass operation: early versus late operation. Ann Thorac Surg 1989; 48:757–763.
49. Gardner TJ, Stuart S, Greene PS, Baumgartner WA. The risk of coronary bypass surgery for patients with postinfarction angina. Circulation 1989; 79(Suppl I):I-79–80.
50. Kennedy JW, Ivey TD, Misbach G, et al. Coronary artery bypass graft surgery early after acute myocardial infarction. Circulation 1989; 79(Suppl I):I-73–78.
51. Kouchoukos NT, Murphy S, Philpott T, Pelate C, Marshall WB Jr. Coronary artery bypass grafting for postinfarction angina pectoris. Circulation 1989; 79(Suppl I):I-68–72.
52. Naunheim KS, Kesler KA, Kanter KR, et al. Coronary artery bypass for recent infarction: predictors of mortality. Circulation 1988; 78(Suppl I):I-122–128.
53. Rogers WJ, Smith LF, Oberman A, et al. Surgical vs nonsurgical management of patients after myocardial infarction. Circulation 1980; 62(Suppl I):I-67–74.
54. Theroux P, Waters DD, Halphen C, et al. Prognostic value of exercise testing soon after myocardial infarction. N Engl J Med 1979; 301:341–345.
55. Brunken R, Tillisch J, Schwaiger M, et al. Regional perfusion, glucose metabolism, and wall motion in patients with chronic electrocardiographic Q wave infarctions: evidence for persistence of viable tissue in some infarct regions by positron emission tomography. Circulation 1986; 73:951–963.
56. Brown KA, O'Meara J, Chambers CE, Plante DA. Ability of dipyridamole-thallium-201 imaging one to four days after acute myocardial infarction to predict in-hospital and late recurrent myocardial ischemic events. Am J Cardiol 1990; 65:160–167.
57. Alderman EL, Bourassa MG, Cohen LS, et al. Ten-year followup of survival and myocardial infarction in the randomized coronary artery surgery study. Circulation 1990; 82:1629–1646.
58. Talley JD, Jones EL, Weintraub WS, King SB III. Coronary artery bypass surgery after failed elective percutaneous transluminal coronary angioplasty: a status report. Circulation 1989; 79(Suppl I):I-126–131.
59. Detre K, Holubkov R, Kelsey S, et al. Percutaneous transluminal coronary angioplasty in 1985–1986 and 1977–1981. The National Heart, Lung, and Blood Institute Registry. N Engl J Med 1988; 318:265–270.
60. Ferguson TB Jr, Muhlbaier LH, Salai DL, Wechsler AS. Coronary bypass grafting after failed elective and failed emergent percutaneous angioplasty. J Thorac Cardiovasc Surg 1988; 95:761–772.
61. Hinohara T, Simpson JB, Phillips HR, Stack RS. Transluminal intracoronary reperfusion catheter: a device to maintain coronary perfusion between failed coronary angioplasty and emergency coronary bypass surgery. J Am Coll Cardiol 1988; 11:977–982.
62. Kereiakes DJ, Topol EJ, George BS, et al. Favorable early and

long-term prognosis following coronary bypass surgery therapy for myocardial infarction: results of a multicenter trial. Am Heart J 1989; 118:199–207.

63. Barner HB, Lea JW IV, Naunheim KS, Stoney WS Jr. Emergency coronary bypass not associated with preoperative cardiogenic shock in failed angioplasty, after thrombolysis, and for acute myocardial infarction. Circulation 1989; 79(Suppl I):I-152–159.

64. Anderson JL, Battistessa SA, Clayton PD, et al. Coronary bypass surgery early after thrombolytic therapy for acute myocardial infarction. Ann Thorac Surg 1986; 41:176–183.

65. Lolley DM, Enerson DM, Rams JJ, Long ET, Rycyna JL, Bauersfeld SR. Should coronary artery bypass be delayed following successful direct coronary artery streptokinase thrombolysis during evolving myocardial infarction? J Vasc Surg 1986; 3:330–337.

66. Akins CW. Early and late results following emergency isolated myocardial revascularization during hypothermic fibrillatory arrest. Ann Thorac Surg 1987; 43:131–137.

67. Flameng W, Sergeant P, Vanhaecke J, Suy R. Emergency coronary bypass grafting for evolving myocardial infarction. J Thorac Cardiovasc Surg 1987; 94:124–131.

68. Bolooki H. Emergency cardiac procedures in patients in cardiogenic shock due to complications of coronary artery disease. Circulation 1989; 79(Suppl I):I-137–148.

69. Pennington DG. Comment: emergency management of cardiogenic shock. Circulation 1989; 79(Suppl I):I-149–151.

70. London RE, London SB. Rupture of the heart. Circulation 1965; 31:202–208.

71. Bates RJ, Bentler S, Resnekov L, Anagnostoupolos CE. Cardiac rupture: challenge in diagnosis and management. Am J Cardiol 1977; 40:429–437.

72. Pifarre R, Sullivan HJ, Grieco J, et al. Management of left ventricular rupture complicating myocardial infarction. J Thorac Cardiovasc Surg 1983; 86:441–443.

73. McMullan MH, Kilgore TL Jr, Dear HD Jr, Hindman SH. Sudden blowout rupture of the myocardium after infarction: urgent management. J Thorac Cardiovasc Surg 1985; 89:259–263.

74. Roberts WC, Morrow AG. Pseudoaneurysm of the left ventricle. Am J Med 1967; 43:639–644.

75. Vlodaver Z, Coe JI, Edwards JE. True and false left ventricular aneurysms; propensity for the latter to rupture. Circulation 1975; 51:567–572.

76. Stewart S, Huddle R, Stuard I, Schreiner BF, DeWeese JA. False aneurysm and pseudo-false aneurysm of the left ventricle: etiology, pathology, diagnosis and operative management. Ann Thorac Surg 1981; 31:259–265.

77. Abrams DL, Edelist A, Luria MH, Miller AJ. Ventricular aneurysm. Circulation 1963; 27:164–169.

78. Schlichter J, Hellerstein HK, Katz LN. Aneurysm of the heart: a correlative study of 102 proved cases. Medicine 1954; 33:43–86.

79. Cosgrove DM, Loop FD, Irarrazaval MJ, et al. Determinants of long-term survival after ventricular aneurysmectomy. Ann Thorac Surg 1978; 26:357–363.
80. Likoff W, Bailey CP. Ventriculoplasty: excision of myocardial aneurysm. JAMA 1955; 158:915–920.
81. Cooley DA, Collins HA, Morris GC Jr, Chapman DW. Ventricular aneurysm after myocardial infarction: surgical excision with use of temporary cardiopulmonary bypass. JAMA 1958; 167:557–560.
82. Daggett WM, Guyton RA, Mundth ED, et al. Surgery for postmyocardial infarct ventricular septal defect. Ann Surg 1977; 186:260–271.
83. Jatene AD. Left ventricular aneurysmectomy. J Thorac Cardiovasc Surg 1985; 89:321–331.
84. Walker WE, Stoney WS, Alford WC Jr, Barrus GR, Glassford DM, Thomas CS Jr. Results of surgical management of acute left ventricular aneurysms. Circulation 1980; 62(Suppl I):I-75–78.
85. Akins CW. Resection of the left ventricular aneurysm during hypothermic fibrillatory arrest without aortic occlusion. J Thorac Cardiovasc Surg 1986; 91:610–618.
86. Couper GS, Bunton RW, Birjiniuk V, et al. Relative risks of left ventricular aneurysmectomy in patients with akinetic scars versus true dyskinetic aneurysms. Circulation 1990; 82(Suppl IV):IV-248–256.
87. Mundth ED, Buckley MJ, DeSanctis RW, Daggett WN, Austen WG. Surgical treatment of ventricular irritability. J Thorac Cardiovasc Surg 1973; 66:943–951.
88. Harken AH, Horowitz LN, Josephson ME. Comparison of standard aneurysmectomy and aneurysmectomy with directed endocardial resection for the treatment of recurrent sustained tachycardia. J Thorac Cardiovasc Surg 1980; 80:527–534.
89. Guiraudon G, Fontaine G, Frank R, Escande G, Etievent P, Cabrol C. Encircling endocardial ventriculotomy: a new surgical treatment for life-threatening ventricular tachycardias resistant to medical treatment following myocardial infarction. Ann Thorac Surg 1978; 26:438–444.
90. Thomas A. AICD sudden therapy survival rate: 98% at one year. In: AICD Technology and Therapy Advances, St. Paul, MN, CPI, 1st quarter, 1988, pp 5–6.
91. Vlodaver Z, Edwards JE. Rupture of ventricular septum or papillary muscle complicating myocardial infarction. Circulation 1977; 55:815–822.
92. Selzer A, Gerbode F, Kerth WJ. Clinical hemodynamics and surgical considerations of rupture of the ventricular septum after myocardial infarction. Ann Thorac Surg 1973; 16:598–609.
93. Swithinbank JM. Perforation of the interventricular septum in myocardial infarction. Br Heart J 1959; 21:562–566.
94. Sanders RJ, Kern WH, Blount SG. Perforation of the interventricular septum complicating myocardial infarction. Am Heart J 1956; 51:736–748.
95. Cooley DA, Belmonte BA, Zeis LB, Schnur S. Surgical repair of

ruptured interventricular septum following acute myocardial infarction. Surgery 1957; 41:930–937.

96. Stinson EB, Becker J, Shumway NE. Successful repair of post-infarction ventricular septal defect and biventricular aneurysm. J Thorac Cardiovasc Surg 1969; 58:20–24.

97. Daggett WN, Burwell LF, Lawson DW, Austen WG. Resection of acute ventricular aneurysm and ruptured interventricular septum after myocardial infarction. N Engl J Med 1970; 283:1507–1508.

98. Kitamura S, Mendez A, Kay JH. Ventricular septal defect following myocardial infarction: experience with surgical repair through a left ventriculotomy and review of literature. J Thorac Cardiovasc Surg 1971; 61:186–199.

99. Javid H, Hunter JA, Najafi H, Dye WS, Julian OC. Left ventricular approach for the repair of ventricular septal perforation and infarctectomy. J Thorac Cardiovasc Surg 1972; 63:14–24.

100. Daggett WM, Buckley MJ, Akins CW, et al. Improved results of surgical management of postinfarction ventricular septal rupture. Ann Surg 1982; 196:269–277.

101. Sanders RF, Neuberger KT, Ravin A. Rupture of posterior papillary muscles: occurrence of rupture of posterior muscle on posterior myocardial infarction. Dis Chest 1957; 31:316–323.

102. Austen WG, Sanders CA, Averill JH, Friedlich AL. Ruptured papillary muscle: report of a case with successful mitral valve replacement. Circulation 1965; 32:597–601.

103. Salomon NW, Stinson EB, Griepp RB, Shumway NE. Patient-related risk factors as predictors of results following isolated mitral valve replacement. Ann Thorac Surg 1977; 24:519–530.

104. Cohn LH. Surgical treatment of acute myocardial infarction. Chest 1988; 93:13S–16S.

Chapter 10

Advanced Mechanical Circulatory Support After Acute Coronary Ischemia and Infarction

D. Glenn Pennington, Marc T. Swartz,
and Keith S. Naunheim

Introduction

Ischemic heart disease is the most common cause of cardiac failure and cardiac death in the United States. Most patients with coronary artery disease can be treated effectively with drugs, percutaneous transluminal coronary angioplasty (PTCA), coronary artery bypass grafting (CABG), or cardiac transplantation. Despite these interventions, a significant number of patients with ischemic heart disease develop cardiogenic shock. Many of them respond well to pharmacological and intra-aortic balloon pump (IABP) therapy. However, many continue to deteriorate and require a more advanced form of circulatory support. Over the last two decades, considerable

Lazar HL (editor): *Current Therapy for Acute Coronary Ischemia,* © Futura Publishing Co., Inc., Mount Kisco, NY, 1993.

progress has been made in the development and clinical application of mechanical circulatory support devices, with a yield of a variety of devices with differing characteristics of function and application. However, in general all circulatory support devices currently in use are designed to provide hemodynamic stabilization until further intervention can be carried out, until the natural heart recovers, or until a donor heart can be located for transplantation. In this chapter, we review the clinical experience of patients with ischemic heart disease who required advanced mechanical circulatory support. The discussions in this chapter are centered around three patient groups:

1. those who suffered an acute myocardial infarction (AMI) or acute hemodynamic deterioration resulting in cardiogenic shock. Most of them were supported initially with femoro-femoral extracorporeal membrane oxygenation (ECMO). Some underwent subsequent coronary artery grafting or insertion of a more sophisticated device, while some were maintained on ECMO in the hope that their heart would recover
2. patients who required support to be weaned from cardiopulmonary bypass after cardiac surgery and those who deteriorated in the immediate postoperative period
3. patients with end-stage ischemic cardiomyopathy and those who suffered a severe AMI requiring support until cardiac transplantation could be performed.

Some of the data included in this chapter was obtained from the American Society of Artificial Internal Organs (ASAIO)–International Society of Heart and Lung Transplantation (ISHLT) combined registry for the clinical use of mechanical ventricular assist devices (VAD) and total artificial hearts (TAH) maintained at Pennsylvania State University. Since participation in this registry is voluntary, all patients receiving advanced mechanical circulatory support are not included. Furthermore, complications are not precisely defined in the registry, resulting in some nonuniform data that must be taken in context.

Patient Selection

Patient selection for advanced circulatory support is one of the most difficult issues faced by clinicians because of high procedure-related morbidity rates and the large costs in terms of personnel and resources. Predictors of survival are being identified, and the hemodynamic criteria used to initiate circulatory support are being redefined. The traditional hemodynamic criteria used to determine a patient's eligibility for mechanical circulatory support were derived from the studies of Norman and associates.[1] These criteria include a cardiac index of less than 1.8 liters/min/m^2, elevated systemic vascular resistance (usually >2100 dynes/sec/cm^5), systolic arterial blood pressure less than 90 mm Hg, left and/or right atrial pressure >20 mm Hg, and decreased urine output despite the use of significant pharmacological support and an IABP if appropriate. However, these hemodynamic criteria should not be strictly enforced. The definition of cardiogenic shock and the decision to implement advanced mechanical support should be based on both objective and subjective criteria. Therefore, the exact criteria to define cardiogenic shock or maximal therapy should be evaluated appropriately for each patient. The precise hemodynamic criteria for the insertion of devices employed in this chapter are not known, but it is doubtful that they always fulfilled the criteria noted above.

Patient selection criteria varies somewhat, depending on where and under what circumstances the patient develops cardiogenic shock. For example, the factors determining whether or not a patient is supported after a failed PTCA in the cardiac catheterization laboratory may differ from the considerations in a postcardiotomy patient who cannot be weaned from cardiopulmonary bypass. Limited experience suggests that age greater than 65 years is a predictor of lower survival rates in patients supported to allow recovery of the natural heart as well as those supported while waiting for cardiac transplantation.[2,3] The presence of persistent renal insufficiency, coagulopathy, and uncontrolled infections were additional risk factors.[4–6] Patients should be excluded if they have major organ dysfunction, which would limit survival after their cardiac problem is resolved. Specific patient selection criteria for the different groups will be discussed in the following sections.

Extracorporeal Membrane Oxygenation

Since the late 1950s, technology has been available to support patients in cardiogenic shock with cardiopulmonary bypass (CPB).[7]

Arteriovenous ECMO has been used to resuscitate patients when conventional therapy has failed.[8–12] ECMO can be instituted within 20 to 40 minutes in almost any hospital environment. This technique is advantageous in many situations due to its rapid and simple insertion as well as its ability to provide cardiac as well as pulmonary support. Femoro-femoral CPB allows hemodynamic stabilization, which can provide time for further evaluation and additional therapy if appropriate. ECMO circuits have been adapted to portable carts that can be transported easily to various hospital departments. Most ECMO perfusion circuits consist of a membrane oxygenator, roller or centrifugal pump, and heat exchanger. Several methods of cannulation are available, including chest cannulation using venous return from the right atrium and arterial inflow through an ascending aortic cannula. Femoral vessel cannulation can be performed using percutaneous or cutdown techniques to cannulate the femoral artery and vein.[8,9] In instances in which ECMO is not to be used more than a few hours, proximal and distal venous and arterial cannulation should be performed. ECMO systems currently require continuous intravenous heparin. However, in the future, heparin-coated surfaces, which would eliminate the need for systemic heparin, may be available.

Since 1985 we have supported 37 patients with resuscitative ECMO at St. Louis University. There were 28 men and 9 women who ranged in age from 40 to 78 years (mean 56 years). Thirty-two patients had cardiac arrest at the time of ECMO insertion, and five had suffered acute severe hemodynamic deterioration. All patients were intubated and mechanically ventilated and 35 had IABPs. ECMO was initiated in the cardiac catheterization laboratory in 13 patients (9 with failed PTCA and 4 undergoing catheterization), in the medical intensive care unit in 13 patients, in the surgical intensive care unit in 10 patients, and in the emergency room in 1 patient. There were four survivors in the failed PTCA group (4/9) and four survivors in the postcardiotomy group (4/10). Bleeding was the most common complication, occurring in 20 patients. Bleeding problems were aggravated by the use of continuous heparin. Of eight patients who developed renal failure requiring dialysis during or after ECMO, none survived. Only one patient developed an ECMO-related infection. There were no incidences of thromboembolism. Durations of support ranged from 2 hours to 5.1 days (mean 1 day). Flows ranged from 1.45 to 5 liters/min (mean 3.08 liters/min). Twenty-five patients were weaned, with eight survivors. This 22% survival rate is comparable to the results reported from other centers (Table 1).[9–12]

Several studies have documented the physiological effects of ECMO on normal and ischemic hearts.[13, 14] In these studies, ECMO decreased right ventricular (RV) preload and afterload, but increased left ventricular (LV) afterload and LV wall stress, resulting in a net increase in myocardial oxygen consumption. Laboratory investigations indicate that LV pressure increases with ECMO flow. ECMO decompresses the right heart and decreases RV afterload, but the LV often is not decompressed and frequently must contend with increased afterload. Some information about LV function during ECMO has been obtained from postoperative pediatric patients in whom cannulation was almost always performed through the sternotomy incision. In several instances, right atrial-aortic ECMO did not lower left atrial pressures, necessitating placement of left atrial or LV cannulae.[15] For these reasons, it seems preferable to keep the period of ECMO as short as possible, especially in patients with myocardial ischemia who have had femoro-femoral insertion without the possibility of left heart decompression.

Our initial goals with resuscitative ECMO are to provide vital organ perfusion and rapidly reverse ischemic organ dysfunction. If the patient has irreversible myocardial damage, the hope is that vital organ function can be preserved until the switch to a more sophisticated device can be undertaken to support the patient until cardiac transplantation can be carried out. Myocardial recovery sufficient to allow weaning from ECMO occurs in approximately 60% of the patients, with 16% to 32% surviving (Table 1). [9–12] As technology improves and better patient selection criteria are developed, the results should improve.

Table 1

Reported Results of Resuscitative ECMO

Author	Year	Reference	# Patients	# Survived	% Survived
Phillips et al.	1989	9	22	5	23
Raithel et al.	1989	11	28	6	21
Reichman et al.	1990	10	38	6	16
Moore et al.	1991	12	53	17	32

Postcardiotomy Support

A small but persistent percentage of patients undergoing surgical revascularization develop postoperative cardiogenic shock. The need for IABP support in elective cardiac surgical cases ranges from 1% to 7%, and survival rates in these IABP patients range from 45% to 60%.[1,16–18] The incidence of VAD support in patients undergoing cardiac surgery is 0.1% to 0.8%, with survival ranging from 29% to 50% in some of the larger series. [19–22] The overall survival rate for patients undergoing postcardiotomy VAD insertion is 23%.[2] From these data, it seems that most postcardiotomy shock patients are supported with drugs and/or an IABP and that a significant percentage die of cardiac failure. A randomized trial is necessary to determine if these patients would benefit from VADs or whether they have irreversible injuries.

Since 1981 44 patients have been supported with assist devices at St. Louis University after cardiac surgical procedures, and 37 after surgical revascularization. These 37 patients represent 0.7% of all the patients undergoing CABGs during this interval at our center. There were 30 men and 7 women who ranged in age from 40 to 75 years (mean 58 years). The number of bypass grafts per patient ranged from 2 to 6, with a mean of 3.9. Nine patients had centrifugal pumps and 28 had Pierce-Donachy Thoratec (Thoratec Medical Corporation, Berkeley, CA) VADs. Sixteen patients were supported with left VADs (LVADs), 16 with bilateral ventricular assist devices (BVADs), and 5 with right VADs (RVADs). Duration of support ranged from 2 hours to 17 days (mean 3.8). Assist device flow rates were 1 to 2.88 liter/m^2/min (mean 1.96). Bleeding occurred in 19 patients, 8 of whom were re-explored. Nine patients developed postoperative renal failure requiring dialysis (no survivors). Five patients had thrombus form in the pump; three of these five suffered a thromboembolic event during the period of support (one survivor). Twelve patients had infections (positive culture) while on the device but only one was clearly device related. Fifteen patients were weaned (40%) with 10 patients being discharged (27%). There were three late deaths at 8, 24, and 53 months. One late death was cardiac related.

Patients undergoing surgical revascularization with or without other procedures are at some risk to develop postoperative cardiogenic shock. Patients undergoing isolated CABG have the best survival, whereas those with postinfarction ventricular septal defect fare the worst (Table 2). Factors influencing survival that can be

Table 2

Operative Procedure Before Mechanical Circulatory Support*

Procedure	Number of Patients	Percent Weaned	Percent Discharged
CABG	338	45.0	21.8
CABG and valve repair or replacement	55	32.3	21.0
Aneurysm repair and CABG	38	39.3	13.2
Ventricular septal defect (post-AMI) ± other procedure	16	43.8	12.5

*ASAIO-ISHLT Registry.
CABG = coronary artery bypass grafting.

evaluated before VAD insertion in the postcardiotomy group are listed in Table 3. Most of these factors have been identified in retrospective studies.[2,23,24] Any combination of these factors likely would further reduce survival. It is critical to determine whether the operative procedure was successful. Patients with unsuccessful operations, such as those with little or no flow through bypass grafts, should be excluded from temporary mechanical circulatory support, since their likelihood of recovery is minimal. If the patient is a potential candidate for cardiac transplantation, support may be initiated as a bridge to transplantation. An acute perioperative myocardial infarction within 24 to 48 hours of operation has been shown to reduce greatly the opportunity for cardiac recovery.[23] Although the diagnosis of intraoperative myocardial infarction is difficult to make in the operating room, the diagnosis of myocardial infarction may be known in some patients before operation.

Table 3

Predevice Risk Factors: Postcardiac Surgery

1. Unsuccessful operation
2. Pre- or intraoperative myocardial infarction
3. Biventricular failure
4. Multiple previous infarctions or history of congestive heart failure
5. Age >65 yr
6. Uncontrollable bleeding while on cardiopulmonary bypass

The presence of biventricular failure also is a factor that reduces the likelihood of survival.[24] In patients with biventricular failure who receive only univentricular support, biventricular failure greatly influences survival. Even with biventricular support, patients suffering biventricular failure have a decreased chance of survival when compared with those suffering only univentricular failure (Table 4). This difference in survival apparently is related to the extent of myocardial damage rather than complications associated with biventricular support.[25]

One of the strongest predictors of survival is age. The overall survival rate for patients younger than 59 years undergoing postcardiotomy VAD support is 34%. However, data from the ASAIO-ISHLT Registry suggests that patients older than 70 years have a survival rate of only 10%.[2] This is in contrast to a recent report by Wareing and Kouchoukos suggesting that age greater than 65 years may not be such a critical predictor of survival.[26] This information is especially useful to clinicians since it is a parameter that can be evaluated before VAD insertion and becomes more important considering that the mean age of patients undergoing elective surgical cardiac procedures has been increasing throughout the last decade.

Intraoperative bleeding so severe that a critical level of systemic perfusion cannot be maintained while on CPB is a relative contraindication to VAD support. In these patients, postoperative bleeding may be excessive even after neutralization of heparin. Bleeding is due to multiple cannulation sites and the extended duration of CPB, which often results in development of a coagulopathy.

Table 4

Postcardiotomy Support Results Based on the Type of Support*

Type of Support	# Patients	Weaned	Discharged
LVAD	349	167 (47.9%)	95 (27.2%)
RVAD	86	33 (38.4%)	20 (23.3%)
BVAD	226	82 (36.3%)	37 (16.4%)†
Total	661	282 (42.7%)	152 (23.0%)

*ASAIO-ISHLT Registry.
†p = 0.003 by Chi-square on discharge; BVAD vs. LVAD.
LVAD = left ventricular assist device; RVAD = right ventricular assist device; BVAD = biventricular assist device.

Patients who require VADs to be weaned from CPB in the operating room appear to have better survival rates than those who are weaned from CPB and returned to the intensive care unit in borderline condition only to deteriorate and require VAD insertion sometime later. Data for this type of application are not available from the ASAIO-ISHLT Registry; however, in our experience at St. Louis University, only 1 of 10 (10%) patients who required VADs within 6 hours to 10 days of the initial operation survived. This is opposed to a 38% survival rate (13/34) in our patients who had VADs inserted at the time of operation. This decreased survival probably is due to longer periods of hypoperfusion and delays in insertion of the VAD.

Several other factors that might influence survival should be evaluated before VAD insertion. Sustained intraoperative ventricular arrhythmias are a negative prognostic indicator if a stable rhythm cannot be maintained. However, intermittent episodes of ventricular tachycardia or fibrillation before device insertion do not predict survival.[27] Preoperative controlled bacterial endocarditis (sterile blood cultures) should not be a contraindication for mechanical circulatory support since patients in the postcardiotomy and bridge-to-transplant groups have been successfully supported, despite bacteremia. Patients having reoperations for coronary artery disease traditionally have been thought to have a decreased chance of survival. The best available information on patients with reoperations requiring VAD support comes from the Thoratec postcardiotomy experience. These data show that 16 of 79 (20.2%) patients survived VAD support after their first CABG while 5 of 23 (21.17%) patients who were similarly supported after reoperation survived. At St. Louis University we have inserted VADs in five postcardiotomy patients after reoperation with one survivor. This 20% survival rate is less than our overall survival rate of 33%, but is not statistically different from the 23% survival rate reported by the ASAIO-ISHLT Registry. From this small group, it seems that reoperation is not an absolute contraindication to VAD support.

Since most cardiac surgical procedures are performed electively, it is doubtful whether many of the potential VAD candidates would suffer from complications that would exclude them for VAD support. Patients undergoing emergency cardiac procedures may suffer renal or hepatic dysfunction, coagulopathy, or severe infectious complications preoperatively. If such patients cannot be weaned from CPB or

Table 5

Complications Postcardiac Surgery*

	Died (n = 440)		Survived (n = 153)		Level of Significance
	#	%	#	%	
Bleeding	196	45	65	42	NS
Renal failure	169	38	18	12	p < 0.001
Respiratory failure	90	20	25	16	NS
Infection	52	12	23	15	NS
Perioperative myocardial infarction	61	14	11	7	NS
Neurological	67	15	13	8	NS
Embolus	34	8	12	8	NS
Thrombus in system	23	5	8	5	NS
Hemolysis	27	6	8	5	NS
Cannula obstruction	16	4	0	0	NS
Mechanical failure	7	1.5	2	1.3	NS

*ASAIO-ISHLT Registry.
NS = not significant.

if they deteriorate soon after arrival to the intensive care unit, mechanical circulatory support may reverse the acute hemodynamic deterioration; however, survival rates in this group undoubtedly would be very low. The incidence of postoperative complications for postcardiotomy patients is shown in Table 5. Renal failure is the only factor that significantly influenced survival.

The ideal patient for postcardiotomy mechanical circulatory support is difficult to identify; however, those younger than 70 years who have no history of congestive heart failure or recent myocardial infarction and who have had a successful operation have the best chance of survival. If the patient is a cardiac transplant candidate, the presence of an AMI or an unsuccessful operation is less critical.

Bridge to Transplantation

Over the last 10 years, there have been significant improvements and growth in the field of cardiac transplantation and associated mechanical circulatory support. Many cardiac transplantation centers are partially compensating for the shortage of donor hearts by the development of programs to mechanically support the circulation of deteriorating patients before cardiac transplantation.[28-30] In this group, the purpose of mechanical circulatory support is to stabilize and possibly improve the patient's hemodynamic situation while the search for a donor organ is underway. Better patient selection and improved patient management have led to increasing survival rates and the wider use of mechanical assist devices as bridges to transplantation.

Patient selection is one of the most important determinants of successful bridging to transplantation.[31] Patient selection criteria are evolving and predictors of survival are being investigated. The goal is to provide bridge-to-transplant survival rates that are equivalent to those of the overall transplant population. Transplant candidates with hemodynamic deterioration should be treated initially with pharmacological therapy and an IABP if appropriate. If the IABP does not provide adequate support within a few hours of insertion, a more sophisticated device should be considered. The traditional hemodynamic criteria should not be the only factors determining whether a patient will be supported, or even to decide the correct time to intervene. Factors such as the amount of pharmacological support needed to maintain stability, the anticipated length of waiting period before a donor heart will be located, and the clinical impression of whether the patient is improving or deteriorating should be considered. The patient's past history and previous hospital admissions should be evaluated. Patients who have had frequent hospital admissions for congestive heart failure should be considered for immediate assist device insertion since their cardiac failure is becoming less responsive to conventional therapy. Some cardiac transplant candidates have a history of chronic illness and gradual decompensation, but in many deterioration is abrupt and sudden death is common. Patients who have been evaluated and listed previously for cardiac transplantation are the best candidates for bridging since their past history is well known. This group should be followed closely and treated aggressively.

Patients who suffer massive AMIs and develop cardiogenic shock also are potential candidates for bridging to transplantation. This patient group often is in better general condition than those who have chronic cardiomyopathy since they have not suffered the malnutrition, inanition, and multiorgan consequences of chronic heart failure. If the cardiogenic shock can be reversed before the development of major organ dysfunction, these patients often make good candidates for transplantation. This group often is admitted in cardiogenic shock to the emergency room, intensive care unit, or cardiac catheterization laboratory. Under these circumstances, at this point it is often difficult or impossible to determine whether the myocardial injury is reversible. Temporary resuscitative systems such as femoro-femoral ECMO may be necessary to stabilize them until cardiac catheterization and other studies can be performed. Once the diagnosis has been established, surgical repair of reversible lesions or placement of a more sophisticated device can be undertaken as a bridge to transplantation. As of April 1992, 19% of the patients bridged to transplantation with the Novacor (Novacor Medical Corp., Oakland, CA) LV assist systems (LVAS) had AMI as the etiology of their cardiogenic shock. A significant number of patients bridged to transplantation with the Thoratec VAD developed cardiogenic shock after an AMI, and the results in this group also were quite favorable.[32] However, patients should be excluded if they suffer renal failure requiring dialysis, uncontrollable sepsis, or are older than 65 years. Other pre-existing conditions such as coagulopathy, cerebral injury, or liver failure are considered contraindications to both mechanical circulatory support and cardiac transplantation.

A small percentage of patients who develop cardiogenic shock after cardiac surgery are potential candidates for bridging to transplantation. There are several strong predictors of irreversible myocardial damage in this patient population. The presence of an acute perioperative myocardial infarction and the development of severe biventricular failure have been shown to be highly predictive of nonsurvival.[23,24] The presence of both these conditions usually is indicative of irreversible myocardial damage and justifies the use of a mechanical device to bridge the patient to transplantation. This patient population can be supported for 7 to 10 days during which time myocardial recovery can be evaluated. If there is no sign of myocardial recovery within 10 days, it is reasonable to list them for transplantation. Unfortunately, many postcardiotomy patients develop complications that eliminate them as candidates for transplantation. For this reason, postcardiotomy patients represent a small percentage of the total patient population who have been successfully bridged to transplantation. Bridging is an option for high-risk patients and can be a planned alternative for patients undergoing elective cardiac procedures. We have performed CABG with VAD standby on 12 high-risk (ejection fraction <30%) patients who were referred for cardiac transplantation. If these patients required VADs to be weaned from CPB, the plan was to bridge them to transplantation after a period of time sufficient to evaluate myocardial recovery (7–14 days). None of this group required a VAD and all were discharged.

Since 1984, 40 patients have been supported at St. Louis University with advanced mechanical circulatory support devices as a bridge to cardiac transplantation. Twenty-two patients had ischemic heart disease, 12 with chronic ischemic cardiomyopathy (9 had previous CABGs), and 10 who had suffered an AMI resulting in cardiogenic shock. There were 21 men and 1 woman ranging in age from 34 to 63 years (mean 51 years). Twenty patients were supported with drugs and an IABP before assist device insertion. Six patients also were supported with ECMO before being switched to a Thoratec VAD (five patients) or Novacor LVAS (one patient). Sixteen patients were intubated. Fourteen patients were supported with Thoratec VADs, six with Novacor LVAS, one with a Symbion J-7 TAH, and one with ECMO alone. Duration of support ranged from 0.2 to 440 days (mean 48). Device flows averaged 2.84 liters/m^2/min. Fourteen patients developed infections during the period of support, eight of which were device related. Seven of these 14 patients were successfully transplanted. Seven patients had bleeding problems (three re-explored). Four patients were dialyzed for renal failure, none of whom were transplanted or survived. Eleven patients were transplanted successfully and discharged. One patient was weaned from an LVAD without transplantation after 53 days of support and discharged with normal LV function. Table 6 shows multicenter results of bridging to transplantation.

Table 6

Results of Bridging to Transplantation*

Device	# Patients	Transplanted	Discharged after Transplant	Longest Successful Implant (Days)
Thoratec VAD	166	108 (65%)	90 (84%)	225
Abiomed BVS	135	98 (72%)	40 (40%)	27
Novacor LVAS	102	60 (58%)	53 (88%)	370
Thermocardiosystems VAS	58	35 (60%)	29 (83%)	324
Symbion TAH	162	118 (73%)	85 (72%)	45

*Data obtained from ASAIO-ISHLT Registry, manufacturers, and investigators.

Description of Available Devices

Several types of mechanical circulatory support devices currently are in use (Table 7). Pneumatic sac type pumps (Fig. 1), implantable LVAS (Fig. 2), and TAH (Fig. 3) are systems that were specially designed for perfusion periods of greater than 7 days. Other systems such as centrifugal (Fig. 4) and roller pumps were designed initially for short-term (several hours) use during cardiac operations. Centrifugal pumps have been used successfully to support the circulation for days, and even several weeks, although their reliability decreases with prolonged support.

The most important factors governing the use of these devices is their availability and cost. Investigational devices such as pneumatic VADs, LVASs, and TAHs have been available to only a limited number of institutions because of federal regulatory restrictions. The investigational devices also are considerably more expensive than commercially available pumps. Since roller and centrifugal pumps are commercially available and inexpensive, many centers have extended their applications to several days or even weeks. Because of the diversity of device characteristics, it is important to fit the device to the specific indication.[33] When deciding the type of mechanical support device to be used, it is important to consider the type of ventricular failure present, whether the device provides biventricular support, the cannulation options, and the need for anticoagulation. The hospital site where the device is to be applied also may be a determinant of the type of device to be used. For example, patients who develop cardiogenic shock or cardiac arrest in the cardiac catheterization laboratory require rapid resuscitation with an ECMO system using femoro-femoral cannulation. The more sophisticated systems such as the pneumatic VAD, LVAS, or TAH require a sternotomy and in some cases full cardiopulmonary bypass for insertion. Such devices are inappropriate for urgent resuscitation, since the delay associated with transporting the patient to the operating room to insert the device may jeopardize vital organ function. Centrifugal and paracorporeal pneumatic devices often are used for postcardiotomy support since they provide biventricular support and allow multiple pump inflow cannulation options. Implantable LVASs are less appropriate for postcardiotomy use since they require LV apex cannulation and provide only LV support. A limited clinical experience has been obtained using the Hemopump (Johnson & Johnson Interventional System Co., Nimbus

Table 7

Description of Mechanical Circulatory Support Devices

Device	Investigational*	Position	Anticoagulation Preferred			Duration
			Support	Required	Application	
Biomedicus	No	Extracorporeal	Rt,L,B	Moderate	P,B-Tx	Short-intermediate term
Sarns/Centrimed	No	Extracorporeal	Rt,L,B	Moderate	P,B-Tx	Short-intermediate term
ECMO	No	Extracorporeal	B	Full	R	Short-term
Abiomed BVS	Yes	Extracorporeal	Rt,L,B	Moderate	P,B-Tx	Short-intermediate term
Pierce-Donachy VAD	Yes	Paracorporeal	Rt,L,B	Low	P,B-Tx	Intermediate-long term
Sarns Pulsatile VAD	Yes	Paracorporeal	Rt,L,B	Low	P,B-Tx	Intermediate-long term
Hemopump	Yes	Internal	L	Moderate	R,P	Short-intermediate term
Novacor LVAS	Yes	Internal	L	Low	B-Tx	Intermediate-long term
Thermocardiosystems LVAS	Yes	Internal	L	Low	B-Tx	Intermediate-long term

*Investigational device exemption required from Food and Drug Administration.
BVS = biventricular support system; ECMO = extracorporeal membrane oxygenation; LVAS = left ventricular assist system; VAD = ventricular assist device; Rt = right; L = left; B = biventricular; R = resuscitative; P = postcardiotomy; B-Tx = bridge to transplantation.

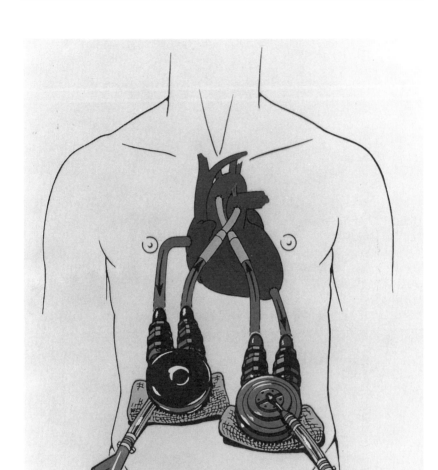

Figure 1: Thoratec biventricular assist devices showing right atrial to pulmonary artery and LV to aortic cannulation.

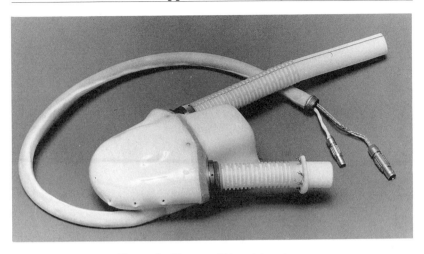

Figure 2: Novacor LV assist system.

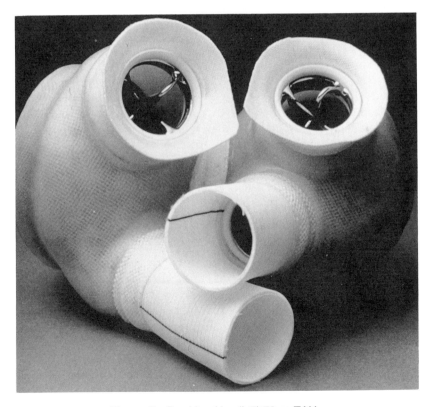

Figure 3: Symbion (Jarvik 7) 70-cc TAH.

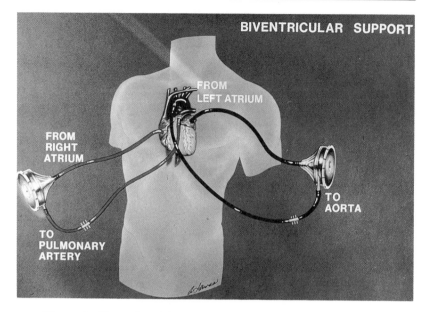

Figure 4: Biomedicus biventricular support with atrial pump inflow.

Medical, Inc., Rancho Cordova, CA) in both acute myocardial infarction and postcardiotomy cardiogenic shock patients.[34] The Hemopump provides only LV support and cannot be implanted in patients with significant aorto-iliac disease.

Clinical Problems

Biventricular Failure

Biventricular failure is a common occurrence in patients with postcardiotomy shock and those being bridged to transplantation.[24,30,32] Moreover, some patients who receive isolated circulatory support for RV or LV failure subsequently develop failure of the unassisted ventricle. Failure of the unassisted ventricle usually occurs soon after device placement, but can occur anytime within the first 24 to 48 hours of support. This ventricular failure may be camouflaged by the presence of ventricular arrhythmias, cardiac tamponade, or bleeding. The recognition and treatment of severe biventricular failure is essential to any type of mechanical circulatory support.

The development of RV failure in patients who seem to have isolated LV failure at the time of device insertion is not completely understood, but is now more easily recognized. There are several theories to explain the development of RV failure, including biventricular infarctions or ischemia, progressively increasing pulmonary vascular resistance as a result of blood transfusions and/or CPB (postcardiotomy patients), global ischemic injury due to inadequate myocardial preservation (postcardiotomy patients), or a shift in the interventricular septum as a result of LV decompression.[24,35] Since there is a risk of RV failure in virtually all patients receiving LV support, it is essential that biventricular support be provided if needed.

Bleeding

A large percentage of patients who receive assist devices develop bleeding complications requiring re-exploration or extensive transfusion (Table 5). There are many factors responsible for bleeding including multiple cannulation sites, the need for heparinization with some systems, and the development of coagulopathies. Surprisingly, post–device implant bleeding is not always a predictor of survival. Analysis of our experience in 80 patients who received either the Thoratec, Novacor, or Jarvik-7 devices demonstrated no significant difference in total chest tube drainage and CPB time between survivors and nonsurvivors in the postcardiotomy group. However, there was a significant difference in the total chest tube drainage between survivors and nonsurvivors in the bridge-to-transplant group. Postimplant bleeding may not be a lethal complication in most patients, but a few die from device-related bleeding. Bleeding also may be partially responsible for the development of later complications such as infection and/or renal failure. The incidence and severity of bleeding in our experience has decreased over the last decade in part due to extensive efforts to establish hemostasis in the operating room. Topical hemostatic agents are used liberally. We make a very large effort to wire the sternum in all cases. We routinely transfuse platelets if the platelet count falls below $100,000/mm^3$ and administer fresh frozen plasma to establish normal prothrombin time and partial thromboplastin time as soon as possible.

Renal Failure

Renal failure develops in approximately 30% of all the patients supported with mechanical circulatory support devices. Renal failure may develop despite normal preoperative renal function.[4] The cause of renal failure usually is attributed to the period of hypoperfusion before device insertion, long CPB times, extensive transfusions, and hemolysis. If renal failure persists after insertion of the device, ultrafiltration and hemodialysis can be used to maintain fluid balance and lower blood urea nitrogen, creatinine, and potassium levels. Despite these interventions, the patient usually is volume overloaded, suffering metabolic instability, and at an increased risk for infection. The need for anticoagulation with dialysis may lead to the resumption of bleeding complications. Under these circumstances, it is difficult to provide optimal conditions for myocardial recovery or to stabilize a patient effectively before transplantation. In our experience, the development of refractory renal failure during assist device support was highly predictive of nonsurvival. Of 174 adults undergoing mechanical circulatory support at St. Louis University, 41 required hemodialysis, of whom none survived.

Infection

Infection rates are high in patients requiring advanced mechanical circulatory support.[6,36,37] Risk factors for infection in this group of patients include long operative procedures, extensive transfusions, prolonged invasive monitoring, immobility, and bleeding requiring reoperation. The presence of transcutaneous cannulas increases the risk of infection. The development of prosthetic material–related infections is related more to the amount of time the device is in place rather than the number of cannulas.[25,37] All currently available systems require at least one percutaneous power cable or several cannulas that communicate directly with a pump pocket or the mediastinum.

Respiratory Insufficiency

Respiratory insufficiency is another common complication that develops in patients requiring assist device support. The etiology of the respiratory failure is multifactorial and includes LV failure, long CPB times, volume loading and transfusions, prolonged intubation, and immobility. Respiratory failure often is aggravated by the presence of untreated biventricular failure, renal failure, bleeding, and infection. Once the device is in place, attempts should be made to maintain the cardiac filling pressures as low as possible but still provide adequate perfusion. Unfortunately, assist devices are not as efficient as the natural heart. Frequently it is necessary to volume load the patients to obtain adequate pump outputs. This is particularly true in patients with atrial cannulation. Frequent diuresis and early patient mobilization can help to reduce the incidence of pulmonary complications.

Thromboembolism

All the currently available mechanical support devices carry a risk of thrombus formation within the device and subsequent thromboembolism. Standardized anticoagulation protocols for the different types of devices have not been developed. Patients with mechanical circulatory support devices are at risk for both bleeding and thromboembolism. Once the postoperative bleeding is controlled, heparin may be given and the activated clotting times maintained between 140 and 160 seconds. The instance of thromboembolism can be reduced by optimizing flow through the device. Patients supported longer than 2 weeks can be maintained on oral antiplatelet and/or anticoagulant drugs with a low risk of thromboembolism.[38]

Weaning

In those patients in whom recovery of the natural heart is anticipated, weaning should begin when the hemodynamics have been stable for 12 to 24 hours. The first step is to reduce pharmacological support, particularly the inotropic drugs. Low dose vasodilators such as nitroprusside or hydralazine often are necessary. For the first 12 to 24 hours the highest possible assist device flows are maintained while attempting to keep the atrial pressures at approximately 10 to 15 mm Hg with a mean aortic pressure of 70 to 75 mm Hg. During this period, pump flow should be maintained at 2.2 liters/m^2/min or greater. After the first stable 24 hours, pump on–pump off data should be obtained with the device temporarily turned off.[39] Left and right atrial pressure, pulmonary and systemic arterial pressure, cardiac output, and mixed venous oxygen saturation should be measured and compared with similar data obtained with the device on. If the patient is able to maintain atrial pressures less than 15 mm Hg and a cardiac index greater than 2 liters/m²/min with the device off, the weaning process may begin. A continuous heparin drip, if not already infusing, should be started to maintain the activated clotting time at 140 to 160 seconds with a partial thromboplastin time of 1.5 times control. Flow through the device should be decreased gradually. During the weaning period, inotropic support should not be increased to high levels in order to compensate for decreases in device flows. If the flow reduction leads to hemodynamic deterioration, the flow should be returned to the preweaning levels and weaning suspended for 12 to 24 hours. As soon as the patient is able to maintain preweaning hemodynamics on a low dose of inotropic support, the device can be removed. Additional studies such as nuclear multigated acquisition scans or echocardiography can be used to evaluate ventricular recovery. In our experience, a ventricular ejection fraction >30% is a good indicator that the ventricle will be able to maintain adequate perfusion. Most recovery patients who are weaned have durations of support of less than 1 week. Support for longer than 1 week does not necessarily preclude myocardial recovery. A few patients thought to be cardiac transplant candidates exhibited myocardial recovery and return of normal ventricular function after as long as 79 days of support.[40]

Discussion

The rationale for the use of temporary circulatory support is to stabilize the patient to allow time for myocardial recovery, or to support the patient until a donor heart can be located. The first line of treatment for cardiogenic shock is pharmacological and IABP support, which is adequate in many patients. However, there clearly is a subpopulation who require more advanced support. Ischemic injuries so severe that they do not respond to conventional therapy most likely will not resolve within a short period of time. Some cardiogenic shock patients have myocardial injuries severe enough to preclude myocardial recovery while recovery may be possible in others. It is difficult if not impossible to differentiate between these two groups in an acute setting. Therefore, the overall survival rate for this group probably will not exceed 60% to 70% for the foreseeable future. Survival rates for patients who receive assist devices for cardiogenic shock after AMI are difficult to determine since so few patients in this group have been supported. The overall survival rate from the ASAIO-ISHLT Registry for patients who receive VADs for postcardiotomy shock is 23%. However, some centers have reported survival as high as 40%. In the bridge-to-transplant patient population, the percentage of patients with VADs who undergo cardiac transplantation ranges from 50% to 75%, with an overall survival after transplantation of approximately 60% (Table 6). However, in individual series of devices the survival rate of transplanted patients may be as high as 80% to 85%.[29,30]

Several factors have led to improvements in survival rates. We now recognize the frequency and importance of biventricular failure. Survival rates in patients with biventricular failure who receive only univentricular support have been discouraging. However, there is now a better understanding of the importance of providing biventricular support if biventricular failure is present. A considerable amount of work has been done and more is underway to determine the etiology of RV failure. Improvements in device insertion techniques and methods of cannulation also have contributed to improved survival. Femoro-femoral cannulation is the preferred technique in patients suffering cardiac arrest since it can be performed rapidly under local anesthesia in virtually any environment. Atrial cannulation is the accepted method of cannulation for VADs in patients in whom recovery of the myocardium is expected, while ventricular apex cannulation is becoming generally preferred in the bridge-to-transplant population.

The ability to supply complete circulatory support or complete decompression of the assisted ventricle varies. Some devices provide adequate support without native heart ejection, depending on the type of device used and the method of cannulation. In general, complete ventricular unloading and maximal decrease in myocardial oxygen consumption have not been our primary goals. Our initial concern has been the restoration and maintenance of perfusion to the vital organs. This is true for patients being supported until their natural heart recovers and in those awaiting cardiac transplantation. In our patients supported for myocardial recovery, at least 50% were weaned from VAD support because they were able to maintain adequate cardiac outputs without the VAD. However, only 35% of these patients survived. Many of these postweaning deaths were due to noncardiac complications such as renal and respiratory insufficiency or infections.

Two important factors in deciding the clinical efficacy of advanced circulatory support are the length of survival and the functional status of survivors of VAD support. Numerous studies have documented long-term survival and excellent functional status in a large percentage of postcardiotomy shock patients supported with VADs.[41,42] A recent report indicated that long-term survival and functional status of patients bridged to cardiac transplantation was similar to those undergoing conventional heart transplantation.[43]

Circulatory support has proven to be an effective method of treatment for some patients with severe ventricular failure. Thus far, this technology has had a small impact on overall cardiac surgical survival rates. In the future, it is anticipated that efficacy and reliability of these techniques will reach a level sufficient to encourage physicians to implant these devices earlier in high-risk patients. If permanent LVASs prove successful, the mortality associated with ischemic cardiomyopathy could be reduced, and the natural course of chronic ischemic cardiac disease significantly altered.

References

1. Norman JC, Cooley DA, Igo SR, et al. Prognostic indices for survival during postcardiotomy intra-aortic balloon pumping. J Thorac Cardiovasc Surg 1977; 74:709–720.
2. Miller CA, Pae WE, Pierce WS. Combined registry for the clinical use of mechanical ventricular assist devices: postcardiotomy cardiogenic shock. Trans Am Soc Artif Intern Organs 1990; 36:43–46.
3. Miller CA, Pae WE, Pierce WS. Combined registry for the clinical use of mechanical ventricular assist pumps and the total artificial heart in conjunction with heart transplantation: fourth official report—1989. J Heart Transplant 1990; 9:453–458.
4. Kanter KR, Swartz MT, Pennington DG, et al. Renal failure in patients with ventricular assist devices. Trans Am Soc Artif Intern Organs 1987; 33:426–428.
5. Al-Mondhiry H, Pierce WS, Richenbacher W, Bull A. Hemostatic abnormalities associated with prolonged ventricular assist pumping: analysis of 24 patients. Am J Cardiol 1984; 53:1344–1348.
6. Didisheim P, Olsen DB, Farrar DJ, et al. Infections and thromboembolism with implantable cardiovascular devices. Trans Am Soc Artif Intern Organs 1989; 35:54–70.
7. Stuckey JH, Newman MM, Dennis C, et al. The use of the heart lung

machine in selected cases of acute myocardial infarction. Surg Forum 1957; 8:342–344.

8. Pennington DG, Merjavy JP, Codd JE, et al. Extracorporeal membrane oxygenation for patients with cardiogenic shock. Circulation 1984; 70(Suppl I):130–137.

9. Phillips SJ, Zeff RH, Kongtahworn C, et al. Percutaneous cardiopulmonary bypass: application and indication for use. Ann Thorac Surg 1989; 47:121–123.

10. Reichman RT, Joyo CI, Dembitsky WP, et al. Improved patient survival after cardiac arrest using a cardiopulmonary support system. Ann Thorac Surg 1990; 49:101–105.

11. Raithel SC, Swartz MT, Braun PR, et al. Experience with an emergency resuscitation system. Trans Am Soc Artif Intern Organs 1989; 35:475–477.

12. Moore CH, Rubin JM, Schnitzler RN, Canon DS, Arpin A. Experience and direction using cardiopulmonary support in fifty-three consecutive cases. Trans Am Soc Artif Intern Organs 1991; 37:M340–342.

13. Martin GR, Short BL. Doppler echocardiographic evaluation of cardiac performance in infants on prolonged extracorporeal membrane oxygenation. Am J Cardiol 1988; 62:929–934.

14. Bavaria JE, Ratcliffe MB, Gupta KB, et al. Changes in left ventricular systolic wall stress during biventricular circulatory assistance. Ann Thorac Surg 1988; 45:526–532.

15. Raithel SC, Pennington DG, Boegner E, Fiore A, Weber TR. Extracorporeal membrane oxygenation in children following cardiac surgery. Circulation 1992; 86(Suppl 5): 305–310.

16. Bolooki H, ed. Clinical Application of Intra-aortic Balloon Pump. 2 ed. Mount Kisco, NY: Futura Publishing Co. 1984; pp 373–394.

17. DiLello F, Mullen DC, Flemma RJ, et al. Results of intra-aortic balloon pumping after cardiac surgery: experience with the Percor balloon catheter. Ann Thorac Surg 446; 46:442–446.

18. Pennington DG, Swartz MT, Codd JE, Merjavy JP, Kaiser GC. Intra-aortic balloon pumping in cardiac surgical patients: a nine year experience. Ann Thorac Surg 1983; 36:125–131.

19. Golding LR, Jacobs G, Groves LL, et al. Clinical results of mechanical support of the failing left ventricle. J Thorac Cardiovasc Surg 1982; 83:597–601.

20. Joyce LD, Kiser JC, Eales F, et al. Experience with the Sarns centrifugal pump as a ventricular assist device. Trans Am Soc Artif Intern Organs 1990; 36:619–622.

21. Pennington DG, Joyce LD, Pae WE, Burkholder JA. Patient selection. Ann Thorac Surg 1989; 47:77–81.

22. Pennington DG, McBride LR, Swartz MT, et al. Use of the Pierce-Donachy ventricular assist device in patients with cardiogenic shock after cardiac operations. Ann Thorac Surg 1989; 47:130–135.

23. Pennington DG, McBride LR, Kanter KR, et al. The effect of perioperative myocardial infarction on survival of postcardiotomy patients supported with ventricular assist devices. Circulation 1988; 78(Suppl III):110–115.

24. Pennington DG, Merjavy JP, Swartz MT, et al. The importance of biventricular failure in patients with postoperative cardiogenic shock. Ann Thorac Surg 1985; 39:16–26.
25. Pennington DG, Reedy JE, Swartz MT, et al. Univentricular versus biventricular assist device support. J Heart Lung Transplant 1991; 10:258–263.
26. Wareing TH, Kouchoukos NT. Postcardiotomy mechanical circulatory support in the elderly. Ann Thorac Surg 1991; 51:443–447.
27. Moroney D, Swartz MT, Reedy JE, et al. Importance of ventricular arrhythmias in recovery patients with ventricular assist devices. Trans Am Soc Artif Intern Organs 1991; 37:516–517.
28. Joyce LD, Johnson K, Cabrol C, et al. Results of the first one hundred patients who received Jarvik total artificial hearts as a bridge-to-cardiac transplantation. Circulation 1989; 80(Suppl III):III-192–III-201.
29. Farrar DJ, Hill DJ, Gray LA, et al. Heterotopic prosthetic ventricles as a bridge-to-cardiac transplantation. N Engl J Med 1988; 318:333–340.
30. Portner PM, Oyer PE, Pennington DG, et al. Implantable electrical ventricular assist system: bridge to transplantation and the future. Ann Thorac Surg 1989; 47:142–150.
31. Reedy JE, Swartz MT, Pennington DG, et al. Bridge to cardiac transplantation—importance of patient selection. J Heart Transplant 1990; 9:473–481.
32. Farrar DJ, Lawson LH, Litwak P, Cederwall G. Thoratec VAD system as a bridge to heart transplantation. J Heart Transplant 1990; 9:415–422.
33. Pennington DG, Swartz MT. Selection of circulatory support devices. Heart Fail 1988; 4(1):5–9.
34. Wampler RK, Frazier OH, Lansing AM, et al. Treatment of cardiogenic shock with the hemopump left ventricular assist device. Ann Thorac Surg 1991; 52:506–513.
35. Farrar DJ, Compton PG, Dajee H, Fonger JD, Hill JD. Right heart function during left heart assist and the effects of volume loading in a canine preparation. Circulation 1984; 70:708–716.
36. Griffith BP, Kormos RL, Hardesty RL, et al. The artificial heart: infection-related morbidity and its effect on transplantation. Ann Thorac Surg 1988; 45:409–414.
37. McBride LR, Ruzevich SA, Pennington DG, et al. Infectious complications associated with ventricular assist device support. Trans Am Soc Artif Intern Organs 1987; 33:201–202.
38. Szukalski E, Reedy JE, Pennington DG, Swartz MT, McBride LR, Miller LW. Oral anticoagulation in patients with ventricular assist devices. Trans Am Soc Artif Intern Organs 1990; 36(3):700–713.
39. Termuhlen DF, Swartz MT, Pennington DG, et al. Predictors for weaning patients from ventricular assist devices. Trans Am Soc Artif Intern Organs 1988; 34:131–139.
40. Dembitsky WP, Moore CH, Holman WL, et al. Successful mechanical circulatory support for noncoronary shock. J Heart Lung Transplant 1992; 11:129–135.

41. Pae WE, Pierce WS, Pennock JL, Campbell DB, Waldhausen JA. Long-term results of ventricular assist pumping in postcardiotomy cardiogenic shock. J Thorac Cardiovasc Surg 1987; 93:434–441.
42. Pennington DG, Bernhard WF, Golding LR, et al. Long-term follow-up of postcardiotomy patients with profound cardiogenic shock treated with ventricular assist devices. Circulation 1985; 72(Suppl II):II-216–II-226.
43. Reedy JE, Pennington DG, Miller LW, et al. Status I heart transplant patients; conventional vs ventricular assist device (VAD) support. J Heart Lung Transplant 1992; 11(Pt. 1):246–252.

Chapter 11

Cardiac Transplantation and Mechanical Bridge to Transplantation for Acute Coronary Ischemia

Matthew M. Cooper and Eric A. Rose

Introduction

The incidence of cardiogenic shock after acute myocardial infarction (AMI) has decreased as a result of more effective medical and thrombolytic therapy applied during the evolution of infarction.[1] Percutaneous transluminal coronary angioplasty (PTCA) and urgent surgical revascularization predominantly, as well as repair of concomitant left ventricular aneurysm (LVA), postinfarction ventricular septal defect (VSD), and intervention for mitral regurgitation secondary to ischemic papillary muscle rupture, to lesser degrees, have contributed to decreased mortality from cardiogenic shock.[1] Despite this array of interventions in conjunction with the use of intra-aortic balloon counterpulsation, cardiogenic shock continues to be associated with high mortality.[2]

Lazar HL (editor): *Current Therapy for Acute Coronary Ischemia,* © Futura Publishing Co., Inc., Mount Kisco, NY, 1993.

The focus of this chapter, cardiac transplantation for acute coronary ischemia, necessarily requires discussion of bridge-to-transplant efforts with mechanical circulatory assistance. Temporary mechanical circulatory assistance may afford stabilization after AMI and allow diagnostic testing (i.e., cardiac catheterization). Correctable lesions can then be addressed by PTCA or operation and the device weaned at the time of operation or thereafter. For those patients unable to be weaned from support or in whom there exists pathology not amenable to a conventional surgical approach, transplantation becomes the final consideration.[3]

What follows is a highly selective review in which only cardiogenic shock after acute coronary ischemia or AMI is included. Patients with ischemic cardiomyopathy related to a distant myocardial infarction and those with postcardiotomy cardiogenic shock were excluded. Postcardiotomy patients including those status post–myocardial infarction or failed PTCA who were surgically revascularized and then unable to be weaned from cardiopulmonary bypass (CPB) also were excluded in order to focus on the direct impact of mechanical assistance and transplantation with regard to the treatment of acute ischemia. Postcardiotomy ventricular failure may be multifactorial and related to preoperative left ventricular (LV) status, including presence or absence of unstable myocardial ischemia, possible complications during induction of anesthesia, duration of aortic cross-clamping, inadequate myocardial preservation or revascularization, reperfusion injury, and physiological adequacy of CPB and metabolic management.[1,4] Inclusion of these patients might tend to confound conclusions reached from analysis of a "purer" population. Patients requiring mechanical assist because of postoperatively documented perioperative myocardial infarction also were excluded.

Finally, this is predominantly a discussion of clinical results. Techniques of implantation and the technical merits of particular devices are well described elsewhere. Therefore, discussion of these aspects of bridge-to-transplant strategies is avoided except in the case of techniques of support worth particular consideration in patients with acute coronary ischemia. Such limited technical discussion is possible because, barring relatively infrequent mechanical failures, there appears to be little question of the ability of the various devices to support the circulation to a greater or lesser extent. Patient survival and outcome are then determined by the patient's state before device implantation (e.g., degree of multiorgan failure). Furthermore, problems encountered in such patients during periods of mechanical support and post-transplant also are related to patient condition before device implantation. These factors support "early" implantation to halt the progression of pre-existing organ failure with potential to decrease the incidence of associated infection.[5]

Patient Selection:
General Considerations

The initial consideration in institution of mechanical circulatory assist involves some estimation of the reversibility or irreversibility of myocardial failure. The next logical consideration is that of available and applicable options should native cardiac function prove irrecoverable and includes cardiac transplantation, placement of a permanent assist device, or withdrawal of support.[6]

Patients with apparently severe, irreversible LV dysfunction may in reality have large areas of reversibly "stunned" myocardium for which mechanical support of significant duration may be required to allow sufficient time for eventual myocardial recovery.[7] The possibility of delayed myocardial recovery suggests that a delay in selected cases before proceeding to transplantation may be warranted. Recovery from stunning after ischemic insult and associated impairment of oxygen utilization efficiency and increase in myocardial oxygen consumption[8] may be facilitated by adenosine or alternative substrate administration. Positron emission tomography scanning (PET) may be useful in evaluating potentially functional myocardium and assist in the decision to proceed to transplantation.

Accepted contraindications to transplantation other than those considered to be reversible after restoration of adequate cardiac output with mechanical assist warrant exclusion of patients from consideration for device implantation.[9–12] Relatively mild degrees of renal insufficiency (creatinine >2.5 mg/dl before device insertion is highly predictive of nonsurvival) and hypoxia, and superficial infection may be improved sufficiently on support to make the patient a viable transplant recipient.[9] Patients in whom contraindications develop during the bridging period and whose condition cannot be stabilized also are ultimately excluded from receiving transplants.[13]

Given these considerations, mechanical assistance may be appropriate even in stable patients to prevent progressive multiorgan dysfunction.[9,14] In particular, even if a patient is stable on intra-aortic balloon pumping (IABP) or extracorporeal membrane oxygenation (ECMO) but unweanable after 24 to 48 hours, consideration of early institution of more sophisticated support also may be appropriate.[9] The lack of reliable criteria upon which to base such decisions makes the process quite difficult.

The timing of device implantation, although critical for optimization of multiorgan function, also is important for several related reasons. Early implantation of assist in the setting of AMI would favor maximal salvage of jeopardized myocardium.[15] Early implantation of assist devices, use of biventricular support, and increased operator experience have all been associated with increased patient survival.[16] Increased experience contributed to improved survival also through better patient selection, the use of more sophisticated (i.e., sac devices) as opposed to centrifugal support, and appropriate timing for termination of support.[16]

The urgency of device implantation may preclude the usual and adequate investigation of pulmonary hemodynamics and pulmonary vascular resistance (PVR).[10] The PVR may be altered during mechanical support and may be difficult to assess accurately before proceeding to transplantation.[10]

Physiological age has an important influence on ultimate survival. Data from the Combined Registry with respect to *chronological* age in the postcardiotomy setting[17] lists survival as 21% to 31% for those <65 years of age, 12% >65, and 6% >70. The advanced age of many patients presenting with AMI may preclude consideration for transplantation as well as device insertion. Should mechanical support be instituted, the ultimate goal would be weaning from assist or consideration for placement of a permanent device.

Coronary artery disease may be part of a generalized atherosclerosis involving the kidneys, brain, and abdominal aorta.[18] Coincident severe hypertension, diabetes mellitus, or hyperlipidemia may all pose potential risk factors for subsequent transplantation.[18]

The extremes of size also may pose problems depending on the particular assist device selected. While few if any limitations exist with respect to roller and centrifugal pump systems, pneumatic devices are limited by size and stroke volume of the device and inlet and outlet cannula size and length.[11,17] Pae[17] notes that pneumatic devices cannot be used practically in any patient weighing <~40 kg and with a body surface area of <1 m^2. Patients of large size, on the other hand, may have problems with short inlet cannula length.

While significant psychosocial problems or substance abuse of any type are usual contraindications to transplantation, the need for mental and psychosocial stability is intensified in those patients considered for bridging with a mechanical assist device.[18,19]

Finally, but certainly not least in importance, is the issue regarding the presence of preformed antibodies to human leukocyte antigens in potential device/transplant recipients. The presence of these antibodies at particular defined levels is considered by some groups[11,19] to be a contraindication for device placement as the ability to transplant the recipient is less likely and therefore the likelihood of prolonged support is increased. This is a debatable point discussed in detail later. At this point it should be raised for consideration that this subgroup of potential transplant recipients may be precisely those for which mechanical bridge devices may have their greatest utility. Mechanical assist has been used successfully to bridge such a patient with a high level of preformed antibodies.[20]

Patient Selection: Specific Criteria

Selection criteria for implantation of mechanical assist devices has developed by extension from postcardiotomy experience. Coronary artery disease in the presence or absence of LVA is the most common pathology in this group.[21]

Inclusion criteria employed at Columbia-Presbyterian Medical Center (CPMC) are listed in Table 1. Of particular note is the requirement that potential device recipients fulfill the requirements for usual transplant recipients. This includes determination that the heart disease is not amenable to medical or surgical therapy with equivalent results to transplantation, prognosis of survival is otherwise limited, and PVR is <5 Wood units.[19] Some groups require a somewhat lower cardiac index for consideration (<1.8 liter/min/ m^2),[22,23] whereas others would consider individuals with cardiac indices in the range of 2.0 to 2.5 liter/min/m^2 in the face of clinical indications, including mental obtundation, rising serum creatinine, cool extremities, evidence of hepatic congestion, and mixed venous oxygen saturation $<50\%$.[24] Additional measured and calculated

---

Table 1

Inclusion and Exclusion Criteria Employed at Columbia-Presbyterian Medical Center for the Use of Thermedics Heart-Mate 2000 LVAD as a Bridge to Cardiac Transplantation

---

Inclusion Criteria
 1. Left atrial or pulmonary capillary wedge pressure >20 mm Hg
 2. Systemic arterial pressure <80 mm Hg
 3. Cardiac index <2.0 L/min/m²
 4. *Patient must be a candidate for cardiac transplantation*
Exclusion Criteria
 1. Body surface area <1.5 m²
 2. Age >70 yr
 3. Chronic renal failure
 4. Severe emphysema
 5. Severe chronic obstructive pulmonary disease
 6. Unresolved pulmonary infarction
 7. Severe pulmonary hypertension
 8. Severe hepatic disease
 9. Cerebral vascular disease with cerebral impairment
 10. Severe gastrointestinal malabsorption
 11. Active systemic infection
 12. Severe blood dyscrasia
 13. Metastatic cancer
 14. Diffuse, severe peripheral vascular disease
 15. Repeated prosthetic valve replacement as a result of infection
 16. Long-term high dose steroid therapy
 17. Positive HIV test
 18. Refractory anuria
 19. Blood urea nitrogen >100 (units)
 20. Creatinine >5.0 (units)
 21. Intractable ventricular tachycardia
 22. Severely compromised right heart function coupled with high PVR (i.e., RVEDP >15 mm Hg, PA systolic <50 mm Hg with a PVR >5 Wood units)
 23. Prolonged (i.e., hr) or multiple attempts to stabilize the circulation with pharmacological methods without improvement in hemodynamic function
 24. Prolonged (i.e., >30 min) unsuccessful attempts to resuscitate the fibrillating or arrested heart

---

LVAD = left ventricular assist device; HIV = human immunodeficiency virus; PVR = pulmonary vascular resistance; RVEDP = right ventricular end-diastolic pressure; PA = pulmonary artery.

inclusion criteria utilized by other groups have included systemic vascular resistance >2100 dynes sec/cm^5 and urine output <20 mL/hr with optimized preload, maximal drug therapy, metabolic balance, and IABP,[9,17] left ventricular work index <1500 g/mm^2 [LVWI = CI × (MAP − PCWP) × 13.6].[2] More specific indices of right ventricular (RV) failure include low cardiac output and systemic hypotension with left atrial (LA) pressure <15 mm Hg despite right atrium (RA) loading to a pressure of 25 mm Hg.[22]

Exclusion Criteria

Renal failure severe enough to require renal dialysis is considered an absolute contraindication to device placement because of experience that it precludes survival in this group.[25] Active gastrointestinal or intracranial bleeding, heparin antibody thrombocytopenia, multiorgan and in particular liver failure as it contributes to coagulopathy also are contraindications to device placement and subsequent transplantation.[14,17] It should be mentioned that with the increasing interest and implementation of mechanical assist without CPB, the presence of problems related to heparin antibodies may decline in importance.

As an aid in selection and exclusion of patients, a scoring system was developed based on a retrospective study of patients being evaluated for transplantation.[9] Risk factors that negatively influenced survival in the mechanically supported group included pulmonary insufficiency requiring an inspired oxygen fraction of >0.7, intubation for >5 days, and cardiac arrest necessitating cardiopulmonary resuscitation (CPR) within 24 hours of evaluation. The severity of the score also correlated with duration of support. Not surprisingly, age <50 was compatible with survival.[9]

Several considerations are of increased importance when considering placement of particular devices. For example, a previous sternotomy is considered by some groups to be a contraindication to implantation of a total artificial heart (TAH) because of an additional risk of bleeding from lysed adhesions when anticoagulated.[11] When considering use of the Hemopump (Johnson & Johnson Interventional System Co., Nimbus Medical, Inc., Rancho Cordova, CA), aortic valvular or aneurysmal disease, the presence of a valve prosthesis, aorto-iliac occlusive disease, or significant blood dyscrasia are all considered particularly exclusionary.[26]

Lessons from Postcardiotomy Use

Experience accrued through postcardiotomy use of mechanical assist has yielded several widely substantiated principles that apply in the setting of AMI. Patients "crashing" when first evaluated usually ultimately do not do well.[17] More specifically, a retrospective analysis of the experience in St. Louis with postcardiotomy use of mechanical assist showed that perioperative myocardial infarction has a negative impact on survival.[21] Twenty-seven percent of survivors and 63% of nonsurvivors postcardiotomy had proven or likely diagnosis of myocardial infarction pre- or perioperatively. Only 1 of 11 survivors had both positive electrocardiographic (ECG) and enzymatic changes consistent with perioperative AMI. These results by extension suggest a level of expectation for use of mechanical assist devices as bridges after AMI. Similar disappointing survival has been reported by others in association with perioperative AMI. In one report only 6 of 18 patients survived,[16] whereas in another postcardiotomy series, no survivor had evidence of myocardial infarction as determined by MB fraction/enzymes, although several had new Q waves on ECG.[27]

Some ray of promise is suggested by small series such as that of Keon et al.,[28] in which three patients with cardiogenic shock after myocardial infarction who could not be weaned from CPB post–coronary artery bypass grafting (CABG) were all successfully bridged to transplant. All three patients were discharged, although one expired at 1 month of rejection.

Postcardiotomy use of mechanical assist also has demonstrated the negative impact on survival of severe renal failure. In one report, only one of nine patients with renal failure severe enough to require dialysis survived.[21] A potential partial explanation for such high mortality in the presence of renal failure is suggested by experimental results using radioactive microspheres in dogs, which showed that left ventricular assist device (LVAD) plus dopamine support may not be able to normalize organ flows completely during cardiogenic shock.[29] This was particularly true for the kidney in which renal blood flow could be recovered maximally to only 83% of control.

Similarly, major infection portends poor survival in the postcardiotomy setting. Only one of eight such patients survived in one series.[21] The duration of support appeared to be a factor in infection and thereby supported initiation of weaning efforts after 24 hours of stabilization.[21]

Mechanical Assist Devices

General Comments

Ideally, the particular device employed should be tailored to the patient's needs. The availability of multiple systems affords flexibility in selection. As a general rule, the success of transplantation after mechanical support is more dependent on patient selection than choice of device with certain restrictions.[25] The simplest and least invasive application is attempted first unless it is clearly evident that the patient needs more extensive support. Patients with the possibility of myocardial recovery or those who are expected to need mechanical support of short duration usually are treated with an IABP or centrifugal pump. Many groups emphasize the value of early institution of LV assist in the case of therapeutic failure of an IABP and the possible need to go directly to LV assist if an IABP is unable to be inserted for technical reasons, or if the cardiac index is <1.0.[3]

The expected duration of support is a key consideration in the choice of mechanical systems in that with longer predicted support, pneumatic systems are preferable to centrifugal systems, which are plagued by hemolysis and the need to change pump heads regularly.[19,30] Those patients with end-stage single ventricular dysfunction may be considered for univentricular assist. If recovery is still considered possible, a heterotopic device is a reversible step.[31,32] However, patients with irreversible biventricular failure with expected prolonged need may be considered for implantation of a TAH.[33] In this regard, however, use of bilateral ventricular assist devices (BVAD) may be preferable to use of a TAH since the potential exists for implantation of the former without CPB and associated anticoagulation.[34] A further consideration in the use of the TAH is the potential for extensive adhesion formation, which may occur soon after implantation and could complicate device explanation as well as implantation of a donor organ.[5] In addition, if patient size is insufficient to preclude hindrance of systemic and pulmonary venous return for a TAH, bilateral heterotopic ventricular assist may be indicated.[35]

An extremely important pearl mentioned by several authors[2,12,27,36–39] with regard to implantation of mechanical assist is the necessity of checking for a patent foramen ovale and closing it if one is present. This can prevent potentially fatal hypoxemia due to right-to-left shunting during LV assist. Intraoperative echocardiography at the time of LVAD placement has been useful in this regard.[16]

Counterpulsation

Intra-aortic balloon counterpulsation is used widely as a first-line intervention because of ease of insertion. However, the IABP has limited potential to stabilize hemodynamics in the most severely affected patients as some LV contractility is necessary.[2,40] This is the reason that most patients in severe cardiogenic shock still die despite IABP support. In addition, ventricular arrhythmias may preclude adjunctive use of the IABP.[30] A clear role has yet to be defined in the acute setting for use of *extra*-aortic counterpulsation systems of both prosthetic and autologous skeletal muscle design.[41-45]

Extracorporeal Membrane Oxygenation

By and large, patients placed on ECMO for severe respiratory failure are contraindicated for ventricular assist device (VAD) placement.[16] Prolonged ECMO has been shown to be suboptimal for bridging for periods >24–48 hr. If a patient is in need of support for longer periods, consideration should be given to placement of a more sophisticated long-term device.[25] Transfer from ECMO to VAD support has the potential to reduce bleeding and infectious complications.[9] This may preclude the progression from development of an adult respiratory distress syndrome (ARDS) to the resultant increase in transpulmonary gradient and pulmonary vascular resistance (PVR) to exclusion from transplant candidacy.

Ventricular Assist Devices

VADs are of two types, centrifugal or pneumatic, and are designed to be placed in either a heterotopic or orthotopic (TAH) position. Before insertion, some assessment of the potential for myocardial recovery should be performed. The amount of potentially salvageable myocardium may be estimated with PET scanning with results that may lead to consideration of conventional surgical alternatives or PTCA.

The potential for myocardial recovery also has implications for technique of VAD implantation. With possible stunning after AMI, atrial rather than ventricular cannulation may be preferred to avoid additional injury to the LV.[21,37] Total capture of cardiac output usually is possible with atrial cannulation.[46] In addition, freshly infarcted LV tissue may hold sutures too poorly to allow secure cannulation.[39] In-flow cannula obstruction and increased bleeding problems after apical cannulation have contributed to the death of at least one patient.[46] LV cannulation immobilizes the heart and makes it more difficult to check for sources of bleeding.[46]

Need for RVAD/Biventricular Assist

It is widely perceived that the use of an LVAD may unmask RV failure. Indeed, it has been shown experimentally that the underlying pathological process is the dominant factor in determining RV function during LVAD support.[47] Alteration in ventricular geometry with LV unloading by an LVAD in a normal heart did not significantly alter RV performance characteristics.[48]

While patients with compromised RV function can be supported by isolated left univentricular support, those patients with an elevated PVR or infarction in the right coronary distribution may require biventricular support.[39] While patients with severe right heart failure and pulmonary hypertension in the face of high *fixed* PVR are not candidates for orthotopic heart transplantation and, therefore, not candidates for mechanical support,[12] patients with normal or near-normal PVR may derive sufficient reduction in pulmonary artery pressure and RV afterload with LV assist to effectively provide simultaneous RV support as well.[12] A further indication for biventricular support may be in an effort to avoid potential morbidity associated with persistent elevation in central venous pressure as in a passive Fontan-type circulation.[30] It has been noted that apparent RV failure in the face of isolated LV assist may be related to pulmonary vasospasm and may be effectively treated with prostaglandin E_1 (PGE_1) rather than RV mechanical assist.[30] There has been a renewed interest in pulmonary artery balloon counterpulsation to treat the RV component of biventricular dysfunction as an alternative to RV assist.[49] The utility of this technique has yet to be widely established. Certainly, accurate monitoring of indicators of bilateral ventricular function is necessary to assess correctly the need for biventricular support.[1] Studies of pressure-volume response of the RV during LVAD support utilizing sonomicrometry and transesophageal echocardiographic measurements may lead to elucidation of clear criteria on which to base selection of patients who require biventricular support.[24]

Minimal if any added morbidity including that related to infection, thrombotic complications, or mechanical problems has been experienced with biventricular as compared with left univentricular support and, therefore, should not be a real factor when deciding between single and biventricular support.[13,50]

In contrast to transplant candidates with cardiomyopathy and biventricular failure who may require biventricular support, patients with acute infarction may have only left ventricular involvement and, thereby, require only single ventricular support.[31] The presence of biventricular failure in patients with potentially recoverable myocardial function, however, is a negative predictor of survival in that it suggests more extensive damage.[50] Kormos et al.[24] distinguish biventricular failure in the chronically dilated and accommodated heart from the situation with acute ischemia where the contribution of the septum and thus performance of both ventricles can be affected. The authors suggest that a high incidence of right heart failure in the presence of LV support may reflect the role of ischemia. They further suggest that, in the context of acute infarction where both ventricles are at risk, there may be a role for the TAH.

Three systems of mechanical assist are of particular note with regard to possible emergent use in patients after AMI because of the relative ease and rapidity of institution. These include percutaneous cardiopulmonary support (CPS), the Nimbus Hemopump (Johnson & Johnson Interventional System Co., Nimbus Medical, Inc., Rancho Cordova, CA), and mechanical ventricular actuation. These are discussed in the following sections.

Percutaneous Cardiopulmonary Support System

The collective reported experience with percutaneous CPS relevant to the setting of acute coronary ischemia numbers 45 patients[4,51-53] (Table 2). The experience is not a pure one with respect to survival with mechanical assist independent of some other intervention, however (i.e., PTCA and/or CABG). Nonetheless, it

Table 2

Collected Relevant Experience with Percutaneous CPS After AMI

# Pts	Cardiac Arrest	Support	Intervention	Survival # (%)	Ref #
5	—	Roller	PTCA	0/5 (0%)	30
5	—	Centrifugal	—	0/5 (0%)	10
7	—	Centrifugal	PTCA/CABG	3/7 (43%)	10
7	7	—	PTCA/CABG	3/7 (43%)	33
19	19	Centrifugal	—	0/19 (0%)	47
2	—	Roller	—	1/2 (50%)	47
			Overall Survival	7/45 (16%)	

CPS = cardiopulmonary support; AMI = acute myocardial infarction; Pts = patients; PTCA = percutaneous transluminal coronary angioplasty; CABG = coronary artery bypass grafting.

proves informative with respect to projections of survival. Experience has been with both portable roller and centrifugal systems. All patients were in cardiogenic shock after AMI with a variable number also reported to be in frank cardiac arrest. Survival is clearly dismal (16% overall), particularly if the patients were in cardiac arrest. This is despite the selective application of single or repetitive PTCA, and surgical revascularization either for "failed" PTCA or after a "successful" angioplasty. The largest series, that of Hartz et al.,[53] documented the rapid institution of CPS. Of the total series of 29 patients, 10 of 29 (34%) were placed on CPS within 15 minutes of arrest, 9 of 29 (31%) within 15 to 30 minutes, and 10 of 29 at or after 30 minutes (34%). This is clearly a prompt response yet with disappointing results. Doubt is cast on the effectiveness of this approach given current criteria for patient selection. Perhaps even earlier utilization before any intervention in the catheterization laboratory may lead to improved survival.

Hemopump

The Hemopump, a rotating turbine passed retrograde into the LV via the aortic valve, is potentially one of the most useful devices for patients with acute decompensation/cardiogenic shock secondary to coronary ischemia. The system allows for ventricular recovery from myocardial stunning and is capable of hemodynamic support equivalent to an LVAD but with the ease of insertion and associated risks closer to those of the IABP. The Hemopump can provide up to 3.5 L of flow without the need for LV contribution or synchronization. Unlike the IABP, the Hemopump is capable of supporting patients in refractory ventricular fibrillation or tachycardia. The potential risks of a major surgical procedure required for LVAD insertion as well as the risks of anticoagulation if CPB is necessary for insertion are avoided.[2]

In a multi-institution study,[2] the Hemopump was inserted successfully in 41 of 53 patients (77%). These 41 patients were supported for a mean time of 52.8 hours (range 1–194 hr). Cardiogenic shock was due to AMI in 17 of 41 (42%). The device usually is placed via surgical exposure of the common femoral or external iliac artery and could not be inserted in 12 patients because of severe atherosclerosis of the iliofemoral system, small native femoral artery (especially in women), and inability to cross the aortic valve. Four of the patients (33%) in whom the device could not be inserted were in the AMI group. Patients with cardiogenic shock due to AMI had a 30-day survival of 41% (7/17) compared with 24% for postcardiotomy shock and 29% for other causes. The survival of the noninsertion group was 17% (2/12) overall with 0% (0/4) surviving after AMI. The Hemopump was used successfully in one additional patient who sustained an AMI due to left anterior descending artery (LAD) dissection during PTCA.[54] After successful CABG the Hemopump was used to wean the patient from bypass and was then removed. The patient ultimately did well. These are very encouraging results when compared with survival using CPS but also may reflect differences in patient selection criteria.

Use of the Hemopump was associated with some elevation in plasma-free hemoglobin and some decrease in platelet count (more severe in those postcardiotomy than after AMI); however, there was no morbidity or mortality related to intravascular hemolysis or spontaneous bleeding, respectively. Aspiration of mural thrombus resulted in loss of mechanical assist and death in one patient and must be considered when contemplating use in patients with an AMI who may have mural thrombus. No leg ischemia was observed in this series, although there was a pump-related thromboembolic rate of 2.4%, and a total incidence of 9.6%.

Mechanical Ventricular Actuation

To avoid the potential technical difficulty of device implantation as well as hemorrhagic and thromboembolic complications, Lowe and colleagues from Duke University have recently championed direct mechanical ventricular actuation.[55] This system provides biventricular assist that can be instituted quickly (in 3–5 min) via a left anterior thoracotomy and has no direct blood contact or need for anticoagulation. An elliptical cup of variable material is attached to both ventricles by a continuous vacuum at the apex of the cup. Once the cup is in position, positive and negative pneumatic forces operate a diaphragm within the cup to "actuate" the ventricles into their normal systolic and diastolic configurations. Cardiac output ranging from 80% to 130% of control may thereby be achieved despite ventricular fibrillation or asystole.

The initial reported experience[55] included two patients in refractory cardiogenic shock after an AMI. One patient had a superimposed idiopathic dilated cardiomyopathy. The first patient underwent unsuccessful thrombolytic therapy and PTCA and ultimately deteriorated despite placement of an IABP. Cardiac arrest occurred before device insertion. During the subsequent 45-hour period of support, ventricular fibrillation persisted. Despite the ventricular fibrillation, an essentially normal cardiac output was maintained, although a technical problem required insertion of a new device at the bedside. The patient remained neurologically unresponsive after the cardiac arrest and was pronounced brain dead and the device removed after 45 hours. The other patient, also in refractory cardiogenic shock, underwent device placement in <3 minutes. "Skin-to-skin," the operation required only 38 minutes. Immediately improved hemodynamics and stabilization allowed discontinuation of all inotropic support and successful transplantation after 56 hours of support. The patient is apparently alive and well more than 1 year later.

The authors cite the potential advantages of this technique with regard to avoidance of vascular connections, rapidity of implantation, restoration of physiological pulsatile flow rates even in the fibrillating heart, and avoidance of elaborate set-up, support team, or training. Further study is required to determine the appropriate niche for this device. Certainly, its potential use in the setting of acute coronary ischemia as temporary support or a bridge to either other devices or transplantation is exciting.

Transplantation

Complete recovery of function and replenishment of myocardial adenosine triphosphate (ATP) stores after myocardial stunning may take days or even weeks and what appears initially to be an irreversibly injured ventricle may regain function if supported long enough.[46,56] In addition, experimental results suggest that perfusion of the coronary circulation with adenosine-enriched blood may accelerate recovery of ischemic myocardium and shorten time required for biventricular assist.[57] This prompts the question as to when the decision regarding transplantation should be made. Should it be made at the time of device placement or with failure to wean? The latter approach may be the more appropriate for use after acute infarction if definite irreversibility is not established.

The demonstrated reliability of the newer mechanical assist devices allows patients to remain on assist long enough for organ recovery to take place rather than proceeding to transplant under suboptimal conditions.[30] In fact, patients may not be listed as priority candidates in order to allow pulmonary edema, renal insufficiency, coagulopathy, mental obtundation, etc., to resolve or stabilize.[11,14,30,37,58] While on mechanical support patients may make nutritional gains, lose edema, improve pulmonary toilet, and enhance their condition by exercise.[25] Time may be allowed for high levels of antihuman leukocyte antigen (HLA) antibodies to decline. It is clear that the better the preoperative condition the more benign the postoperative course.[5] In this regard it has been suggested that LVAD support also may allow transpulmonary gradient and PVR to decline from high-risk levels to the more successful range.[24]

What if organ function has not fully recovered on mechanical support when a donor becomes available?[10] Do you proceed to transplantation? Certainly there are those who believe that dysfunction of noncardiac organs should not preclude transplantation if dysfunction is secondary to low flow and therefore reversible.[31] In addition, organ dysfunction also can develop while on mechanical support and can potentially preclude transplant candidacy.

Results

General and Combined Registry

The success of the bridge-to-transplant strategy depends on careful patient selection.[10,12,21,58] Improved success as measured by increased survival to and from ultimate transplantation has occurred as experience has accrued. Critical to such success has been earlier institution of mechanical assist and more aggressive treatment of biventricular failure, including biventricular assist.[21] By and large candidates for mechanical assist should meet criteria for transplantation, although mild degrees of end-organ dysfunction expected to improve with increased cardiac output may be accepted.

Postoperative bleeding has been a significant limiting complication in the use of mechanical assist.[12,14,19,21,59-62] This has been true predominantly in the group of patients who are postcardiotomy or after PTCA where previous systemic anticoagulation is contributory. Use of assist in the setting of AMI without prior anticoagulation and the increasing ability and interest in instituting assist without the use of CPB should significantly reduce bleeding-related morbidity and limitation in the future. Sternal closure, if possible, after implantation also may decrease postoperative bleeding and, in addition, may allow extubation if otherwise possible if a delay to transplantation is expected.[21]

After bleeding, infection has been a significant limiting factor in patient survival.[61,62] In particular, infection has correlated directly with duration of support but may not be strictly device related.[12,17,37] In one postcardiotomy experience, patients supported ≤48 hours had no infection whereas the incidence was 70% in those supported for 3 to 21 days.[37] Of those infected, 30% survived as compared with 70% of noninfected patients.

Mediastinal infection has been a more dominant problem with orthotopic than heterotopic devices apparently unrelated to ascending infection along drive lines but rather related to pericardial dead space associated with removal of the native heart and the placement of a large foreign body.[10,11] Improvement of the nutritional state during prolonged mechanical support also may help to reduce infection rate.[37]

Of particular importance for the present discussion is the demonstration, again from the postcardiotomy experience, that perioperative myocardial infarction is an important deterrent to survival in patients receiving mechanical bridge support.[62] However, the direct implication of this to the setting of the AMI patient who is not postcardiotomy is unclear.

Results from the Combined Registry of mechanical ventricular assist[63] indicate that the age distribution for circulatory support in conjunction with heart transplantation paralleled that seen with isolated heart transplantation. Not surprisingly, the best results in terms of percentage of patients undergoing transplantation and ultimate discharge were at the youngest end of the age spectrum (age 7–20 years) in which 79% were transplanted and 82% discharged from the hospital. The poorest results were at the oldest end of spectrum with values of 53% and 50% respectively (age >60 years). The older age groups would be expected to be represented more heavily in those patients with AMI considered for mechanical assist. The rates of transplantation were equal regardless of the type of support employed. However, outcome favored univentricular support over the TAH (Table 3). For patients receiving LV support, the rates of transplantation and hospital discharge were similar with regard to electric, pneumatic, or centrifugal devices (Table 4). There was a trend for patients supported with centrifugal devices to fare less well. However, this did not reach statistical significance. Analysis of patients treated with biventricular assist suggested that the use of hybrid systems, as compared with two identical centrifugal or pneumatic devices, led to overall inferior results and nearly reached statistical significance. The best results of biventricular assist were still inferior, however, to that of isolated univentricular support.

The overall operative mortality from the Registry for orthotopic transplantation after mechanical support is 18% compared to roughly 10% for nonassisted patients.[63] Breakdown of the mortality showed a range from 9% after univentricular assist to 18% after paracorporeal biventricular assist, to 23% after support with the TAH. Statistical significance was reached only when comparing pretransplant univentricular versus TAH support. Actuarial survival inclusive of operative mortality for all patients after mechanical bridge to transplant was 65% at 1 and 2 years as compared with 80% for those not requiring pretransplant mechanical assist. However, the 1- and 2-year survival after univentricular assist was 86% and 83%, respectively, and essentially was equivalent to that after nonstaged transplant.

Table 3

Results of Circulatory Support by Device Type: Data from the Combined Registry

	No. of Patients	Transplanted # (%)	Discharged # (%)
RVAD	4	1 (25)	1 (100)
LVAD	122	87 (71)	76 (87)*
BVAD	161	105 (65)	73 (70)†
TAH	189	135 (71)	67 (50)‡
Total	476	328 (69)	217 (66)

*p = 0.003, LVAD vs. BVAD.
†p = 0.002, BVAD vs. TAH.
‡p = 0.000, LVAD vs. TAH.
RVAD = right ventricular assist device; LVAD = left ventricular assist device; BVAD = biventricular assist; TAH = total artificial heart.
From ref. 63.

Table 4

Results of LV Support with Regard to Device Type: Data from the Combined Registry

	No. of Patients	Transplanted # (%)	Discharged # (%)
Electric	39	27 (69)	25 (93)
Pneumatic	54	38 (70)	35 (92)
Centrifugal	26	20 (77)	16 (80)

LV = left ventricular.
From ref. 63.

Transplantation After Mechanical Circulatory Support: Individual Center Results

Recent experience has demonstrated that temporary circulatory support can lead to a success rate after transplantation that is similar to or even possibly superior to that of patients not requiring prior support,[13,25,39,40,61,64–66] although equivalent survival has not been universally demonstrated.[34] This equivalent or possibly enhanced survival is due to the potentially improved multiorgan function of patients maintained on pretransplant mechanical support.

The 1-year survival rate after staged transplantation in the Utah Cardiac Transplant Program (86%) was essentially identical to that after nonstaged transplantation (88%).[19] However, one must be careful in analyzing results with mechanical support that include both IABP and VAD support. Clearly those patients able to be bridged by the IABP alone are a functionally superior group with greater remaining cardiac function than those requiring more extensive hemodynamic support. In the Utah experience, of those patients treated with VADs, 22% died while awaiting transplant, 44% were weaned from support, 33% received transplants, and 78% of the patients survived to discharge. Of the IABP patients, 18% died while awaiting transplant, 79% underwent transplantation, and 96% were discharged from the hospital.

Excellent results also have been reported in similar patients by Farrar et al.[13] The authors reported that 20 of 21 patients (95%) were discharged after transplantation. Eleven of the first 12 patients (92%) were alive at 1 year, the first 3 were alive at 2 years, and their first patient was alive 3 years after transplant.

Standard immunosuppresive regimens have been employed in patients after staged transplantation after mechanical support with an incidence of rejection comparable to nonbridged patients.[19,40,62,65,67] While the complication and infection rate posttransplant appears to be similar in bridged and nonbridged patients,[65] Pifarre et al.[40] reported a higher incidence of infection in the transplanted group with prior mechanical support (52% vs. 23% in the nonbridged group). The infections were predominantly respiratory, urinary tract, and mucocutaneous herpes simplex.

Patient Data: Acute Coronary Ischemia

Dennis and associates are credited with the first use of mechanical assistance in the treatment of cardiogenic shock after AMI in 1957.[68] They employed venoarterial bypass successfully in one patient. Of the next 24 patients in whom this technique was utilized, however, there were no long-term survivors.

It was not until 1978 that the successful use of a mechanical bridge to transplantation was first reported by Reemtsma et al.[69]

The IABP was used to support a 48-year-old patient after a recent massive myocardial infarction for 13 days until transplantation could be successfully performed. The modern era of mechanical bridge support to transplantation for acute ischemia was ushered in by Hill et al.[31] at Pacific Presbyterian Medical Center in San Francisco. They employed a Thoratec Pierce-Donachy (Thoratec Medical Corporation, Berkeley, CA) prosthetic ventricle in a 47-year-old man in refractory cardiogenic shock after anteroseptal AMI. Transplantation was performed 2 days later and after a stormy course related predominantly to his pretransplant state he was discharged 3 months after admission.

A subsequent multicenter experience with the Pierce-Donachy (Thoratec) LVAD in 29 patients has been reported.[13] Of the 29 patients, 7, including Hill's first patient, were staged after an AMI. The mean age was 42 ± 8 years (range 41–53 years). Five of the 7 (71%) were transplanted successfully after an average of 2.2 ± 0.3 days of support (range 1.5–3 days). All but the first patient, who was supported with an LVAD only, received biventricular support. The two patients not transplanted after AMI died after 1 and 12.5 days of support due to hypoxia/aspiration and multiorgan failure/sepsis, respectively.

Multicenter experience with the Novacor Left Ventricular Assist System (Novacor Medical Corp., Oakland, CA) has included 20 patients, 6 of whom were status post-AMI.[12] The mean age was 50 ± 3 years (range 38–59 years) and duration of support 22 ± 11 days (range 4–67 days). Three patients (50%) survived to transplant, although one died 2 hours later due to graft failure. One patient died of multiorgan failure after 5 days of support, one from a fatal air embolus due to a deairing complication after 10 days during concomitant support with a centrifugal RV assist device (RVAD), and one patient after 67 days of support from accidental hemorrhage and disseminated intravascular coagulation. There were no malfunctions or complications related to the use of the Novacor device.

Only one series has been reported to date dealing specifically with the issue of transplantation for AMI.[70] This limited study by Loisance et al.[70] well describes the multilevel approach to treatment that these patients require. In particular, the authors point out that clinical improvement with medical therapy may be only temporary, and that the risk of sudden arrhythmic death even in the face of optimal intravenous inotropic therapy may be independent of the extent of hemodynamic improvement. They further note the usually incomplete recovery of viable ischemic myocardium and the need for an earlier and more aggressive approach to device implantation if no contraindications to transplantation are present. Three of their 10 patients received assist devices including two TAHs and one LVAD. One TAH recipient deteriorated without explanation on day 3 and died. The other two patients were transplanted after 2 and 3 days of support, respectively, and have done well.

The remainder of the successful experience with bridge-to-transplant strategy for AMI has been scattered, although overall encouraging.[11,20,25,32,61,64,71] Experience from Barnes Hospital in St. Louis with centrifugal assist as a bridge after AMI experience resulted in two of three patients being successfully transplanted after a relatively brief period of support (0.5 and 3 days, respectively).[67] Of particular interest was that all three devices were inserted without CPB, obviating the need for full heparinization and potential associated bleeding. The third patient in their series died on LVAD support before required biventricular assist could be instituted.

Conclusions: Future Prospects

Future success of the mechanical bridge-to-transplant approach to the treatment of acute coronary ischemia is critically dependent on the definition and refinement in patient selection criteria. Criteria for selection of the appropriate device or method of support to be utilized in a particular situation also must be refined. Early institution of mechanical assist may afford significant reduction in multiorgan dysfunction and improve salvage.[1,60]

The use of sophisticated mechanical assist devices in the setting of acute coronary ischemia has been relatively limited and will require further application. The larger question posed concerns the distinction between what can be done technologically and what should be done from the standpoint of the individual's expected duration and quality of life and accompanying societal, economic, and limited resource issues. Does our commitment to treat a patient with an AMI necessarily extend our obligation to place a VAD and then to offer a heart transplant if unweanable from mechanical support? Given the limited supply of suitable donor organs, an additional impetus is provided by this group of patients to demonstrate the effectiveness of permanently implantable mechanical assist devices.[66]

With respect to the assorted devices, technical modifications can be expected that may facilitate implantation without the use of CPB[61] and allow percutaneous insertion of devices such as the Hemopump.[26] New and different technology may be required for use of the various devices in the face of anatomical obstacles such as severe peripheral vascular disease. Further study of the rapidly applicable modality of direct mechanical actuation certainly is indicated.[55]

The potential applicability, if any, of biological bridges employing cardiomyoplasty[72,73] or skeletal muscle ventricles[74] in the setting of acute ischemia also is to be addressed. The use of dynamic skeletal muscle patches to replace acutely infarcted ventricular wall[1,72,73] may be of particular interest. Experimental studies have suggested the possibility of using donor cardiac allografts that are of small size or otherwise unsatisfactory for orthotopic replacement or xenografts in a heterotopic position for short-term LV assistance as a bridge to definitive orthotopic transplantation.[74]

An important issue requiring resolution is the place of mechanical assist, either temporary or permanent, in the patient with high cytotoxic antibody reactivity. Is this precisely the group for which long-term or even permanent mechanical assistance be employed? Or should these patients be denied assist devices because of the decreased likelihood of finding a donor match? As assist devices continue to improve, the negative impact of long-term mechanical support must be re-evaluated. In fact, it may be true that patients well supported for longer duration may become superior transplant recipients.

Finally, while the current bridge-to-transplant strategy may achieve long-term survival in a smaller percentage of patients than desired, it certainly allows salvage of patients that otherwise would surely have died.[76] However, as we continue to expand our technological capabilities we must be ever mindful of consideration of the quality of the lives we may be able to sustain.[59]

References

1. Mundth ED. Assisted circulation. In: Sabiston DC, Jr, Spencer FC, eds. Surgery of the Chest. 5th ed. Philadelphia: WB Saunders. 1990; pp 1777–1799.

2. Wampler RK, Frazier OH, Lansing AM, et al. Treatment of cardiogenic shock with the Hemopump left ventricular assist device. Ann Thorac Surg 1991; 52:506–513.
3. Pae WE Jr, Pierce WS. Temporary left ventricular assistance in acute myocardial infarction and cardiogenic shock. Rationale and criteria for utilization. Chest 1981; 79:692–695.
4. Rose DM, Connolly M, Cunningham JN Jr, Spencer FC. Technique and results with a roller pump left and right heart assist device. Ann Thorac Surg 1989; 47:124–129.
5. Emery RW, Joyce LD, Prieto M, Johnson K, Goldenberg IF, Pritzker MR. Experience with the Symbion total artificial heart as a bridge to transplantation. Ann Thorac Surg 1992; 53:282–288.
6. Holman WL, Bourge RC, Kirklin JR. Case report: circulatory support for seventy days with resolution of acute heart failure. J Thorac Cardiovasc Surg 1991; 102:932–933.
7. Ballantyne CM, Verani MS, Short HD, Hyatt C, Noon GP. Delayed recovery of severely "stunned" myocardium with the support of a left ventricular assist device after coronary artery bypass graft surgery. J Am Coll Cardiol 1987; 10:710–712.
8. Bavaria JE, Furukawa S, Kreiner G, et al. Myocardial oxygen utilization after reversible global ischemia. J Thorac Cardiovasc Surg 1990; 100:210–220.
9. Reedy JE, Swartz MT, Termuhlen DF, et al. Bridge to heart transplantation: importance of patient selection. J Heart Transplant 1990; 9:473–481.
10. Hill DJ. Bridging to cardiac transplantation. Ann Thorac Surg 1989; 47:167–171.
11. Griffith BP. Interim use of the Jarvik-7 artificial heart: lessons learned at Presbyterian-University Hospital of Pittsburgh. Ann Thorac Surg 1989; 47:158–166.
12. Portner PM, Oyer PE, Pennington DG, et al. Implantable electrical left ventricular assist system: bridge to transplantation and the future. Ann Thorac Surg 1989; 47:142–150.
13. Farrar DJ, Hill JD, Gray LA, et al. Heterotopic prosthetic ventricles as a bridge to cardiac transplantation. A multicenter study in 29 patients. N Engl J Med 1988; 318:333–340.
14. Brugger JP, Bonandi L, Meli M, Lichtsteiner M, Odermatt R, Hahn CH. SWAT team approach to ventricular assistance. Ann Thorac Surg 1989; 47:136–141.
15. Laschinger JC, Cunningham JN Jr, Krieger K, et al. Delayed institution of pulsatile left atrial/femoral artery bypass: effects on reduction of myocardial infarct size. Surg Forum 1983; 34:258–261.
16. Adamson RM, Dembitsky WP, Reichman RT, Moreno-Cabral RJ, Daily PO. Mechanical support: asset or nemesis? J Thorac Cardiovasc Surg 1989; 98:915–921.
17. Pennington DG, Moderator. Patient Selection. Panel Discussion presented at the Circulatory Support Symposium of the Society of Thoracic Surgeons, St. Louis, MO, Feb 6–7, 1988. Panelists: Joyce LD, Pae WE Jr, Burkholder JA. Ann Thorac Surg 1989; 47:77–81.

18. Lichtlen PR, Herrmann G. Indications for heart transplantation in endstage coronary artery disease. Adv Cardiol 1988; 36:228–245.
19. Marks JD, Karwande SV, Richenbacher WE, et al. Perioperative mechanical circulatory support for transplantation. J Heart Lung Transplant 1992; 11:117–128.
20. Lick S, Copeland JG, Rosado LJ, Sethi G, Smith RG, Cleavinger M. Long-term bridge to transplantation with the Symbion acute ventricular assist device system. Ann Thorac Surg 1991; 52:308–309.
21. Pennington DG, McBride LR, Swartz MT, et al. Use of the Pierce-Donachy ventricular assist device in patients with cardiogenic shock after cardiac operations. Ann Thorac Surg 1989; 47:130–135.
22. Pae WE Jr. Temporary ventricular support. Current indications and results. Trans Am Soc Artif Intern Organs 1987; 33:4–7.
23. Richenbacher WE, Pennock JL, Pae WE Jr, Pierce WS. Artificial heart implantation for end-stage cardiac disease. J Cardiac Surg 1986; 1:3–12.
24. Kormos RL, Borovetz HS, Armitage JM, Hardesty RL, Marrone GC, Griffith BP. Evolving experience with mechanical circulatory support. Ann Surg 1991; 214:471–477.
25. Pennington DG, McBride LR, Kanter KR, et al. Bridging to heart transplantation with circulatory support devices. J Heart Transplant 1989; 8:116–123.
26. Frazier OH, Wampler RK, Duncan JM, et al. First human use of the Hemopump, a catheter-mounted ventricular assist device. Ann Thorac Surg 1990; 49:229–304.
27. Pierce WS, Parr GVS, Myers JL, Pae WE Jr, Bull AP, Waldhausen JA. Ventricular-assist pumping in patients with cardiogenic shock after cardiac operations. N Engl J Med 1981; 305:1606–1610.
28. Keon WJ, Masters RG, Farrell EM, Koshal A. Use of the Jarvik total artificial heart as a bridge to transplantation. Adv Cardiol 1988; 36:270–277.
29. Sukehiro S, Flameng W. Effects of left ventricular assist for cardiogenic shock on cardiac function and organ blood flow distribution. Ann Thorac Surg 1990; 50:374–383.
30. Starnes VA, Oyer PE, Portner PM, et al. Isolated left ventricular assist as bridge to cardiac transplantation. J Thorac Cardiovasc Surg 1988; 96:62–71.
31. Hill JD, Farrar DJ, Hershon JJ, et al. Use of a prosthetic ventricle as a bridge to cardiac transplantation for postinfarction cardiogenic shock. N Engl J Med 1986; 314:626–628.
32. Zumbro GL, Kitchens WR, Shearer G, Harville G, Bailey L, Galloway RF. Mechanical assistance for cardiogenic shock following cardiac surgery, myocardial infarction, and cardiac transplantation. Ann Thorac Surg 1987; 44:11–13.
33. Joyce LD, Emery RW, Eales F, et al. Mechanical circulatory support as a bridge to transplantation. J Thorac Cardiovasc Surg 1989; 98:935–941.
34. Oaks TE, Wisman CB, Pae WE, Pennock JL, Burg J, Pierce WS. Results of mechanical circulatory assistance before heart transplantation. J Heart Transplant 1989; 8:113–115.

35. Copeland JG, Smith R, Icenogle T, et al. Orthotopic total artificial heart bridge to transplantation: preliminary results. J Heart Transplant 1989; 8:124–138.
36. McCarthy PM, Portner PM, Tobler HG, Starnes VA, Ramasamy N, Oyer PE. Clinical experience with the Novacor ventricle assist system. Bridge to transplantation and the transition to permanent application. J Thorac Cardiovasc Surg 1991; 102:578–587.
37. Pierce WS, Moderator. Other postoperative complications. Panel Discussion presented at the Circulatory Support Symposium of the Society of Thoracic Surgeons, St. Louis, MO, Feb 6–7, 1988. Panelists: Gray LA Jr, McBride LR, Frazier OH. Ann Thorac Surg 1989; 47:96–101.
38. Baldwin RT, Duncan JM, Frazier OH, Wilansky S. Patent foramen ovale: a cause of hypoxemia in patients on left ventricular support. Ann Thorac Surg 1991; 52:865–867.
39. Kormos RL, Borovetz HS, Gasior T, et al. Experience with univentricular support in mortally ill cardiac transplant candidates. Ann Thorac Surg 1990; 49:261–272.
40. Pifarre R, Sullivan H, Montoya A, et al. Comparison of results after heart transplantation: mechanically supported versus nonsupported patients. J Heart Lung Transplant 1992; 11:235–239.
41. Li CM, Hill A, Colson M, Desrosiers C, Chiu RC-J. Implantable rate-responsive counterpulsation assist system. Ann Thorac Surg 1990; 49:356–362.
42. Lee KF, Hanan SA, Tuchy GE, et al. Skeletal muscle extraaortic counterpulsation. A true arterial counterpulsation. J Thorac Cardiovasc Surg 1991; 102:757–765.
43. Pattison CW, Cumming DVE, Williamson A, et al. Aortic counterpulsation for up to 28 days with autologous latissimus dorsi in sheep. J Thorac Cardiovasc Surg 1991; 102:766–773.
44. Chachques JC, Grandjean PA, Fischer EIC, et al. Dynamic aortomyoplasty to assist left ventricular function. Ann Thorac Surg 1990; 49:225–230.
45. Zelano JA, Ko W, Lazzaro R, et al. Evaluation of an extraaortic counterpulsation device in severe cardiac failure. Ann Thorac Surg 1992; 53:30–37.
46. Pennock JL, Pierce WS, Wisman CB, Bull AP, Waldhausen JA. Survival and complications following ventricular assist pumping for cardiogenic shock. Ann Surg 1983; 198:469–478.
47. Farrar DJ, Chow E, Compton PG, Foppiano L, Woodward J, Hill JD. Effects of acute right ventricular ischemia on ventricular interactions during prosthetic left ventricular support. J Thorac Cardiovasc Surg 1991; 102:588–595.
48. Elbeery JR, Owen CH, Savitt MA, et al. Effects of the left ventricular assist device on right ventricular function. J Thorac Cardiovasc Surg 1990; 99:809–816.
49. Skillington PD, Couper GS, Peigh PS, Fitsgerald D, Cohn LH. Pulmonary artery balloon counterpulsation for intraoperative right ventricular failure. Ann Thorac Surg 1991; 51:658–660.
50. Pennington DG, Reedy JE, Swartz MT, et al. Univentricular versus

biventricular assist device support. J Heart Lung Transplant 1991; 10:258–263.

51. Reichman RT, Joyo CI, Dembitsky WP, et al. Improved patient survival after cardiac arrest using a cardiopulmonary support system. Ann Thorac Surg 1990; 49:101–105.

52. Phillips SJ, Zeff RH, Kongtahworn C, et al. Percutaneous cardiopulmonary bypass: application and indication for use. Ann Thorac Surg 1989; 47:121–123.

53. Hartz R, LoCicero J III, Sanders JH Jr, Frederiksen JW, Joob AW, Michaelis LL. Clinical experience with portable cardiopulmonary bypass in cardiac arrest patients. Ann Thorac Surg 1990; 50:437–441.

54. Jegaden O, Bastien O, Girard C. Temporary left ventricular assistance with a Hemopump assist device during acute myocardial infarction. J Thorac Cardiovasc Surg 1990; 100:311–313.

55. Lowe JE, Anstadt MP, Van Trigt P, et al. First successful bridge to cardiac transplantation using direct mechanical ventricular actuation. Ann Thorac Surg 1991; 52:1237–1245.

56. Braunwald E. The stunned myocardium: newer insights into mechanisms and clinical implications. J Thorac Cradiovasc Surg 1990; 100:310–311.

57. Demmy TL, Magovern JA, Lao RL, Magovern GJ. Resuscitation of injured myocardium with adenosine and biventricular assist. Ann Thorac Surg 1991; 52:1044–1051.

58. Magovern GJ, Moderator. Weaning and bridging. Panel Discussion presented at the Circulatory Support Symposium of the Society of Thoracic Surgeons, St. Louis, MO, Feb 6–7, 1988. Panelists: Golding LAR, Oyer PE, Cabrol C. Ann Thorac Surg 1989; 47:102–107.

59. Pennington DG, Bernhard WF, Golding LR, Berger RL, Khuri SF, Watson JT. Long-term follow-up of postcardiotomy patients with profound cardiogenic shock treated with ventricular assist devices. Circulation 1985; 72(Suppl II):II-216–226.

60. Pifarre R, Sullivan H, Montoya A, et al. Use of total artifical heart and ventricular assist device as a bridge to transplantation. J Heart Transplant 1990; 9:638–643.

61. Farrar DJ, Lawson JH, Litwak P, Cederwall G. Thoratec VAD system as a bridge to heart transplantation. J Heart Transplant 1990; 9:415–423.

62. Pennington DG, Kanter KR, McBride LR, et al. Seven years' experience with the Pierce-Donachy ventricular assist device. J Thorac Cardiovasc Surg 1988; 96:901–911.

63. Oaks TE, Pae WE Jr, Miller CA, Pierce WS. Combined registry for the clinical use of mechanical ventricular assist pumps and the total artificial heart in conjunction with heart transplantation: fifth official report—1990. J Heart Lung Transplant 1991; 10:621–625.

64. Cabrol C, Solis E, Muneretto C, et al. Orthotopic transplantation after implantation of a Jarvik 7 total artificial heart. J Thorac Cardiovasc Surg 1989; 97:342–350.

65. Birovljev S, Radovancevic B, Burnett CM, et al. Heart transplantation after mechanical circulatory support: four years' experience. J Heart Lung Transplant 1992; 11:240–245.

66. Pennington G. *Discussion of* Kormos RL, Borovetz HS, Armitage JM, Hardesty RL, Marrone GC, Griffith BP. Evolving experience with mechanical circulatory support. Ann Surg 1991; 214:471–477.
67. Bolman RM, Cox JL, Marshall W, et al. Circulatory support with a centrifugal pump as a bridge to cardiac transplantation. Ann Thorac Surg 1989; 47:108–112.
68. Dennis C. *Discussion of* Pennock JL, Pierce WS, Wisman CB, Bull AP, Waldhausen JA. Survival and complications following ventricular assist pumping for cardiogenic shock. Ann Surg 1983; 198:469–478.
69. Reemtsma K, Drusin R, Edie R, Bregman D, Dobelle W, Hardy M. Cardiac transplantation for patients requiring mechanical circulatory support. N Engl J Med 1978; 298:670–671.
70. Loisance D, Deleuze PH, Hillion ML, et al. The real impact of mechanical bridge strategy in patients with severe acute infarction. ASAIO Transactions 1990; 36:M135–M137.
71. Champsaur G, Ninet J, Vigneron M, Cochet P, Neidecker J, Boissonnat P. Use of the Abiomed BVS System 5000 as a bridge to cardiac transplantation. J Thorac Cardiovasc Surg 1990; 100:122–128.
72. Bolman RM, Cox JL, Marshall W, et al. Circulatory support with a centrifugal pump as a bridge to cardiac transplantation. Ann Thorac Surg 1989; 47:108–112.
73. Chachques JC, Grandjean PA, Pfeffer TA, et al. Cardiac assistance by atrial or ventricular cardiomyoplasty. J Heart Transplant 1990; 9:239–251.
74. Magovern GJ, Park SB, Kao RL, Christlieb IY, Magovern GJ Jr. Dynamic cardiomyoplasty in patients. J Heart Transplant 1990; 9:258–263.
75. Hooper TL, Niinami H, Hammond RL, et al. Skeletal muscle ventricles in circulation as true left heart assist devices (abstr.) J Heart Lung Transplant 1992; 11:210.
76. Raza ST, Tam SKC, Sun S-C, et al. Sequentially paced heterotopic heart transplant in the left chest provides improved circulatory support for the left ventricle. A potential biologic bridge to orthotopic transplantation. J Thorac Cardiovasc Surg 1989; 98:266–274.

Index

Abiomed mechanical circulatory support system, 243
Acidosis, reperfusion, 117
Acute coronary insufficiency, coronary sinus intervention, 78–79
Acute coronary ischemia
 adenosine triphosphate, 112
 alpha-ketoglutarate level, 114
 amino acid, 114
 angina, 187–199
 anisoylated plasminogen streptokinase activator, 37–40, 44, 46–47
 aspartate, 126
 calcium, 113–114
 cardiogenic shock, 129–135
 cardioplegia maintenance, 125
 cold blood cardioplegic induction, 124
 coronary artery bypass grafting, 63–64, 74, 79, 111, 116
 coronary sinus intervention, 63–80
 "culprit lesion" percutaneous transluminal coronary angioplasty, 92–94
 diltiazem, 126
 effect of type of reperfusion, 115–120
 electrocardiogram, 42–43
 emergency coronary artery bypass graft surgery, 149–164, 167–181
 free radical, 114–115
 Global Utilization of Streptokinase Trial, 39
 glutamate, 114, 126
 grafting order, 125
 hypoxanthine, 114–115
 inosine, 113
 Krebs' cycle, 114–115
 mechanical assist device, 257–279
 mechanical circulatory support, 229–252, 257–279
 myocardial change, 113–115
 myocardial infarction, 205–220
 myocardial ischemic injury, 1–25
 myocardial necrosis, 167–181
 myocardial protection, 111–135
 neutrophil, 115
 oxalaocetic acid level, 114
 pathophysiology, 1–25
 percutaneous transluminal coronary angioplasty, 63–64, 72, 74–76, 79, 85–106, 111–112, 149–164, 167–181
 plasminogen, 33–43
 postcardiotomy, 264
 recombinant tissue plasminogen activator, 36–56
 regional reperfusion control, 125–126
 reperfusion, 1–25, 111–135
 streptokinase, 37–41, 44, 46–47, 52–53, 55
 surgical revascularization, 187–199
 thrombolysis, 36–39
 thrombolytic therapy, 33–56
 transplantation, 257–279
 warm blood cardioplegic induction, 124–125
Acute coronary occlusion, remote myocardium, 120–123

285

Acute coronary syndromes
  pathogenesis diagram, 87
  pathophysiology, 34–36
Acute myocardial infarction
  aneurysm of left ventricle, 215–217
  aspartate, 126
  cardiogenic shock, 129–135
  cardioplegia maintenance, 125
  cardiorrhexis, 214
  cold blood cardioplegic induction, 124
  diltiazem, 126
  evolving, 212–214
  failed percutaneous transluminal coronary angioplasty, 211–212
  glutamate, 126
  grafting order, 125
  history of surgery for, 206–209
  interventricular septum rupture, 217–219
  left ventricle wall rupture, 214–215
  mechanical complications, 214
  myocardial protection strategy, 123–126
  papillary muscle rupture, 219–220
  percutaneous transluminal coronary angioplasty, 96–105
  plasminogen, 33–43
  postinfarction angina, 209–211
  regional reperfusion control, 125–126
  surgery for, 205–220
  thrombolytic therapy, 33–56
  warm blood cardioplegic induction, 124–125
Adenosine triphosphate
  acute coronary ischemia, 112
  myocardial ischemic injury, 2–3
  reperfusion injury, 17
Age, thrombolytic therapy, 41–42
Alpha-ketoglutarate level, acute coronary ischemia, 114
Amino acid
  acute coronary ischemia, 114
  reperfusion, 117

Anatomy, coronary sinus, 66–67
Aneurysm, left ventricle, 215–217
Angina
  acute coronary ischemia, 187–199
  patient profile with failed percutaneous transluminal coronary angioplasty, 152, 156
  percutaneous transluminal coronary angioplasty, 88–96
  postinfarction, 209–211
  refractory unstable, 187–199
  thrombolytic therapy, 43–44
Angioplasty. See also Percutaneous transluminal coronary angioplasty
Angiotensin-converting enzyme, reperfusion injury, 19–20
Anisoylated plasminogen streptokinase activator, acute coronary ischemia, 37–40, 44, 46–47
Antegrade coronary perfusion, necrosis, 169–172
Antigenicity, thrombolytic agent, 37
Antiplatelet therapy, 54–55
Arrhythmias, reperfusion, 10–11
Arteriovenus anastomosis, coronary sinus, 66–67
Aspartate, acute myocardial infarction, 126
ATP. See Adenosine triphosphate

Balloon pump
  myocardial necrosis, 169, 175
  patient profile with failed percutaneous transluminal coronary angioplasty, 153
  pressure-controlled intermittent coronary sinus occlusion, 76–77
Biomedicus, mechanical circulatory support, 243
Biventricular assist, right ventricle assist device, 267–268
Biventricular failure, mechanical circulatory support, 246–247

Bleeding
mechanical circulatory support, 238, 247
thrombolytic therapy, 45–46
Blood cardioplegic induction, acute myocardial infarction, 124
Bridge, mechanical circulatory support, until transplant available, 238–241, 257–279
Bypass, left-heart, myocardial necrosis, 179

Calcium
acute coronary ischemia, 114
reperfusion, 117
reperfusion injury, 17
Calcium channel blockers, for necrosis after failed percutaneous transluminal coronary angioplasty, 168–169
Calcium level, acute coronary ischemia, 113
Cannula obstruction, mechanical circulatory support, 238
Cardiac transplantation, mechanical circulatory support until donor available, 238–241, 257–279
Cardiogenic shock, acute myocardial infarction, 129–135
Cardioplegia
acute myocardial infarction, 125
reperfusion, 117
Cardiorrhexis, 214
Catheter, retroperfusion, 72–73
Catheter insertion, patient profile with failed percutaneous transluminal coronary angioplasty, 153
Catheterization, coronary sinus, 68–69
Catheterization profile, failed percutaneous transluminal coronary angioplasty, 153
Cerebrovascular accident, coronary artery bypass graft surgery after failed percutaneous transluminal coronary angioplasty, 155, 158

Circulatory support
acute coronary ischemia, 229–252, 257–279
clinical problems with, 246–248
counterpulsation, 266
devices available, 242–246
extracorporeal membrane oxygenation, 231–233, 266
Hemopump, 269–271
mechanical ventricular actuation, 271–272
percutaneous cardiopulmonary support system, 268–269
postcardiotomy support, 234–238
right ventricle assist device, biventricular assist, 267–268
transplantation, 272–273, 275–276
ventricular assist device, 266–267
Clinical problems, with mechanical circulatory support, 246–248
Cold blood cardioplegic induction, acute myocardial infarction, 124
Collagen matrix, reperfusion injury, 19
Collateral blood flow
infarct size correlation chart, 8
myocardial ischemic injury, 7
Complications, percutaneous transluminal coronary angioplasty, 88–89
Congestive heart failure, patient profile with failed percutaneous transluminal coronary angioplasty, 152, 156
Consequences, myocardial ischemia, 2–5
Contraindications, thrombolytic therapy, 44–48
Coronary artery bypass graft surgery. See also Emergent coronary artery bypass graft surgery
after failed percutaneous transluminal coronary angioplasty, 149–164

Coronary artery bypass surgery, acute coronary ischemia, 63–64, 74, 79, 111, 116

Coronary blood flow increase, myocardial necrosis, 169–174

Coronary dissection, patient profile with failed percutaneous transluminal coronary angioplasty, 153

Coronary ischemia. See also Acute coronary ischemia

Coronary occlusion, patient profile with failed percutaneous transluminal coronary angioplasty, 153

Coronary sinus
anatomy of, 66–67
arteriovenus anastomosis, 66–67
catheterization, 68–69
flow dynamics, 67–68
occlusion pressure, 68
physiology, 67–68
pressure-controlled intermittent coronary sinus occlusion, 76–78
retroinfusion, 69–71
synchronized retroperfusion, 70–76
venoluminal anastomosis, 66–67
venovenous anastomosis, 66–67

Coronary sinus intervention
acute coronary insufficiency, 78–79
acute coronary ischemia, 63–80
history of, 64–66

Counterpulsation, mechanical circulatory support, 266

Creatine kinase isoform, infarct size, 9

Creatine kinase level, failed percutaneous transluminal coronary angioplasty, 152

"Culprit lesion" percutaneous transluminal coronary angioplasty, acute coronary ischemia, 92–94

Deferred percutaneous transluminal coronary angioplasty, versus elective percutaneous

transluminal coronary angioplasty, 103–105

Devices, for mechanical circulatory support, 242–246

Diabetes, patient profile with failed percutaneous transluminal coronary angioplasty, 152, 156

Diltiazem
acute myocardial infarction, 126
reperfusion, 117

Direct percutaneous transluminal coronary angioplasty, acute myocardial infarction, 97–101

Dose, thrombolytic agent, 37

Drug. See Medication

ECG. See Electrocardiogram

Elective percutaneous transluminal coronary angioplasty, versus deferred percutaneous transluminal coronary angioplasty, 103–105

Electrocardiogram
acute coronary ischemia, 42–43
patient profile with, 153

Embolus, mechanical circulatory support, 238

Emergent coronary artery bypass graft surgery, following failed percutaneous transluminal coronary angioplasty, 149–164, 167–181

End-diastolic pressure, left ventricular end-diastolic pressure, 68

Endocardium, myocardial ischemic injury, 4–5

Evolving acute myocardial infarction, 126–129, 212–214

Extracorporeal membrane oxygenation, mechanical circulatory support, 231–233, 266

Failed percutaneous transluminal coronary angioplasty
acute myocardial infarction, 211–212

catheterization profile, 153
coronary artery bypass graft surgery after, 149–164
creatine kinase level, 152
emergent coronary artery bypass graft surgery, 149–164, 167–181
myocardial necrosis with coronary artery bypass graft surgery, 159–164
necrosis following coronary artery bypass graft surgery for, 159–164
necrosis following in patients undergoing coronary artery bypass graft surgery, 167–181
patient management, 150–152
patient profiles, 154–158, 160
Fibrin selectivity, thrombolytic agent, 37
Fibrinogen breakdown, thrombolytic agent, 37
Flow dynamics, coronary sinus, 67–68
Free radicals
acute coronary ischemia, 114–115
reperfusion, 117
reperfusion injury, 18–19

Global Utilization of Streptokinase Trial, acute coronary ischemia, 39
Glutamate
acute coronary ischemia, 114
acute myocardial infarction, 126
for necrosis after failed percutaneous transluminal coronary angioplasty, 169
Grafting order, acute myocardial infarction, 125

Half-life, thrombolytic agent, 37
Hemolysis, mechanical circulatory support, 238
Hemopump, mechanical circulatory support, 269–271
Hemorrhage
coronary artery bypass surgery after failed percutaneous transluminal coronary angioplasty, 155, 158
intracranial, thrombolytic therapy, 45
Heparin, 53–54
Hyperglycemia, reperfusion, 117–118
Hyperosmolarity, reperfusion, 117
Hypertension, patient profile with failed percutaneous transluminal coronary angioplasty, 152, 156
Hypotension
thrombolytic agent, 37
thrombolytic therapy, 46–47
Hypoxanthine, acute coronary ischemia, 114–115

Immediate percutaneous transluminal coronary angioplasty, acute myocardial infarction, 101–103
Immunologic complications, thrombolytic therapy, 46–47
Inderal, for necrosis after failed percutaneous transluminal coronary angioplasty, 168–169
Infarct size
creatine kinase isoform, 9
myocardial ischemic injury, 5–9
quantitation, 9
Infarct size correlation chart, collateral flow, 8
Infarction, mechanical circulatory support, 229–252
Infection
mechanical circulatory support, 238, 248–249
sternum, coronary artery bypass graft surgery after failed percutaneous transluminal coronary angioplasty, 155, 158
Injury, reperfusion, 10–25
Inosine, acute coronary ischemia, 113

Internal mammary artery, coronary artery bypass graft surgery for failed percutaneous transluminal coronary angioplasty, 151
Interventricular septum, rupture, 217–219
Intra-aortic balloon pump, necrosis, 169, 175
Intra-aortic balloon pump insertion, patient profile with failed percutaneous transluminal coronary angioplasty, 153
Intracranial hemorrhage, thrombolytic therapy, 45
Irreversible ischemic injury, 4–5
Ischemic myocardium, reperfusion, 9–25

Krebs' cycle
  acute coronary ischemia, 114–115
  reperfusion, 117

Left-heart bypass, myocardial necrosis, 179
Left ventricle
  aneurysm, 215–217
  cardiogenic shock, 129–135
  end-diastolic pressure, 68
  free wall rupture, 214–215
Leukopenia, reperfusion, 118

Mammary artery, coronary artery bypass graft surgery, after failed percutaneous transluminal coronary angioplasty, 151
Mechanical assist device. See Mechanical circulatory support
Mechanical circulatory support
  Abiomed system, 243
  acute coronary ischemia, 229–252, 257–279
  Biomedicus system, 243
  biventricular failure, 246–247
  bleeding, 238, 247
  cannula obstruction, 238
  clinical problems with, 246–248
  counterpulsation, 266

devices available, 242–246
  embolus, 238
  extracorporeal membrane oxygenation, 231–233, 266
  hemolysis, 238
  Hemopump, 243, 269–271
  infection, 238, 248–249
  mechanical ventricular actuation, 271–272
  Novacor system, 243
  patient selection, 230–231
  percutaneous cardiopulmonary support system, 268–269
  perioperative myocardial infarction, 238
  Pierce-Donachy system, 243
  postcardiotomy support, 234–238
  renal failure, 238, 248
  respiratory failure, 238
  respiratory insufficiency, 248–249
  right ventricle assist device, biventricular assist, 267–268
  Sarns/Centrimed system, 243
  Sarns Pulsatile system, 243
  Thermocardiosystem, 243
  thromboembolism, 249
  thrombus, 238
  transplantation, 272–273, 275–276
  ventricular assist device, 266–267
  weaning, 249–250
Mechanical complications, acute myocardial infarction, 214
Mechanical ventricular actuation, mechanical circulatory support, 271–272
Medication, thrombolytic agent, 33–56
Myocardial change, acute coronary ischemia, 113–115
Myocardial infarction, coronary artery bypass graft surgery after failed percutaneous transluminal coronary angioplasty, 155, 158
Myocardial ischemic injury
  adenosine triphosphate, 2–3

collateral flow, 8
creatine kinase isoform, 9
defined, 2
endocardium, 4–5
infarct size, 5–9
irreversible ischemic injury, 4–5
oxygen demand, 7–9
pathophysiology, 2–9
positron emission tomography, 7
reversible ischemic injury, 2–3
single photon emission comput-
    erized tomography, 7
subepicardium, 3
Myocardial metabolic demand, myo-
    cardial ischemic injury, 7–9
Myocardial necrosis
    after failed percutaneous trans-
        luminal coronary angioplasty
        in patients undergoing coro-
        nary artery bypass graft sur-
        gery, 167–181
    antegrade coronary perfusion,
        169–172
    calcium channel blockers, 168–
        169
    coronary blood flow increase, 169–
        174
    glutamate, 169
    inderal, 168–169
    intra-aortic balloon pump, 169,
        175
    Nimbus hemopump, 169, 178–179
    nitroglycerin, 168–169
    percutaneous bypass, 169, 176–
        179
    reduction of after failed percuta-
        neous transluminal coronary
        angioplasty, 168–169
    retrograde coronary sinus perfu-
        sion, 169, 172–174
Myocardial protection strategy,
    acute myocardial infarction,
    123–126
Myocardial rupture, thrombolytic
    therapy, 47–48
Myocardial salvage, reperfusion-
    induced, 9–10
Myocardial stunning, reperfusion
    injury, 14–21

Necrosis
    after failed percutaneous trans-
        luminal coronary angioplasty
        in patients undergoing coro-
        nary artery bypass graft sur-
        gery, 167–181
    antegrade coronary perfusion,
        169–172
    calcium channel blockers, 168–
        169
    coronary blood flow increase, 169–
        174
    following coronary artery bypass
        graft surgery for failed per-
        cutaneous transluminal coro-
        nary angioplasty, 159–164
    glutamate, 169
    inderal, 168–169
    intra-aortic balloon pump, 169,
        175
    Nimbus hemopump, 169, 178–
        179
    nitroglycerin, 168–169
    percutaneous bypass, 169, 176–
        179
    reduction of after failed percuta-
        neous transluminal coronary
        angioplasty, 168–169
    reperfusion injury, 10, 13–14
    retrograde coronary sinus perfu-
        sion, 169, 172–174
Neutrophil, acute coronary isch-
    emia, 115
Nimbus hemopump
    necrosis, 169, 178–179
    for necrosis after failed percuta-
        neous transluminal coronary
        angioplasty, 169
Nitroglycerin, for necrosis after
    failed percutaneous translu-
    minal coronary angioplasty,
    168–169
No-reflow, reperfusion injury, 11–
    13
Nontransmural wave myocardial in-
    farction, thrombolytic ther-
    apy, 43–44
Novacor mechanical circulatory sup-
    port system, 243

Occlusion pressure, coronary sinus, 68
Oxalaocetic acid level, acute coronary ischemia, 114
Oxygen, supply/demand balance, 169, 179–181

Papillary muscle, rupture, 219–220
Pathogenesis diagram, acute coronary syndromes, 87
Pathophysiology
acute coronary syndromes, 1–25, 34–36
myocardial ischemic injury, 2–9
reperfusion, 9–25
unstable angina, 189
Patient data
acute coronary ischemia with mechanical circulatory support, 276–278
failed percutaneous transluminal coronary angioplasty, 154–158, 160
Patient selection
mechanical circulatory support, 230–231
percutaneous transluminal coronary angioplasty, 94–96
Percutaneous bypass, necrosis, 169, 176–178
Percutaneous cardiopulmonary support system, mechanical circulatory support, 268–269
Percutaneous left-heart bypass, necrosis, 179
Percutaneous transluminal coronary angioplasty. See also Failed percutaneous transluminal coronary angioplasty
acute coronary ischemia, 63–64, 72, 74–76, 79, 85–106, 111–112
acute myocardial infarction, 96–105
complications, 88–89
direct, 97–101
immediate, 101–103
patient selection, 94–96

rescue, 103
restinosis, 94
revascularization completeness, 93
thrombolytic therapy, 49–50
unstable angina, 88–96, 191–194
Perioperative myocardial infarction, mechanical circulatory support, 238
Physiology, coronary sinus, 67–68
PICSO technique. See Pressure-controlled intermittent coronary sinus occlusion
Pierce-Donachy mechanical circulatory support, 243
Plasminogen
acute myocardial infarction, 33–43
thrombolytic therapy, 36–39
Plasminogen binding, thrombolytic agent, 37
Positron emission tomography, myocardial ischemic injury, 7
Postcardiotomy support, mechanical circulatory support, 234–238
Postinfarction angina, acute myocardial infarction, 209–211
"Preconditioning" phenomenon, reperfusion injury, 21–25
Pressure-controlled intermittent coronary sinus occlusion, 76–78
balloon pressure correlation chart, 77

Quantitation, infarct size, 9

Recombinant tissue plasminogen activator, acute coronary ischemia, 36–56
Refractory unstable angina
refractory unstable angina, 187–199
revascularization for, 187–199
Remote myocardium, acute coronary occlusion, 120–123
Renal failure, mechanical circulatory support, 238, 248

Reperfusate, composition of, 117–120

Reperfusion
acidosis, 117
acute coronary ischemia, 1–25, 111–135
acute myocardial infarction, 125–126
amino acid, 117
aspartate, 126
calcium, 117
cardioplegia, 117
conditions of, 117
diltiazem, 117, 126
evolving infarction, 126–129
free radical, 117
glutamate, 126
hyperglycemia, 117–118
hyperosmolarity, 117
ischemic myocardium, 9–25
Krebs' cycle, 117
leukopenia, 118
myocardial protection, 111–135
necrotic process, 10
pathophysiology, 1–25
reperfusion-induced myocardial salvage, 9–10
type of, effect on viability, 115–120

Reperfusion catheter, patient profile with failed percutaneous transluminal coronary angioplasty, 153

Reperfusion injury, 10–25
angiotensin-converting enzyme, 19–20
arrhythmias, 10–11
calcium, 17–18
collagen matrix, 19
free radicals, 18–19
myocardial stunning, 14–21
no-reflow, 11–13
"preconditioning" phenomenon, 21–25
superoxide dismutase, 12–13
"therapies" for myocardial stunning, 19–21
thrombolytic therapy, 47–48
vascular damage, 11–13

xanthine oxidase, 18

Rescue percutaneous transluminal coronary angioplasty, 103

Respiratory failure, mechanical circulatory support, 238

Respiratory insufficiency
coronary artery bypass graft surgery after failed percutaneous transluminal coronary angioplasty, 155, 158
mechanical circulatory support, 248–249

Restinosis, percutaneous transluminal coronary angioplasty, 94

Retrograde coronary sinus perfusion, myocardial necrosis, 169, 172–174

Retroinfusion, coronary sinus, 69–71

Retroperfusion, catheter, 72–73

Revascularization
failed percutaneous transluminal coronary angioplasty comparison with unstable angina, 199
immediate outcome with unstable angina, 196–197
intraoperative management with unstable angina, 196
long-term outcome with unstable angina, 197
medical therapy comparison with unstable angina, 198
patient selection with unstable angina, 195
preoperative therapy with unstable angina, 195
for refractory unstable angina, 187–199

Revascularization completeness, percutaneous transluminal coronary angioplasty, 93

Reversible ischemic injury, 2–3

Right ventricle assist device, biventricular assist, 267–268

Risk region, myocardial ischemic injury, 6–7

Role, of surgeon. See Surgeon, role of

Rupture
  interventricular septum, 217–219
  left ventricle wall, 214–215
  papillary muscle, 219–220

Sarns/Centrimed, mechanical circulatory support, 243
Sarns Pulsatile mechanical circulatory support system, 243
Single photon emission computerized tomography, myocardial
  ischemic injury, 7
Stenosis, patient profile with failed
  percutaneous transluminal
  coronary angioplasty, 153
Sternal infection, coronary artery
  bypass graft surgery after
  failed percutaneous transluminal coronary angioplasty,
  155, 158
Streptokinase, acute coronary ischemia, 37–41, 44, 46–47, 52–
  53, 55
Subepicardium, myocardial ischemic injury, 3
Superoxide dismutase, reperfusion
  injury, 12–13
Supply/demand balance, oxygen,
  169, 179–181
Surgeon, role of, acute myocardial
  infarction, 205–220
Surgery, for acute myocardial infarction, history of, 206–209
Surgical revascularization
  failed percutaneous transluminal
    coronary angioplasty com-
    parison with unstable an-
    gina, 199
  immediate outcome with unstable
    angina, 196–197
  intraoperative management with
    unstable angina, 196
  long-term outcome with unstable
    angina, 197
  medical therapy comparison with
    unstable angina, 198
  patient selection with unstable
    angina, 195

preoperative therapy with unstable angina, 195
refractory unstable angina, 187–
  199
Synchronized retroperfusion, coronary sinus, 70–76
Systemic bleeding, thrombolytic
  therapy, 45–46

Thermocardiosystem, mechanical
  circulatory support, 243
Thromboembolism, mechanical circulatory support, 249
Thrombolysis, acute coronary ischemia, 36–39
Thrombolytic agent
  acute coronary ischemia, 36–39
  antigenicity, 37
  dose, 37
  fibrin selectivity, 37
  fibrinogen breakdown, 37
  half-life, 37
  hypotension, 37
  plasminogen binding, 37
  time dependency, 37
Thrombolytic therapy
  acute coronary ischemia, 33–56
  acute myocardial infarction, 33–
    56
  age, 41–42
  antiplatelet therapy, 54–55
  contraindications, 44–48
  coronary artery bypass surgery,
    50–53
  future trends, 53
  heparin, 53–54
  hypotension, 46–47
  immunologic complications, 46–
    47
  intracranial hemorrhage, 45
  myocardial rupture, 47–48
  nontransmural wave myocardial
    infarction, 43–44
  percutaneous transluminal cor-
    onary angioplasty, 49–50
  reperfusion injury, 47–48
  systemic bleeding, 45–46
  unstable angina, 43–44

Thrombus, mechanical circulatory support, 238
Time dependency, thrombolytic agent, 37
Tissue plasminogen activator, 36–39, 53–55
Transplantation
  acute coronary ischemia, 257–279
  after mechanical circulatory support, 275–276
  mechanical circulatory support, 238–241, 257–279

Unstable angina
  defined, 188–189
  pathophysiology, 189
  patient profile with failed percutaneous transluminal coronary angioplasty, 152, 156
  percutaneous transluminal coronary angioplasty, 88–96, 191–194

rationale for medical therapy, 190–191
refractory, 187–199
thrombolytic therapy, 43–44

Vascular damage, reperfusion injury, 11–13
Venoluminal anastomosis, coronary sinus, 66–67
Venovenous anastomosis, coronary sinus, 66–67
Ventricular assist device, mechanical circulatory support, 266–267

Warm blood cardioplegic induction, acute myocardial infarction, 124–125
Weaning, mechanical circulatory support, 249–250

Xanthine oxidase, reperfusion injury, 18